CARDIOVASCULAR DIAGNOSIS BY ULTRASOUND

Transesophageal, Computerized, Contrast, Doppler Echocardiography

DEVELOPMENTS IN CARDIOVASCULAR MEDICINE

VOLUME 22

Series ISBN 90-247-2336-1

CARDIOVASCULAR DIAGNOSIS BY ULTRASOUND

Transesophageal, Computerized, Contrast, Doppler Echocardiography

edited by

PETER HANRATH, M.D., WALTER BLEIFELD, M.D.
Department of Cardiology
Medical Clinic
University Hospital Eppendorf
Hamburg

and

JACQUES SOUQUET, Ph.D.
Advanced Technology Laboratories,
Bellevue WA

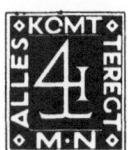

1982
MARTINUS NIJHOFF PUBLISHERS
THE HAGUE / BOSTON / LONDON

Distributors:

for the United States and Canada

Kluwer Boston, Inc.
190 Old Derby Street
Hingham, MA 02043
USA

for all other countries

Kluwer Academic Publishers Group
Distribution Center
P.O. Box 322
3300 AH Dordrecht
The Netherlands

ISBN-13:978-94-009-7605-4 e-ISBN-13:978-94-009-7603-0
DOI: 10.1007/978-94-009-7603-0

CONTENTS

FOREWORD

This volume contains most of the invited lectures presented at the second "International Symposium on the Evaluation of Cardiac Dynamics by Ultrasound" which was held on May 27–28, 1982, in Hamburg.

Main topics of the symposium dealt with new echocardiographic technologies such as the transesophageal technique and digital image processing of echocardiograms, as well as with latest clinical and experimental results in the fields of contrast and Doppler echocardiography, tissue characterization and analysis of left ventricular function.

We are greatly indebted to all participants who kept a very tight schedule in order to have these proceedings available at the time of the meeting. We cordially thank Dr. M. Schlüter for his editorial assistance, Mrs. B. Kratzenberg for her secretarial help, and the Pharma-Schwarz Company for their generous financial support.

Hamburg, May 1982

The Editors

CONTRIBUTORS

ABE, A., First Department of Medicine, Osaka University Medical School, 1–1–50, Fukushima, Fukushima-ku, Osaka 553, Japan.

BACKS, B., Medizinische Universitätsklinik Bonn, Abteilung für Kardiologie, 5300 Bonn, BRD.

BAKER, D.W., Ph.D., Squibb Medical Systems International, 2100 124th Avenue NE, Bellevue, WA 98005, USA.

BIAMINO, G., M.D., Klinikum Steglitz, Kardiologische Abteilung, Hindenburgdamm 30, 1000 Berlin 20, BRD.

BLEIFELD, W., M.D., Abteilung für Kardiologie, Universitätskrankenhaus Eppendorf, Martinistrasse 52, 2000 Hamburg 20, BRD.

BOM, K., Ph.D., Thorax Center, Erasmus University, P.O. Box 1738, 3000 DR Rotterdam, The Netherlands.

BRENNEKE, R., Abteilung Kinderkardiologie und Biomedizinische Technik, Klinikum der Christian-Albrechts-Universität, Schwanenweg 20, 2300 Kiel, BRD.

BRINK, J.A., Cardiac Ultrasound Laboratory, Massachusetts General Hospital, Boston, Massachussetts 02114, USA.

CAHALAN, M.K., University of California, Department of Cardiology, Moffitt 1186, San Francisco, CA 94143, USA.

CANNON, J., Cardiology, Veterans Medical Center, San Antonio, Texas 78284, USA.

CARCIA, E., Cedars-Sinai Medical Center, Halper Research Building, 8700 Beverly Boulevard, Los Angeles, CA 90048, USA.

CIKES, I., M.D., Institute of Cardiovascular Diseases, Kispaticeva 12 – Rebro, 41000 Zagreb, Yugoslavia.

CORALLO, S., M.D., Cardiac Department, University Hospital 'L. Sacco', Milano, Italy.

CUDDEBACK, J.L., Cardiac Ultrasound Laboratory, Massachusetts General Hospital, Boston, Massachusetts 02114, USA.

DiMAGNO, E.P., M.D., Gastroenterology Unit, Mayo Clinic, Saint Mary's Hospital, Rochester, Minnesota 55901, USA.

DISSELHOFF, W., Klinikum Charlottenburg, Abteilung Kardiologie, Spandauer Damm 130, 1000 Berlin 19, BRD.

DUHM, P., Abteilung Kinderkardiologie und Biomedizinische Technik, Klinikum der Christian-Albrechts-Universität, Schwanenweg 20, 2300 Kiel, BRD.

ERBEL, R., Abteilung Innere Medizin I, Medizinische Fakultät, Rhein.-Westfälische Technische Hochschule, Goethestrasse 27/29, 5100 Aachen, BRD.

EUGEL, S., Abteilung für Kardiologie, Universitätskrankenhaus Eppendorf, Martinistrasse 52, 2000 Hamburg 20, BRD.

FRANKLIN, T.D., Cardiac Ultrasound Laboratory, Massachusetts General Hospital, Boston, Massachusetts 02114, USA.

GIBSON, D., M.D., Brompton Hospital, Cardiac Department, Fulham Road, London SW2 6HP, Great Britain.

GRUBE, E., M.D., Medizinische Universitätsklinik Bonn, Abteilung für Kardiologie, 5300 Bonn, BRD.

HAHNE, H.-J., Abteilung Kinderkardiologie und Biomedizinische Technik, Klinikum der Christian-Albrechts-Universität, Schwanenweg 20, 2300 Kiel, BRD.

HANRATH, P., M.D., Abteilung für Kardiologie, Universitätskrankenhaus Eppendorf, Martinistrasse 52, 2000 Hamburg 20, BRD.

HEINTZEN, P.H., M.D., Abteilung Kinderkardiologie und Biomedizinische Technik, Klinikum der Christian-Albrechts-Universität, Schwanenweg 20, 2300 Kiel, BRD.

HISANAGA, K., M.D., Department of Internal Medicine, Mitsubishi Nagoya Hospital, 48 Soto doi – cho, Atsuta -ku, 456 Nagoya, Japan.

HISANAGA, A., Department of Internal Medicine, Mitsubishi Nagoya Hospital, 48 Soto doi – cho, Atsuta -ku, 456 Nagoya, Japan.

HISTAND, M.B., Ph.D., Department of Mechanical Engineering, Colorado State University, Fort Collins, CO 80523.

INOUE, M., First Department of Medicine, Osaka University Medical School, 1–1–50, Fukushima, Fukushima-ku, Osaka 553, Japan.

JONG, N. de, Thorax Center, Erasmus University, P.O. Box 1738, 3000 DR Rotterdam, The Netherlands.

KÖHLER, E., M.D., Medizinische Klinik B der Universität, Moorenstrasse 5, 4000 Düsseldorf, BRD.

KREMER, P., M.D., University of California, Department of Cardiology, Moffitt 1186, San Francisco, CA 94143, USA.

KRONIK, G., M.D., I. Medizinische Universitätsklinik, Allgemeines Krankenhaus, Lazarettgasse 14, A – 1090 Wien, Austria.

KÜBLER, W., Klinikum der Universität, Abteilung III – Kardiologie, Bergheimer Strasse 58, 6900 Heidelberg, BRD.

KUSUKAWA, R., University of California, San Diego, Department of Medicine, A–011, La Jolla, CA 92093, USA.

LANCÉE, C.T., Ph.D., Thorax Center, Erasmus University, P.O. Box 1738, 3000 DR Rotterdam, The Netherlands.

LANGENSTEIN, B.A., Abteilung für Kardiologie, Universitätskrankenhaus Eppendorf, Martinistrasse 52, 2000 Hamburg 20, BRD.

LIGTVOET, C.M., Thorax Center, Erasmus University, P.O. Box 1738, 3000 DR Rotterdam, The Netherlands.

LOGAN SINCLAIR, R.B., Brompton Hospital, Cardiac Department, Fulham Road, London SW3 6HP, Great Britain.

MAEDA, T., First Department of Medicine, Osaka University Medical School, 1–1–50, Fukushima, Fukushima-ku, Osaka 553, Japan.

MARTIN, D., Hopital Beaujou, Service de Cardiologie, Bd de Général Leclerc 100, F – Clichy 92000, France.

MATSUMOTO, M., M.D., First Department of Medicine, Osaka University Medical School, 1–1–50, Fukushima, Fukushima-ku, Osaka 553, Japan.

MATSUZAKI, M., M.D., University of California San Diego, Department of Medicine, 1–011, La Jolla, CA 92093, USA.

MEERBAUM, S., Ph.D., Cedars-Sinai Medical Center, Halper Research Building, 8700 Beverly Boulevard, Los Angeles, CA 90048, USA.

MEHMEL, H.C., Klinikum der Universität, Abteilung III – Kardiologie, Bergheimer Strasse 58, 6900 Heidelberg, BRD.

MELTZER, R.S., Thorax Center, Erasmus University, Postbus 1738, 3000 DR Rotterdam, The Netherlands.

MERX, W., Abteilung Innere Medizin I, Medizinische Fakultät, Rhein.-Westfälische Technische Hochschule, Goethestrasse 27/29, 5100 Aachen, BRD.

OLSHAUSEN, K. von M.D., Klinikum der Universität, Abteilung III – Kardiologie, Bergheimer Strasse 58, 6900 Heidelberg, BRD.

ONG, K., Cedars-Sinai Medical Center, Halper Research Building, 8700 Beverly Boulevard, Los Angeles, CA 90048, USA.

POLSTER, J., Abteilung für Kardiologie, Universitätskrankenhaus Eppendorf, Martinistrasse 52, 2000 Hamburg 20, BRD.

PRASQUIER, R., M.D., Hopital Beaujou, Service de Cardiologie, Bd. de Général Leclerc 100, F – Clichy 92000, France.

REDEL, D.A., M.D., Universitäts-Kinderklinik, Adenauerallee,5300 Bonn, BRD.

REIFART, N., M.D., Klinikum der J.W. Goethe-Universität, Zentrum der Inneren Medizin, Abteilung Kardiologie, Theodor-Stern-Kai 7, 6000 Frankfurt / M. 70, BRD.

RICHARDS, K.L., M.D., Cardiology, Veterans Medical Center, San Antonio, Texas 78284, USA.

ROELANDT, J., M.D., Thorax Center, Erasmus University, Postbus 1738, 3000 DR Rotterdam, The Netherlands.

RUTSCH, W., Klinikum Charlottenburg, Abteilung Kardiologie, Spandauer Damm 130, 1000 Berlin 19, BRD.

SAHN, D.J., M.D., University of Arizona, Health Sciences Center, Department of Pediatrics, Tucson, Arizona 85724, USA.

SANGVI, N.T., Cardiac Ultrasound Laboratory, Massachusetts General Hospital, Boston, Massachusetts 02114, USA.

SCHARTL, M., M.D., Klinikum Charlottenburg, Abteilung Kardiologie, Spandauer Damm 130, 1000 Berlin 19, BRD.

SCHILLER, N.B., M.D., University of California, Adult Noninvasive Laboratories, Moffitt 1186, San Francisco, CA 94143, USA.

SCHLÜTER, M., Ph.D., Abteilung für Kardiologie, Universitätskrankenhaus Eppendorf, Martinistrasse 52, 2000 Hamburg 20, BRD.

SCHMUTZLER, H., Klinikum Charlottenburg, Abteilung Kardiologie, Spandauer Damm 130, 1000 Berlin 19, BRD.

SCHWEIZER, P., M.D., Abteilung Innere Medizin I, Medizinische Fakultät, Rhein.-Westfälische Technische Hochschule, Goethestrasse 27/29, 5100, Aachen, BRD.

SCHWIETZER, U., Klinikum Steglitz, Kardiologische Abteilung, Hindenburgdamm 30, 1000 Berlin 20, BRD.

SEWARD, J.B., M.D., Mayo Clinic, Cardiovascular Diseases and Internal Medicine, Rochester Minnesota 55901, USA.

SOUQUET, J., Ph.D., Advanced Technology Laboratories, Inc., 13208 Northup Way, Bellevue, WA 98008-0639, USA.

TOUCHE, T., Hopital Beaujou, Service de Cardiologie, Bd. de Général Leclerc 100, F – Clichy 92000, France.

VERDOUW, P.D., Thorax Center, Erasmus University, Postbus 1738, 3000 DR Rotterdam, The Netherlands.

VERVIN, P., Hopital Beaujou, Service de Cardiologie, Bd. de Général Leclerc 100, F – Clichy 92000, France.

WELLS, M.K., Ph.D., 205 Cobleigh Hall, Department of Civil Engineering to Engineering Mechanics, Montana State University, Bozman, Montana 59717, USA.

WESSEL, A., M.D., Abteilung Kinderkardiologie und Biomedizinische Technik, Klinikum der Christian-Albrechts-Universität, Schwanenweg 20, 2300 Kiel, BRD.

WEYMAN, A.E., M.D., Cardiac Ultrasound Laboratory, Massachusetts General Hospital, Boston, Massachusetts 02114, USA.

YASUI, K., First Department of Medicine, Osaka University Medical School, 1–1–50, Fukushima, Fukushima-ku, Osaka 553, Japan.

ZWEHL, W., Cedars-Sinai Medical Center, Halper Research Building, 8700 Beverly Boulevard, Los Angeles, CA 90048, USA.

ZYWIETZ, M., Medizinische Universitätsklinik Bonn, Abteilung für Kardiologie, 5300 Bonn, BRD.

CONTRAST ECHOCARDIOGRAPHY OF THE RIGHT AND LEFT HEART

J. Roelandt, R.S. Meltzer

Thoraxcentre, Erasmus University and Academic Hospital Dijkzigt, Rotterdam, the Netherlands.

Contrast echocardiography has become a well-established adjunct to M-mode and two-dimensional echocardiography. Any biologically compatible solution containing microbubbles of air and injected into the circulation makes the blood "echogenic" enabling it to be followed on its way through the cardiac chambers. However, the microbubbles contained in solutions are too large to pass a capillary bed. As a consequence, an echo-contrast effect on the left side of the heart cannot be achieved with peripheral vein injections. Recently, the possibility of transmitting echo-contrast material across the pulmonary capillary bed to the left heart has been demonstrated in animals with experimental contrast agents (see chapter 1). Human application of these agents awaits toxicology studies.
At present, opacification of the left heart requires catheter injections making it an invasive procedure. This explains why its clinical application has been limited.

This chapter aims to review some methodological and clinical aspects of right and left heart contrast echocardiography.

METHODOLOGICAL ASPECTS

Peripheral venous injections

Microbubbles of air present in the injectate or injecting apparatus are the predominant cause of echocardiographic contrast (1). A rapid injection of the microbubble containing solution in a large proximal vein will yield the best contrast effect.
We routinely use a 16 or 18 gauge, 45 mm long intravenous teflon cannula (Venflon^R) which is inserted into an antecubital vein of the left arm in order not to miss an persistent left superior vena cava, which usually drains into an enlarged coronary sinus.
We use 5-10 ml of saline or dextrose 5% solution, which we shake in the syringe with air which is quickly removed prior to injection. The solution can also be aerated by rapidly injecting it in and out of the vial. Occasionally we add 2 ml of carbon dioxide to the solution when insufficient contrast effect is obtained (2). Needles should be avoided since they often damage the wall of the vein during injection and may cause extravasation and hematomas during injection.

In neonates, scalp veins should be avoided because rapid injections cause painful reactions and movements which disturb the recordings. More peripheral (hand) vein injections can be utilized when fluids containing large amounts of microbubbles, such as freshly prepared indocyanine green dye, are injected.

The concentraction of the indocyanine green dye varies according to body weight: 5 mg/ml for patients weighing more than 30 kg, 2.5 mg/ml for those of 10-30 kg, 1.25 mg/ml for those of 5-10 kg, and 0.6 mg/ml for those of less than 5 kg.

Echocardiographic contrast studies are best recorded during held respiration, although phasic flow changes during respiration sometimes yield interesting physiologic information. A Valsalva and/or Müller maneuver with sudden release should be performed in patients suspected of having a small atrial septal defect or patent foramen ovale (3,4).

Central catheter injections

M-mode and two-dimensional contrast echocardiograms can be recorded during a manual catheter flush of 5 to 10 ml of dextrose 5% solution or 1 ml of indocyanine green dye solution in the left heart during cardiac catheterization (5-7). Since multiple views are usually studied several injections are required limiting the use of indocyanine green dye.

Adequate contrast echocardiograms of the left heart can be obtained with pulmonary wedge injections in animals (8,9) and humans (10-12). Reale et al (10) obtained echocardiographic contrast, using different echo-producing substances, in all patients studied using a Swan-Ganz balloon-tipped catheter.

We were less successful with this catheter and saw contrast in only 3 out of 14 patients, while adequate left-sided contrast was produced in 30 out of 38 patients with a Cournand 7F catheter. We further found that injection pressure had to be more than 40 KPa and that a firm occlusive wedge position must be achieved. It is conceivable that the pressure applied during occlusive injections causes deformation of the microbubbles of air, resulting in their passage through the capillary bed rather than their being retained by its "sieve" function (8-12).

Examination techniques

M-mode and two-dimensional contrast echocardiography each have specific advantages and disadvantages for clinical problem solving. M-mode contrast echocardiography yields excellent time resolution and allows accurate analysis of flow related events across the cardiac valves, in the ventricles and in the great arteries; two-dimensional contrast echocardiography is comparable to a tomographic angiogram (echo-ventriculography) and offers advantages when abnormal anatomy and blood flow patterns need to be analyzed. Timing of events from two-dimensional echocardiographic studies is more difficult. As compared with cineangiocardiography, contrast echocardiography

has the advantage of eliminating potential interference from
surrounding and overlying cardiac structures and chambers.
M-mode echocardiographic contrast studies in adults are usually
performed from the parasternal transducer position. The constant
underlying anatomical relationship of the aorta, right pulmonary
artery and left atrium makes the suprasternal notch approach
attractive for evaluation of ventriculo-arterial connections and
right-to-left shunts in infants and children with complex congenital
heart disease (13).

Two-dimensional echocardiographic studies can be performed from four
ultrasonic windows to the heart (parasternal, apical, subcostal and
suprasternal) and the number of cardiac cross-sections which can be
imaged is in principle unlimited (14,15). The diagnostic yield of
two-dimensional echo contrast studies is potentially much higher than
that obtained with M-mode studies but it is a highly demanding method.
Left ventricular contrast echocardiography is mainly performed with
two-dimensional echocardiography in the catheterization laboratory.
Apical views are particularly useful for quantitative left ventricular
studies, since the entire left ventricle from apex to base is commonly
recorded.

ANALYSIS OF CONTRAST ECHOCARDIOGRAMS (TABLE I)

Timing of appearance yields important physiologic and diagnostic
information. Left heart contrast appearing a few cycles after right
heart opacification implies an intracardiac shunt, whereas a
consistent delay of 6-8 cardiac cycles suggests intrapulmonary right-
to-left shunting (16,17).
The timing of echo-contrast appearance in the left heart after peripheral contrast injection in patients with a ventricular septal defect
may help in the assessment of right ventricular hemodynamics (18).
Cyclical opacification of a great artery proves its arterioventricular
connection (13).
In the presence of an intracardiac shunt, the relative intensities of
contrast in the right and left heart contain information on the shunt
size (19).

TABLE I
ANALYSIS OF CONTRAST ECHOCARDIOGRAMS
Timing of appearance
Pattern of opacification
Cyclical opacification
Duration of opacification (clearance time)
Intensity
Slope of trajectories
Negative contrast effect

The slopes of contrast trajectories on M-mode echocardiographic
tracings represent the velocity component of the blood moving in the
direction of, or away from, the transducer, thus providing information
similar to that obtained using pulsed Doppler techniques. This
possibility has been insufficiently utilized but some authors are now
studying intracardiac flow patterns using echo-contrast. A correlation
between invasive measured pulmonary blood velocities and the velocity
of contrast trajectories on M-mode recordings has been demonstrated by
Japanese investigators (20).
Negative contrast effects may be seen whenever echo-contrast free
blood passes into a contrast filled cavity and can be used to diagnose
left-to-right shunts using peripheral venous injection (21,22).

CLINICAL APPLICATIONS OF CONTRAST ECHOCARDIOGRAPHY

The clinical applications of contrast echocardiography are listed in
table II.

TABLE II
CLINICAL APPLCIATIONS OF CONTRAST ECHOCARDIOGRAPHY
- Structure identification (M,2-D)
- Diagnosis (or exclusion) of shunts
    Localization (2-D)
    Direction shunting blood flow (M,2-D)
    Timing (M)
- Complex congenital heart disease (2-D)
- Valvular insufficiency
    Venous injections: tricuspid and pulmonic (M)
    Catheter injections: aortic and mitral (M,2-D)
- Intracavitary and transvalvular flow patterns
    (2-D)
- Videodensitometric analysis of echo contrast (2-D)
- Improved quantitation of left ventricle (2-D)

M,2-D: indication for which points M-mode or two-dimensional
echocardiography offer relative advantages.

STRUCTURE IDENTIFICATION

Contrast echocardiography was originally used for identifying cardiac
structures on M-Mode echocardiograms (23) and later for two-dimensional
echocardiography (14,24). Specific structures where contrast echocardiography has aided in correct identification include: the aortic
root and valve cusps (25), the endocardium of the left ventricle (26),
the coronary sinus (27), the interatrial septum (23), left main
coronary artery (28), the interatrial baffle after Mustard's operation
for transposition of the great arteries (29) and the pericardial space
during   pericardiocentesis   (30).

Goldberg (31) used the contrast technique to validate the underlying anatomy of heart and great vessels from the suprasternal transducer position. Right-sided heart structures are delineated by echocardiographic contrast, which allows identification of the endocardium of the anterior heart wall, interventricular septum, and better delineation of the right ventricular outflow tract, areas often obscured by non-structural echoes.

A persistent left superior vena cava entering the right atrium through a dilated coronary sinus may simulate the pattern of pericardial effusion on M-mode echocardiograms. This anomaly is readily identified by a left arm contrast injection (27,32).

Peripheral contrast injections can aid in the correct identification of other structures, such as the Eustachian valves, at the level of the inferior vena cava - right atrial junction (33); space-occupying lesions in the right atrium and ventricle if they have poor echo-reflective characteristics (34).

Direct catheter injections of echo contrast have been used to identify the common pulmonary venous chamber in patients with total anomalous pulmonary venous return (35), patent ductus arteriosus (36), and the ascending and descending thoracic aorta.

DIAGNOSIS (AND EXCLUSION) OF SHUNTS

Since echocardiographic contrast is entirely removed from the circulation by the pulmonary capillary bed (8), the appearance of contrast in the left heart after a peripheral venous injection is diagnostic for a right-to-left shunt. The pattern and appearance time of the echo-contrast in the left heart are determined by the level of the shunt and the relative pressures in the cardiac chambers. Shunts as small as 5% can be detected by contrast echocardiography (37). Recently, it has been shown that pulmonary wedge injections can yield left heart contrast which may be used to demonstrate left-to-right shunts without left heart catheterization (10-13)(figure 1). Catheter injections of echocardiographic contrast into the left atrium or ventricle make a left-to-right shunt directly visible (38)(figure 2). This method is helpful in demonstrating additional muscular septal defects, which are easily overlooked in the presence of complex congenital heart disease.

The small right-to-left shunt present in early systole in an uncomplicated atrial septal defect (39) can be used to diagnose a shunt at atrial level by peripheral contrast echocardiography (see chapter 3 by Dr G. Kronik)(40-46).

Although there is some bidirectional flow across a ventricular septal defect, peripheral venous contrast studies often fail to show the right-to-left shunting in the absence of pulmonary hypertension. Right-to-left shunting of contrast material occurs when the right ventricular systolic pressure approaches 50% of the systolic systemic pressure (47,48).

6

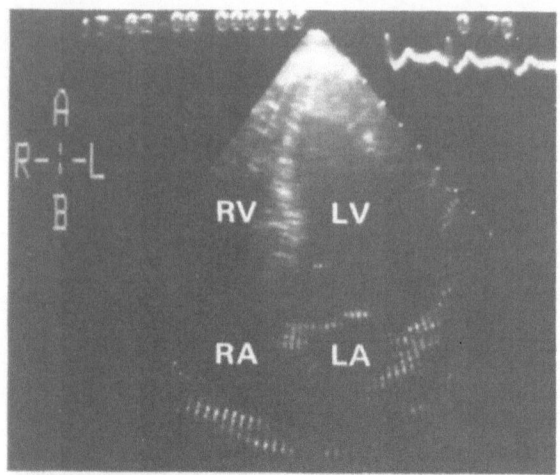

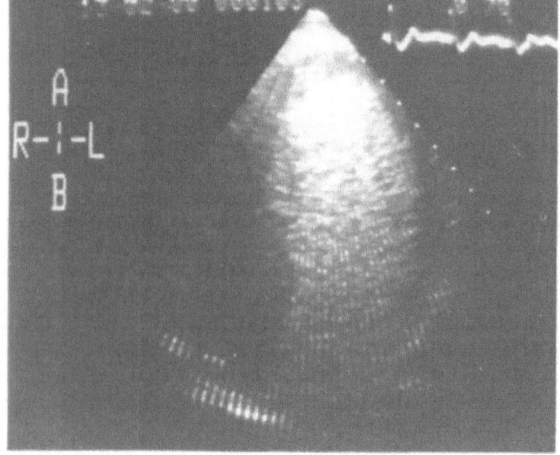

Figure 1: Stop-frame, apical four-chamber views obtained from a patient with a normal left ventricle immediately before (upper panel) and after pulmonary wedge injection of echocardiographic contrast (lower panel). The echo contrast fills both the left atrium (LA) and left ventricle (LV), of which the cavity contour becomes clearly delineated. A: apical; B: basal; L: left; R: right; RA: right atrium and RV: right ventricle.

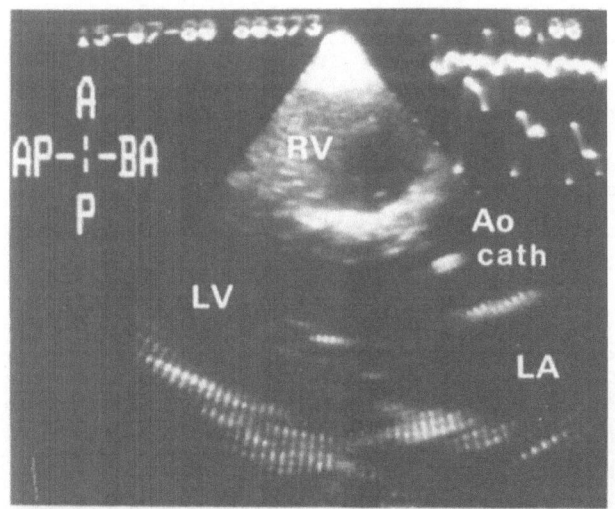

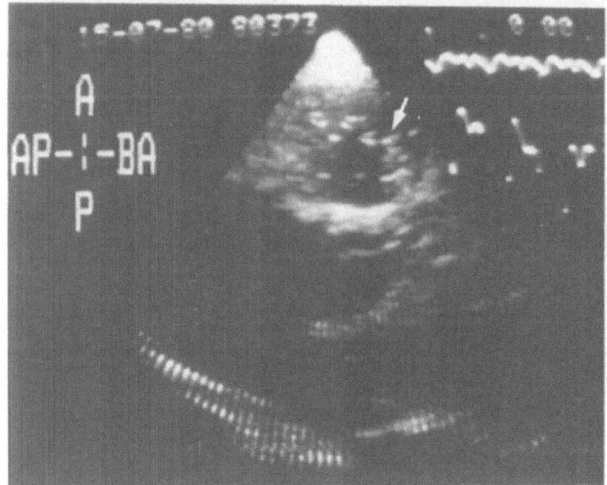

Figure 2: Parasternal long axis views of a patient with a small ventricular septal defect before (upper panel) and after (lower panel) catheter injection of echo contrast in the left ventricular outflow tract. Echoes appears in the right ventricular outflow tract (arrow) proving the existence of a small left-to-right shunt. A: anterior; AP: apical; BA: basal; P: posterior; Ao: aorta; cath: catheter; LA: left atrium; LV: left ventricle; RV: right ventricle.

The shunting occurs in protodiastole during isovolumic relaxation of the left ventricle. With increasing pressure, specific patterns of right-to-left shunting blood-flow can be observed (17). In uncomplicated ventricular septal defects, right-to-left shunting may occasionally be observed during Valsalva maneuver or ventricular premature beats (49).
In some cases with post-infarction ventricular septal defect, contrast echoes may be seen passing from the right to the left ventricle, possibly as a result of inequalities in relaxation between both ventricles (figure 3).

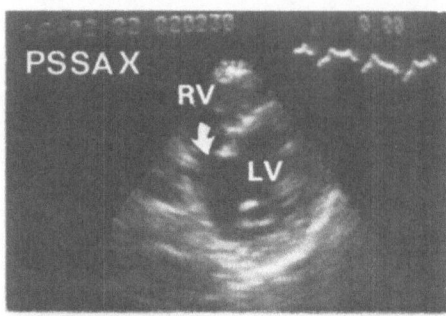

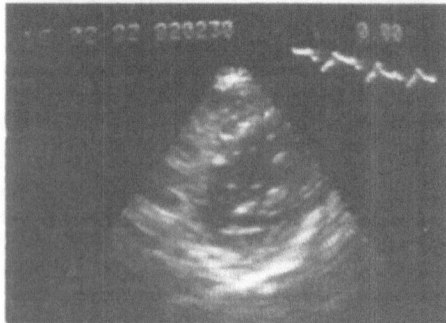

Figure 3: Parasternal short axis views of a patient with postinfarction ventricular septal defect (see arrow). After contrast injection in the right atrium via a Swan--Ganz catheter contrast echoes fill the right ventricle (RV) and appear in the left ventricle (LV) via the defect.

Negative contrast effect, however may be more sensitive for detecting uncomplicated and post-infarct ventricular septal defects.
Intracardiac catheter injections were performed by Cooperberg et al (50) to study a sinus of Valsalva aneurysm which had ruptured into the right ventricle. We recently visualized a pseudoaneurysm of the left ventricle (figure 4). Based on negative contrast effect, the diagnosis of a sinus of Valsalva aneurysm rupture into the right atrium can be made using peripheral injections (51).

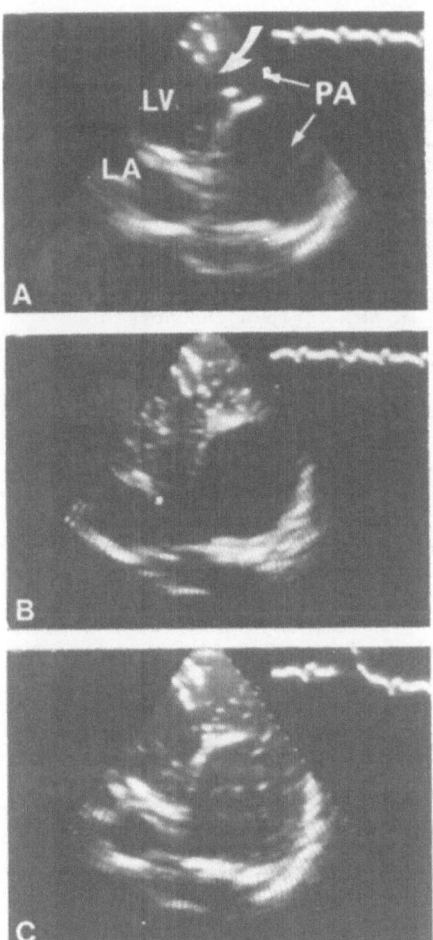

Figure 4: Apical views of the left ventricle (LV) and left atrium (LA) foreshortened to the left in the four-chamber plane. The patient had a large postmyocardial infarction pseudoaneurysm (PA). The defect in the lateral LV wall is indicated by the arrow in panel A. Echo-contrast injected in the left ventricle passes via the defect into the anterior part of the PA (panel B) and subsequently opacifies it completely (panel C). The echo-contrast remained circulating in the PA during many cardiac cycles after it had disappeared from the LV.

COMPLEX CONGENITAL HEART DISEASE

Using information obtained by peripheral contrast injections from both
the parasternal and suprasternal transducer positions, it is possible
ot determine the position of the great vessels and their ventriculo-
atrial connections (47). Together with the ability to detect and
localize shunts, contrast echocardiography offers important advantages
to the pediatric cardiologist who needs to analyze complex congenital
heart disease (52), particularly in the case of critically ill
neonates with cardiorespiratory problems (53). The more complex the
defect, the more likely is the existence of lesionspecific echocardiographic anatomy and blood-flow patterns. Using different views one can
observe the timing of the contrast appearance in the various chambers
and structures.
Characteristic contrast echocardiographic patterns have been described
in univentricular hearts with either one of two atrioventricular
valves (54), tricuspid atresia (55), truncus arteriosus (56),
straddling tricuspid valve and "double inlet" left ventricle (57).
Direct left ventricular echo-contrast injections are now increasingly
used in the catheterization laboratory. The method is a superior
technique to angiography for the detailed assessment of the interventricular septum and blood flow patterns in the presence of atrioventricular canal defects (58) and for the demonstration of small
muscular septal defects (59). Left ventricle to right atrium shunts
have been demonstrated with left ventricular contrast injections.

DIAGNOSIS OF VALVULAR INSUFFICIENCY

Contrast echocardiography has become a useful technique in detecting
right-sided valvular insufficiency. Analysis of the timing - more
specifically the moment of appearance of the contrast bolus in the
inferior vena cava (IVC) after an aupper extremity vein injection -
allows the examiner to diagnose or exclude tricuspid valve
insufficiency. If contrast appears in the inferior vena cava
synchronous with the v-wave of the atrial pressure curve, the
diagnosis of tricuspid insufficiency can be made with a great degree
of accuracy (60)(figure 5).
Two-dimensional echocardiography has been used (61) but may lead to
false positive diagnoses because timing of the contrast appearance is
less accurate than with M-mode recordings (60).
Contrast is frequently seen to appear synchronous with the a-wave
(presystolic) or in no definite relation to the cardiac cycle: this
does not suggest tricuspid insufficiency. This pattern is frequently
seen in normals during deep inspiration; in the presence of an atrial
septal defect; in conditions affecting right ventricular filling, such
as pulmonary stenosis, constrictive pericarditis, tricuspid stenosis,
pulmonary hypertension, cardiomyopathies; during rhythm disturbances.

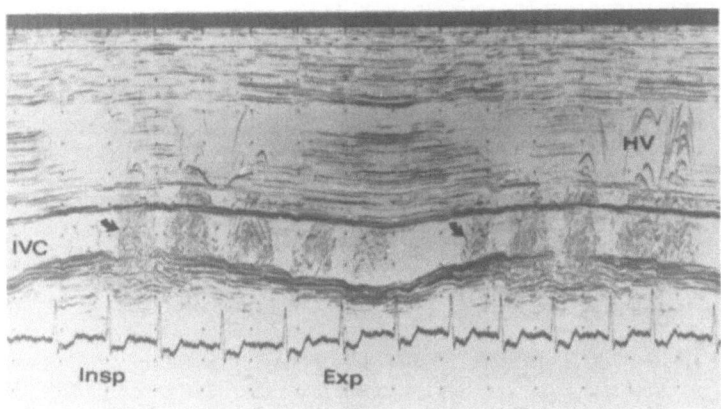

Figure 5: M-mode echocardiogram showing the inferior vena cava (IVC) and a "v-wave synchronous" appearance of echo-contrast (see arrows). This pattern is diagnostic for tricuspid insufficiency. Note the increase of contrast intensity during inspiration (Carvallo's sign) as the regurgitant flow increases.

Since no ideal method of diagnosing tricuspid insufficiency is available, contrast echocardiography may gain clinical importance. Specific echo contrast patterns across the pulmonary valve have been reported in pulmonary insufficiency, but their sensitivity and specificity remain a subject for further study (62). Following up these observations, we were able to demonstrate a specific echo contrast flow pattern over the pulmonary valve in patients with pulmonary hypertension. The pattern explains the highly specific mid-systolic closure of this valve commonly seen in these patients (63). These studies confirmed experimental work by Tahara et al (64), who demonstrated the temporal relationship between the pulmonary valve echogram, the pressure gradient and flow over the valve.

Demonstration of left-sided valvular insufficiency requires catheter injection and thus cardiac catheterization. However, it is a sensitive method for the detection (or exclusion) of valvular insufficiency, since regurgitant volumes as small as 10% of the forward stroke volume can be detected (65). Aortic insufficiency can be detected with a high degree of sensitivity by injecting its appearance in the left ventricle during diastole. Mitral regurgitation is demonstrated by detecting left atrial contrast during systole after left ventricular injection. The clearance time of echo contrast from the left ventricle in these conditions is prolonged but cannot be used, however, to quantitate regurgitation reliably.

USEFULNESS OF CONTRAST ECHO-VENTRICULOGRAPHY (TABLE III)

Echo-ventriculography can be considered in situations where contra-indications to radiographic contrast agents (allergy, renal insufficiency) or ionizing radiation (pregnancy) exist.

TABLE III
ADVANTAGES OF ECHO-VENTRICULOGRAPHY
- Multiple injections and cardiac views for analysis
- High sensitivity for detection of shunts and valvular insufficiency
- No adverse effects:
  no toxic contrast (allergy, renal failure)
  no ionizing energy (pregnancy)
- Avoidance of arrhythmias
- Lower cost

It is not yet fully realized that two-dimensional echocardiography may be an efficient imaging technique for guiding and proper positioning of catheter during catheterization procedures and thus reducing fluoroscopic control to a minimum. Selective contrast echocardiography is also useful in determining proper catheter location prior to selective angiography, especially when the amount of contrast material which may be injected is limited. Further advantages are that multiple injections can be performed and many different cardiac views can obtained for analysis, since entirely nontoxic contrast agents are used, and that hand injections of small amounts of fluid do not cause the premature beats frequently seen during standard cardiac angio-graphy.

STUDY OF SPECIFIC BLOOD FLOW PATTERNS

The non-contrast blood flowing from the left atrium into the left ventricle after its opacification with echo contrast by central catheter injection allows observation of transmitral blood flow. The negative contrast shadow delineates the functional mitral valve orifice. This is demonstrated in figure 6 obtained from a patient with mitral valve stenosis. The functional dimension is visualized by the echo-free blood entering the left ventricle after its opacification and is smaller than the anatomical dimension of the valve orifice which is visualized during the baseline study. Intracavitary blood flow patterns produced by tricuspid and mitral valve prostheses can be imaged after peripheral and pulmonary wedge injections. Occasionally one may observe a circulating vortex of echo contrast within an ischemic aneurysm in patients with coronary artery disease and it is conceivable that this pattern in part may explain the formation of a laminated thrombus present in most of these patients.

Left ventricular contrast echocardiography may thus allow a new type of study on local flow, turbulence and stasis, which promises to become more useful in the future if transpulmonary echo contrast transmission becomes available.

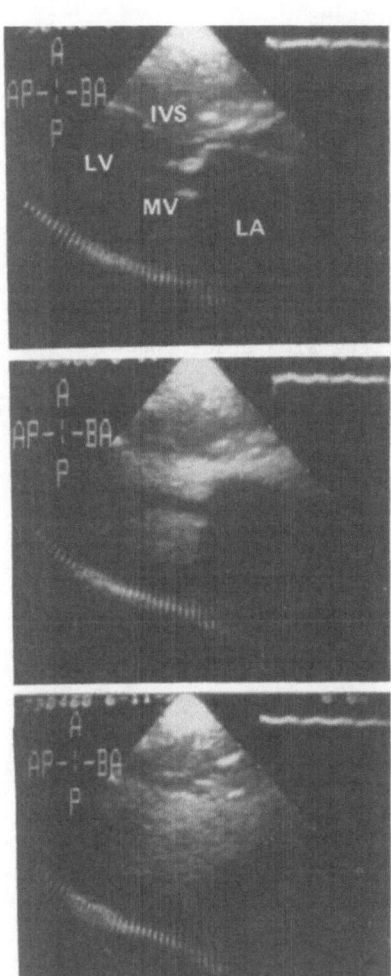

Figure 6: Stop-frame photographs of parasternal long axis views of a patient with mitral valve stenosis before (upper panel) and after injection of echo contrast via a catheter in the left ventricle. The middle panel shows a frame recorded during diastole. The negative shadow caused by the non contrast blood flowing from the left atrium into the ventricle visualizes the transmitral blood flow pattern. During systole (lower panel), the echo contrast does not pass into the left atrium, excluding mitral incompetence. A: anterior; AP: apical; BA: basal; P: posterior; IVS: interventricular septum; LA: left atrium; LV: left ventricle; MV: mitral valve.

14

VIDEODENSITOMETRIC ANALYSIS OF CONTRAST ECHOCARDIOGRAMS

Bommer et al (66) described in 1978 a method of obtaining dilution
curves of echocardiographic contrast by videodensitometry. The
dilution curves were reproducible on multiple echocardiographic
contrast injections to an accuracy of 15%. Time course of decay
enabled separation of normal patients from those with low cardiac
output and/or tricuspid regurgitation. Echo contrast indicator
dilution curves of the left ventricle were subsequently performed in
dogs and good correlations with cardiac output measurements were found
(67-69). We have used an image processing computer to analyze video
recordings of contrast injections in order to follow the decay of
density after left ventricular and pulmonary wedge injections in 17
patients (figure 7). A meaningful calculation of the area under the
curve could not be made because of limitations due to video "overload"
immediately after injection.
The decay phase, however, was found to be exponential and had
characteristics of indicator-dilution curves, as predicted
theoretically. Our preliminary data indicate that R-wave gating may
allow estimation of ejection fraction (70).
Hagler et al (19) used computer-based videodensitometric techniques to
analyze video recordings of left ventricular contrast echocardiograms
for quantitating left-to-right shunts.

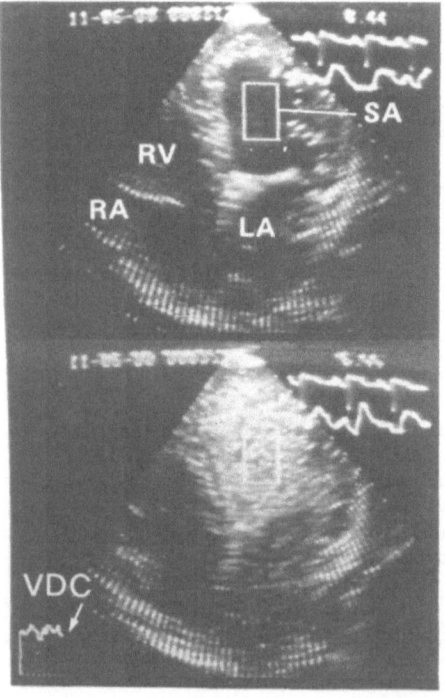

Figure 7: Apical
four-chamber views
with a rectangular
sample area (SA) for
measuring the
videodensity within
the left ventricular
cavity (upper
panel). During
contrast studies, a
curve of the
cumulated video-
density (VDC) is
simultaneously
displayed on the
videoscreen (lower
panel). LA: left
atrium; RA: right
atrium; RV: right
ventricle.

QUANTITATION OF LEFT VENTRICULAR VOLUMES

Feigenbaum et al (26) utilized left ventricular injections of indocyanine green dye to differentiate the endocardium from other echoes
within the cavity. Even when using newer equipment, non-structural
echoes often obscure the endocardial boundaries and make proper
delineation of the left ventricular cavity difficult or even
impossible, especially in the apical area. It is conceivable that
opacification of the left ventricular cavity with echocardiographic
contrast would improve border recognition.
Improved cavity delineation by echocardiographic contrast may increase
the accuracy of left ventricular volume determination from two-
dimensional images (figure 8). All studies published so far on
comparison of left ventricular volumes determined by angiocardiography
and two-dimensional echocardiography have demonstrated a systematic
underestimation of volumes by the echo method. We therefore made
recordings of the left ventricle in four views at mitral level; apical
4-chamber and long axis views) before and during left ventricular
injections of dextrose 5% in water in 13 patients. Long axis length
and surface area within the endocardial contours were measured from
stop-frame images, independently from recordings with and without
contrast, using a lightpen system and a digital computer. These
measurements were repeated by the same investigator one month later.

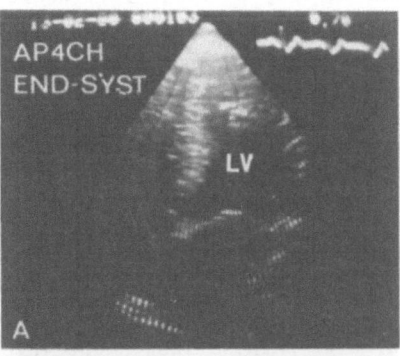
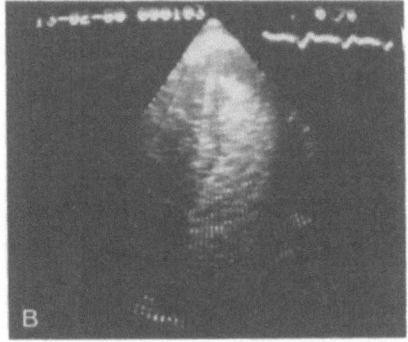

Figure 8: Apical four-chamber
views ((AP4CH) at end-systole
before (panel A) and after
(panel B) opacification of the
left ventricle (LV) with echo-
contrast. The endocardial
contour is blurred by non-
structural echoes in the
apical area and lateral segments
are not seen because of
"drop-outs". These area's
are delineated by echo-contrast
and the accuracy of surface
area measurements will be
improved.

Both long axis length and the surface area were significantly larger with contrast than without (p 0.001). The use of echo contrast improved the accuracy of these measurements but reduced the reproducibility, showing a raised intra-observer variability. This is not surprising as echo contrast improves border recognition in areas with non-structural echoes and endocardial drop-outs but obscures the endocardium in the areas where it is clearly visible during the baseline study. Clearly more work must be done in this area using contrast together with non-contrast echocardiography if reliable routine left ventricular measurements are to be achieved.

FUTURE DIRECTIONS OF CONTRAST ECHOCARDIOGRAPHY

Development of a contrast agent yielding adequate contrast during routine studies has a high priority for research and specially designed microbubbles may be used in the future to provide a more reliable and quantifiable contrast effect. Utilizing contrast agents which allow an injectate of constant mass, indicator dilution curves from videodensitometric analysis of two-dimensional echocardiograms may enable actual measurement of cardiac output (67-71). Transmission of echocardiographic contrast through capillary beds may be an attainable objective (see chapter by Roelandt et al), which would enhance our ability to image left heart structures.

CONCLUSIONS

Contrast echocardiography is a rapidly developing field and will undoubtedly play an increasing role in the daily practice of cardiology in the future. Its definitive breakthrough will probably come with the availability of a reliable, quantifiable and nontoxic contrast agent able to pass the lung capillary bed. Close cooperation between academic institutions and industry is likely to lead to the development of hardware and software configurations necessary for examination and analysis of contrast studies. Integration of the data thus obtained on blood flow with those on structure and function may lead to a multi-purpose instrument which can provide answers to many clinical questions and replace invasive procedures in a large number of cardiac patients.

REFERENCES

1. Meltzer RS, Tickner EG, Sahines TP, Popp RL: The source of
    ultrasound contrast effect. J Clin Ultrasound 8: 121, 1980.
2. Meltzer RS, Serruys PW, Hugenholtz PG, Roelandt J: Intravenous
    carbon dioxide as an echocardiographic contrast agent. J Clin
    Ultrasound 9: 127, 1981.
3. Kronik G, Slany J, Mösslacher H: Contrast M-mode echocardiography
    in diagnosis of atrial septal defects in acyanotic patients.
    Circulation 59: 372, 1979.
4. Kronik G, Mösslacher H, Schmoliner R, Hutterer B: Kontrast
    Echokardiographie bei Patienten mit kleinen interatrialen
    Kurzschlussverbindungen (offenes Foramen Ovale). Wien Klin
    Wochenschrift 92: 290, 1980.
5. Seward JB, Tajik AJ, Hagler DJ, Ritter DG: Peripheral venous
    contrast echocardiography. Am J Cardiol 39: 202, 1977.
6. Seward JB, Tajik AJ, Spangler JG, Ritter DG: Echocardiographic
    contrast studies. Mayo Clin Proc 50: 163, 1975.
7. Feigenbaum H, Stone JM, Lee DA, Nasser WK, Chang S: Identifi-
    cation of ultrasound echoes from the left ventricle by use of
    intracardiac injections of indocyanine green. Circulation 41:
    615, 1970.
8. Meltzer RS, Sartorius OEH, Lancée CT, Verdouw PD, Essed CE,
    Serruys PW, Roelandt J: Transmission of ultrasonic contrast
    through the lungs. Ultrasound in Med & Biol 7: 377, 1981.
9. Bommer WJ, Mason DT, DeMaria AN: Studies in contrast echocardio-
    graphy: development of new agents with superior reproducibility
    and transmission through lungs. Circulation 59 and 60 (Suppl II):
    II-17, 1979.
10. Reale A, Pizzuto F, Gioffré PA, Nigri A, Romeo F, Martuscelli E,
    Mangieri E, Scibilia G: Contrast echocardiography: transmission
    of echoes to the left heart across the pulmonary vascular bed.
    Eur Heart J 1: 101, 1980.
11. Meltzer RS, Tickner EG, Popp RL: Why do the lungs clear ultra-
    sonic contrast ? Ultrasound in Med & Biol 6: 263, 1980.
12. Meltzer RS, Serruys PW, McGhie J, Verbaan N, Roelandt J:
    Pulmonary wedge injections yielding left sided echocardiograpic
    contrast. Brit Heart J 44: 390, 1980.
13. Mortera C, Hunter S, Tynan M: Contrast echocardiography
    and the suprasternal approach in infants and children. Eur J
    Cardiol 9/6: 437, 1979.
14. Tajik AJ, Seward JB, Hagler DJ, Mair DD, Lie JJ: Two-dimensional
    real-time ultrasonic imaging of the heart and great vessels.
    Technique, image orientation, structure identification and
    validation. Mayo Clin Proc 53: 271, 1978.
15. Meltzer RS, Meltzer C, Roelandt J: Sector scanning views in
    echocardiography: a systematic approach. Eur Heart J 1: 379,
    1980.
16. Shub C, Tajik AJ, Seward JB, Dines DE: Detecting intra-pulmonary
    right-to-left shunt with contrast echocardiography. Mayo Clin
    Proc 51: 81, 1976.

18

17. Hernandez A, Strauss AW, McKnight R, Hartman AFjr: Diagnosis of pulmonary arteriovenous fistula by contrast echocardiography. J Pediatr 93: 258, 1978.
18. Serwer GA, Armstrong BE, Anderson PAW, Sherman D, Benson DWjr, Edwards SB: Use of contrast echocardiography for evaluation of right ventricular hemodynamics in the presence of ventricular septal defects. Circulation 58: 327, 1978.
19. Hagler DJ, Tajik AJ, Seward JB, Mair DD, Ritter DG, Ritman EL: Videodensitometric quantitation of left-to-right shunts with contrast sector echocardiography. Circulation 57 and 58 (Suppl II): II-70, 1978.
20. Shiina A, Kondo K, Nakasone Y, Tsuchiya M, Yaginuma T, Hosada S: Contrast echocardiographic evaluation of changes in flow velocity in the right side of the heart. Circulation 63: 1408, 1981.
21. Weyman AE, Wann S, Caldwell RL, Hurwitz RA, Dillon JC, Feigenbaum H: Negative contrast echocardiography: a new technique for detecting left-to-right shunts. Circulation 59: 498, 1979.
22. Feigenbaum H: Echocardiography, 3rd edition, Lea & Febiger, Philadelphia, 1981, p 362.
23. Gramiak R, Nanda NC: Structure identification in echocardio-graphy. In: Gramiak R and Waag RC (editors), Cardiac Ultrasound. St.Louis, CV Mosby, 1975, p 29.
24. Sahn DJ, Williams DE, Shackelton S, Friedman WF: The validity of structure identification for cross-sectional echocardiography. J Clin Ultrasound 2: 201, 1974.
25. Gramiak R, Shah PM: Echocardiography of the aortic root. Invest Radiol 3: 356, 1968.
26. Feigenbaum H, Stone JM, Lee DA, Nasser WK, Chang S: Identifi-cation of ultrasound echoes from the left ventricle by use of intracardiac injections of indocyanine green. Circulation 41: 615, 1970.
27. Snider RA, Ports TA, Silverman NH: Venous anomalies of the coronary sinus: Detection by Mmode, two-dimensional and contrast echocardiography. Circulation 60: 721, 1979.
28. Weyman AE, Feigenbaum H, Dillon JC, Johnston KW, Eggleton RC: Noninvasive visualization of the left main coronary artery by cross-sectional echocardiography. Circulation 54: 169, 1976.
29. Nanda NC, Stewart S, Gramiak R, Manning JA: Echocardiography of the intra- atrial baffle in dextro-transposition of the great vessels. Circulation 51: 1130, 1975.
30. Chandraratna PAN, Langevin E, O'Dell R: Echocardiographic contrast studies during pericardiocentesis. Ann Int Med 87: 199, 1977.
31. Goldberg B: Suprasternal ultrasonography. JAMA 215: 245, 1971.
32. Stewart JA, Fraker TD, Slosky DA, Wise NK, Kisslo JA: Detection of persistent left superior vena cava by two-dimensional contrast echocardiography. J Clin Ultrasound 7: 357, 1979.
33. Nanda NC, Gramiak R (editors): Two-dimensional contrast echocardio-graphy. In: Clinical Echocardiography, St.Louis, CV Mosby, 1978, p 425.
34. Kisslo JA: Usefulness of M-mode and cross-sectional echocardio-graphy for analysis of right-sided heart disease. In: Lancée CT (ed), Echocardiology, Martinus Nijhoff, the Hague, 1979, p 37.

35. Paquet M, Gutgesell H: Echocardiographic features of total anomalous pulmonary venous connection. Circulation 51: 599, 1975.
36. Allen HD, Sahn SJ, Goldberg SJ: New serial contrast technique for assessment of left-to-right shunting patent ductus arteriosus in the neonate. Am J Cardiol 41: 288, 1978.
37. Pieroni DN, Varghese J, Freedom RM, Rowe RD: The sensitivity of contrast echocardiography in detecting intracardiac shunts. Cath & Cardiovasc Diagn 5: 19, 1979.
38. Roelandt J, Meltzer RS, Serruys PW: Contrast echocardiography of the left ventricle. In: Rijsterborgh H (ed), Echocardiology, Martinus Nijhoff, the Hague, 1981, p 219.
39. Levin AR, Spach MS, Boineau JP: Atrial pressure-flow dynamics in atrial septal defect (secundum type). Circulation 37: 476, 1968.
40. Serruys PW, Van den Brand M, Hugenholtz PG, Roelandt J: Intra-cardiac right-to-left shunts demonstrated by two- dimensional echocardiography after peripheral vein injection. Brit Heart J 42: 429, 1979.
41. Fraker TD, Harris PJ, Behar VS, Kisslo JA: Detection and exclusion of interatrial shunts by two-dimensional echocardio-graphy and peripheral venous injections. Circulation 59: 379, 1979.
42. Valdez-Cruz LM, Pieroni DR, Roland JMA, Varghese PH: Echocardio-graphic detection of intracardiac right-to-left shunts following peripheral vein injection. Circulation 54: 588, 1976.
43. Bourdillon PDV, Foale RA, Richards AF: Identification of atrial septal defect by cross-sectional contrast echocardiography. Brit Heart J 44: 401, 1980.
44. Serruys PW, Hagemeijer F, Bom AH, Roelandt J: Echocardiologie de contraste en deux dimensions et en temps réel. 2: Applications cliniques. Arch Mal Coeur 71: 611, 1978.
45. Serruys PW, Hagemeijer F, Roelandt J: Echocardiological contrast studies with dynamically focussed multiscan. Acta Cardiologica 34: 283, 1979.
46. Lunde P, Abrahamsen AM: Contrast shunting through a patent foramen ovale in a patient with pulmonary stenosis. Eur J Cardiol 12: 129, 1980.
47. Roelandt J, Serruys PW: Real-time cross-sectional contrast echocardiography. In: Bleifeld W, Effert S, Hanrath P, Mathey D (editors), Evaluation of Cardiac Function by Echocardiography, Springer-Verlag, Berlin, 1980, p 152.
48. Serruys PW, Vletter WB, Hagemeijer F, Ligtvoet CM: Bidimensional real-time echocardiological visualization of a ventricular right-to-left shunt following peripheral vein injection. Eur J Cardiol 6/2: 99, 1977.
49. Meltzer RS, Schwartz J, French J, Popp RL: Ventricular septal defect noted by two-dimensional echocardiography. Chest 76: 455, 1979.
50. Cooperberg P, Mercer EN, Mulder DS, Winsberg F: Rupture of a sinus Valsalva aneurysma: report of a case diagnosed pre-operatively by echocardiography. Radiology 113: 117, 1974.
51. Nakamura K, Suzuki S, Satomi G: Detection of ruptured aneurysm of sinus of Valsalva by contrast two-dimensional echocardiography. Brit Heart J 45: 219, 1981.

52. Seward JB, Tajik AJ, Hagler DJ: Contrast echocardiography in the assessment of acyanotic and complex congenital heart disease: peripheral venous, invasive, and unique applications. In: Meltzer RS and Roelandt J (editors), Contrast echocardiography, Martinus Nijhoff, the Hague, 1982 (in press).

53. Sahn DJ, Allen HD, George W, Mason M, Goldberg SJ: The utility of contrast echocardiographic techniques in the care of critically ill infants with cardiac and pulmonary disease. Circulation 56: 959, 1977.

54. Seward JB, Tajik AJ, Hagler DJ, Giugliani ER, Gan GT, Ritter DG: Contrast echocardiography in common (single) ventricle: angiographic anatomic correlation. Am J Cardiol 39: 217, 1977.

55. Seward JB, Tajik AJ, Hagler DJ, Ritter DG: Echocardiographic spectrum of tricuspid atresia. Mayo Clin Proc 53: 100, 1978.

56. Assad-Morell JL, Seward JB, Tajik AJ, Hagler DJ, Giuliani ER, Ritter DG: Echo-phonocardiographic and contrast studies in conditions associated with systemic arterial trunk overriding the ventricular septum. Circulation 53: 663, 1976.

57. Kato H, Yoshioka F: Echocardiographic approach for atrioventricular malalignment and related conditions. J Cardiogr 8: 521, 1978.

58. Hagler DJ, Tajik AJ, Seward JB, Mair DD, Ritter DG: Real-time wide-angle sector echocardiography: atrioventricular canal defects. Circulation 59: 140, 1979.

59. Seward JB, Tajik AJ, Hagler DJ: Two-dimensional contrast echocardiography. In: Lündstrom NR (ed), Pediatric Echocardiography - cross-sectional, M-mode and Doppler, Elsevier/North Holland Biomedical, Amsterdam, 1980, p 239.

60. Meltzer RS, Van Hoogenhuyze DCA, Serruys PW, Haalebos MMP, Roelandt J: Diagnosis of tricuspid regurgitation by contrast echocardiography. Circulation 63: 1093, 1981.

61. Lieppe W, Behar VS, Scallion R, Kisslo JA: Detection of tricuspid regurgitation with two-dimensional echocardiography and peripheral vein injections. Circulation 57: 128, 1978.

62. Gullace G, Savoia MT, Ravizza P, Locatelli V, Addamiano R, Ranzi C: Contrast echocardiographic features of pulmonary hypertension and regurgitation. Brit Heart J 46: 369, 1981.

63. Meltzer RS, Valk NK, Vermeulen HWJ, Piérard LA, Ten Cate FJ, Roelandt J: Contrast echocardiography to diagnose pulmonary hypertension and explain the hemodynamic significance of the early closure sign. Circulation 64 (Suppl IV): IV-47, 1981.

64. Tahara M, Tanaka H, Nakao S, Yoshimura H, Sakurai S, Tei C, Kashima T, Kanehisa T: An experimental study on the mechanism of mid-systolic semiclosure of the pulmonary valve echogram in pulmonary hypertension. J Cardiogr 10: 199, 1980.

65. Kerber RE, Kioschos JM, Lauer RM: Use of an ultrasonic contrast method in the diagnosis of valvular regurgitation and intracardiac shunts. Am J Cardiol 34: 722, 1974.

66. Bommer W, Neef J, Neumann A, Weinert L, Lee G, Mason DT, DeMaria AN: Indicator-dilution curves obtained by photometric analysis of two-dimensional echo-contrast studies. Am J Cardiol 41: 370, 1978 (abstract).

67. DeMaria AN, Bommer W, Riggs K, Dajee A, Miller L, Mason DT: In vivo correlation of cardiac output and densitometric dilution curves obtained by contrast two-dimensional echocardiography. Circulation 62 (Suppl III): III-101, 1980.
68. DeMaria AN, Bommer W, Razor J, Tickner G, Mason DT: Determination of cardiac output by two-dimensional echocardiography. In: Rijsterborgh H (ed), Echocardiology, Martinus Nijhoff, the Hague, 1981, p 245.
69. DeMaria AN, Bommer WJ, Mason DT: Evaluation of cardiac performance and pressures by ultrasound: past promises and future potentials. Am Heart J 101: 514, 1981.
70. Bastiaans OL, Roelandt J, Piérard L, Meltzer RS: Ejection fraction from contrast echocardiographic videodensity curves. Clin Res 29: 176A, 1981.
71. Meltzer RS, Bastiaans OL, Lancée CT, Piérard LA, Serruys PW, Roelandt J: Videodensitometric processing of contrast two-dimensional echocardiographic data. (Submitted J Ultraound Med & Biol).

DIAGNOSIS OF INTERATRIAL COMMUNICATIONS BY CONTRAST ECHO-
CARDIOGRAPHY
G.KRONIK

INTRODUCTION
Standard M-mode and two-dimensional echocardiography are both
very sensitive methods for the diagnosis of atrial septal defects
(ASD). Right ventricular dilatation with or without abnormal
septal motion and an apparently defective atrial septum can be
demonstrated in virtually all ASD patients (1-4). However, these
signs lack specificity (2-4). Therefore contrast echocardiography
has recently been used for the direct visualization of interatrial right to left (R-L) and left to right (L-R) shunts.

ATRIAL R-L SHUNTS
R-L shunts can be diagnosed by contrast echocardiography, when
contrast echoes appear in the left heart following peripheral
venous injections (5) (=contrast shunting). Normally the microbubbles of gas, which cause the ultrasonic contrast (6) are only
seen in the right heart chambers but they are all cleared during
the passage of the blood through the pulmonary capillary bed (5).
Using contrast echocardiography it has become clear, that
patients with ASD do not only have the well known clinically important L-R shunt but usually also a small accompanying R-L
shunt, even though oxymetry and dye curves may fail to indicate
such a shunt (7-12). This observation is in accordance with earlier angiographic studies by Levin (13).
The sensitivity of contrast echocardiography in detecting this
small accompanying R-L shunt is high. Patients with a hemodynamic
situation that favours such a shunt (Eisenmenger-reaction, ASD
with pulmonic stenosis or Ebstein's disease), virtually always
have positive contrast studies (8-12). Even in uncomplicated
ASD the sensitivity has been reported as high as 73-100 %

(average 82 %) (7-12).

The amount of contrast, which appears in the left heart is very variable in ASD patients, ranging between just a few scattered contrast echoes - which must be carefully looked for - and very obvious left heart opacification (fig.1). Surprisingly the intensity of contrast shunting is not helpful in predicting either right ventricular systolic pressure or the magnitude of the L-R shunt (7-11). Even intense contrast shunting is entirely compatible with an uncomlicated ASD (fig.1) and must not be taken as evidence for inoperable pulmonary hypertension (8,9). Contrast echocardiography does not seem suited for follow up studies in individual patients either, for contrast shunting may be inconstant and variable upon subsequent injections in the same patient (9).

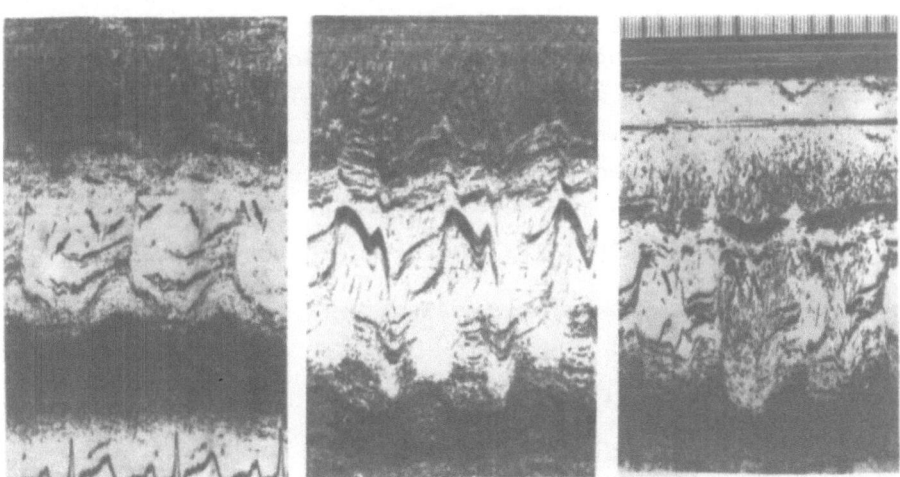

FIGURE 1: Positive contrast studies in 3 patients with uncomplicated ASD. Despite similar hemodynamic findings in these patients, the degree of contrast shunting is very different. Some contrast echoes in the left panel are marked with arrows.

When contrast studies during quiet respiration have been negative, it is worth-while to repeat contrast injections while the patient performs the Valsalva maneuver (8,9). With Valsalva provocation we have noted increased contrast shunting in roughly one fourth of all examined ASD cases and the sensitivity of con-

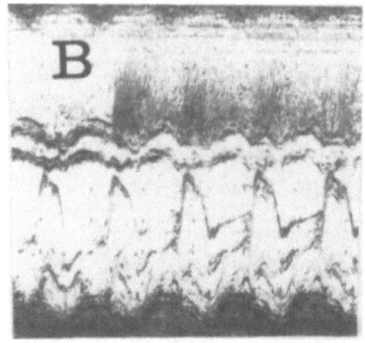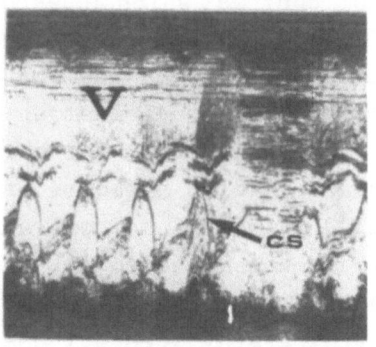

FIGURE 2: Provocation of more intense contrast shunting (CS) by the Valsalva maneuver (V). B = contrast study during basal conditions.

trastechocardiography was improved from 85 to 94 % (9) (fig.2).

The differential diagnosis of a positive contrast study in ASD includes other shunt lesions and the erroneous diagnosis of contrast echoes in the left heart, when in fact none are there. True contrast echoes show a characteristic motion pattern as they are carried by the streaming blood. Confusion of contrast with noise echoes, the "overload" effect or incomplete mitral structures can usually be avoided firstly because bubble echoes look different (fig.3) and secondly by applying stringent criteria for

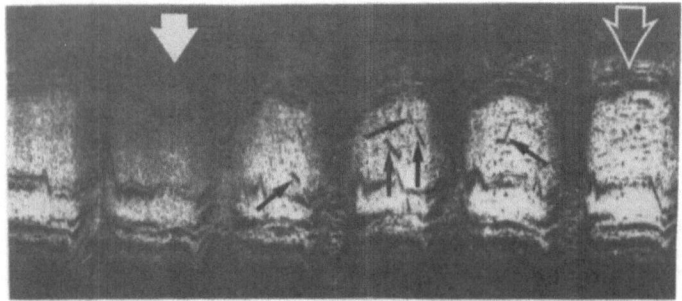

FIGURE 3: Poor quality contrast echocardiogram with contrast shunting, recorded during the Valsalva maneuver in a patient with patent foramen ovale. There is a homogenous veil-like opacification of the left heart due to the "overload" effect (solid white arrow) and there are multiple noise echoes (open white arrow) in the tracing. Nevertheless the typical linear contrast echoes in the left heart (some marked with black arrows) can be recognized.

a positive study. In our laboratory we require at least five
typical contrast echoes in the left heart following one injection
for a positive M-mode study. On two-dimensional studies counting
of contrast echoes is impractical. Very few contrast echoes are
only considered diagnostic, when their way through the left heart
can be clearly followed for some distance. With these criteria
technically false positives have not been a problem in our experience (8,19).

R-L shunts through a ventricular septal defect are easily
recognized by the fact, that the bubble echoes spare the left
atrium and the mitral funnel (14). Contrast shunting of the "ASD
type" (with left atrial and mitral funnel opacification) also
occurs in pulmonary arteriovenous fistula and certain venous
anomalies (15,16), but these lesions are rare and do not resemble
an ASD clinically.

Of greater practical importance is the fact, that a patent
foramen ovale may be sufficient for a positive contrast study (11,
17). We have examined 20 patients with patent foramen ovale but
no clinical or oxymetric evidence of a shunt. Contrast shunting
was demonstrated in 63 %, particularly during the Valsalva
maneuver. Even in the subgroup with normal right heart pressures
23 % had positive contrast studies at rest and 62 % either at
rest or with provocation (17).

This observation underlines the very high sensitivity of contrast echocardiography but detracts from the specificity of a
positive finding. A patient with questionable clinical findings
of an ASD and a positive contrast study may well have only a
patent foramen ovale. Occasionally the diagnosis of a patent
foramen may be clinically useful, for example when paradoxical
embolism is suspected.

ATRIAL L-R SHUNTS
Using two-dimensional echocardiography interatrial L-R shunts
can be visualized with peripheral venous injections. During right
atrial opacification the L-R shunt washes away the contrast
echoes near the defect (fig.4) thus creating a contrast-free area
which is called "negative contrast" or "wash out effect" (10,18,
19).When viewed in real time the wash out effect is accompanied

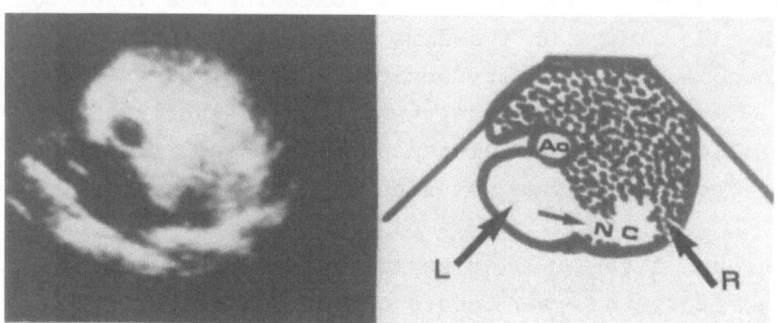

FIGURE 4: "Negative contrast" (NC) effect in a patient with
ASD. The sectioning plane runs through the aorta (Ao) and the
left (L) and right (R) atrium. The small black arrow indicates
the flow direction on the contrast-free left atrial blood
into the right atrium.

by turbulence and the flow direction of the contrast free blood
from the left to the right can be observed.

In most ASD patients the demonstration of the L-R shunt is
technically more difficult than the demonstration of the small
accompanying R-L shunt. The wash-out phenomenon is only seen,
when the sectioning plane crosses right through the defect (19).
In addition the right heart should be densely opacified and
there should not be a massive R-L shunt, so that the left atrial
blood remains contrast-free. The selection of the appropriate
sectioning plane is hampered by the fact that actually intact
parts of the atrial septum often appear defective because of
artifactual echo drop out (3,4,19). Looking for the negative
contrast without knowing the precise localization of the defect
can be cumbersome and the success rate is - among other factors -
also a matter of peristence.

This may at least partly explain the highly variable results
of different investigators. Weyman (18), Gilbert (10) and our
group (19) have reported a sensitivity of about 80 % in uncomplicated ASD. Others have seen the wash out effect in only 0 - 30 %
(11,12). The"negative contrast" effect is rare in servere Eisenmenger-reaction (10).

The width of the negative contrast does not permit conclusions
with respect to the shunt size (10,18,19), for the sectioning

plane may unpredictably cut through a central or a lateral portion of the defect. Surprisingly we have seen the wash out
effect in a few patients with an interatrial communication although no L-R shunt could be demonstrated by oxymetry (19).

The wash out effect that is caused by a L-R shunt must be
differenciated from certain normal phenomena (19). A negative
study is ideally characterized by homogeneous right atrial opacification (fig.5). Inhomogeneous filling, the intermittent

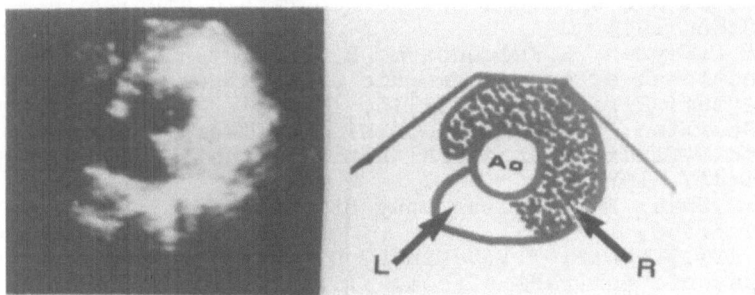

FIGURE 5: Clear and sharp demarcation between the contrast
free left atrium (L) and the homogeneously opacified right
atrium (R). This is the ideal negative finding in patients
without a shunt. Ao = aorta in cross section.

appearance of contrast-free blood and turbulence are typical
findings in conjunction with a L-R shunt. However these findings
are normal in certain parts of the right atrium, for the right
atrium always receives contrast-containing and contrast-free
blood from different sources. When these phenomena are very
prominent but not definite streaming of contrast-free blood
from the left to the right can be demonstrated the contrast
study may be inconclusive with respect to a L-R shunt. It should
be stressed, however, that a typical negative contrast effect
can nevertheless be diagnosed with confidence and provides firm
evidence for an interatrial leak (19).

CONCLUSION
Using all available contrast techniques a R-L or L-R shunt
can be demonstrated in virtually all ASD patients. A negative
contrast study makes the diagnosis of an ASD very unlikely.
However, contrast echocardiography is not helpful in evaluating

the hemodynamic status and positive studies may occur in patients
with only a patent foramen ovale.

REFERENCES

1. Radtke W.E., A.J.Tajik, G.T.Gau, T.T.Schattenberg, E.R.
   Giuliani, R.G.Tancredi: Atrial septal defect: Echocardiographic observations, studies in 120 patients. Ann.Int.Med.
   84:246, 1976
2. Kerber R.E., W.F.Dippel, F.M.Abboud: Abnormal motion of the
   interventricular septum in right ventricular volume overload: experimental and clinical echocardiographic studies.
   Circulation 48:86, 1973
3. Dillon J.C., A.E.Weyman, H.Feigenbaum, R.C.Eggleton, K.John-
   ston: Cross-sectional echocardiographic examination of the
   interatrial septum. Circulation 55:115, 1977
4. Lieppe W., R.Scallion, V.S.Behar, J.A.Kisslo: Two-dimensional
   echocardiographic findings in atrial septal defect.
   Circulation 56:447, 1977
5. Gramiak R., P.M.Shah: Echocardiography of the aortic root.
   Invest.Radiol. 3:356, 1968
6. Meltzer R.S., E.G.Tickner, T.P.Sahines, R.L.Popp: The
   source of ultrasonic contrast effect. J.Clin.Ultrasound
   8:121, 1980
7. Serruys P.W., M.van der Brand, P.G.Hugenholtz, J.Roelandt:
   Intracardiac right to left shunts demonstrated by two-dimensional echocardiography after peripheral vein injection.
   Brit.Heart J. 42,429, 1979
8. Kronik G., J.Slany, H.Mösslacher: Contrast M-mode echocardiography in diagnosis of atrial septal defect in acyanotic
   patients. Circulation 59:372, 1979
9. Kronik G.: Contrast echocardiography in patients with interatrial communications. J.Ultrasound in Med.& Biol. (in press)
10. Gilbert B.M., M.Drobac, H.Rakowski: Contrast two-dimensio-
    nal echocardiography in interatrial shunts. Amer.J.Cardiol
    45:402, 1980 (abstract)
11. Fraker J.D., P.J.Harris, V.S.Behar, J.A.Kisslo: Detection
    and exclusion of interatrial shunts by two-dimensional echo-
    cardiography and peripheral venous injections. Circulation
    59:379, 1979
12. Bourdillon P.D.V., R.A.Foale, A.F.Rickards: Assessment of
    atrial septal defect by cross-sectional echocardiography.
    In: Echocardiology (Martinus Nijhoff Publishers 1979;
    C.T.Lancee editor), p.61,1979
13. Levin H.A., M.S.Spach, J.Boineau, R.V.Cantet, P.Capp, P.H.
    Jewett: Atrial pressure flow dynamics in atrial septal defects
    (secundum type). Circulation 37:476, 1968
14. Seward J.B., A.J.Tajik, D.J.Hagler, D.G.Ritter: Peripheral
    venous contrast echocardiography. Amer.J.Cardiol 39:202,
    1977
15. Lewis A.B., G.F.Gates, P.Stanley: Echocardiography and per-
    fusion scintigraphy in the diagnosis of pulmonary arterio-
    venous fistula. Chest 73,675, 1978

16. Bourdillon P.D., R.A.Foale, J.Sommerville: Persistent left superior vena cava with coronary sinus and left atrial connections. Eur.J.Cardiol 11:227, 1980
17. Kronik G., H.Mösslacher: Positive contrast echocardiograms in patients with patent foramen ovale and normal right heart hemodynamics. Amer.J.Cardiol (in press)
18. Weyman A.E., L.S. Wann, R.L.Caldwell, R.A.Hurwitz, J.C. Dillon, H.Feigenbaum: Negative contrast echocardiography: A new method for the detecting left to right shunts. Circulation 59:498, 1979
19. Kronik G., B.Hutterer, H.Mösslacher: Diagnose atrialer links-rechts Shunts mit Hilfe der zwei-dimensionalen Kontrastechokardiographie. Z.f.Kardiol. 70:138, 1981

OPACIFICATION OF THE LEFT HEART BY PERIPHERAL VENOUS CONTRAST
ECHOCARDIOGRAPHY: ANIMAL EXPERIMENTS

J. Roelandt, R.S. Meltzer, and P.D. Verdouw

Thoraxcentre, Erasmus University and Academic Hospital Dijkzigt,
Rotterdam, the Netherlands.

The echocardiographic contrast effect seen when biologically
compatible solutions are injected peripherally predominantly results
from the presence of microbubbles of air in the injectate and
injecting apparatus (1). Survival time of these microbubbles in the
blood is not very long and the smaller the bubble the faster it
disappears because of surface tension effects (2). In addition,
microbubbles larger than 8 microns do not pass the pulmonary capillary
bed, due to the "sieve effect" of the capillaries (3).
As a consequence, echocardiographic contrast effect on the left side
of the heart can at present only be obtained with pulmonary wedge or
direct left heart catheter injection (4-6), in the absence of intracardiac or intrapulmonary shunting.
Transmission of echo-contrast material through the lungs following a
peripheral venous injection would be of great clinical interest since
it would allow visualization of left-heart flow dynamics, demonstration of left-to-right shunts, eventually improve quantitave
analysis of the left ventricle, and perhaps be useful in arterial
ultrasonography.
Several possible methods can be considered to cause echo transmission
through the lungs. We have tested the following ones in animal
experiments.

Physical cavitation:
A liquid, such as diethyl ether, could be administrated intravenously,
pass through the pulmonary capillary bed and boil on the left side of
the heart yielding a gas phase and echo-contrast (7,8).
Following two control hand injections of saline and a Swan-Ganz
balloon tipped catheter in the right heart, multiple injections of
increasing amounts of diethyl ether (0.5, 1, 1.5, 2 or 3 ml) followed
by a "flush" of saline were made in 10 open-chested pigs. In each, a
Krautkramer-Branson 3.5 MHz transducer was sutured directly onto the
left ventricular epicardium for detecting left-sided echo-contrast.
Two pigs showed left-sided echo-contrast after saline injections and
were excluded from the study because of the possibility of intracardiac or intrapulmonary shunting. Echo-contrast was obtained in six
of the remaining eight animals with injections of 1 ml of diethyl
ether or more.
Injection of 2 ml of diethyl ether caused hypotension in all animals
and occasionally asystole.

Chemical reaction:
A chemical substance, such as hydrogen peroxide, could be injected intravenously, pass through the pulmonary capillary bed and undergo a chemical reaction on the left side of the heart, yielding a gas and therefore echo-contrast (8,9).
Twelve pigs were studied as described above but instead of ether, 0.2 to 5 ml of hydrogen peroxide was injected. Concentrations between 0.75 and 30% were used. Two animals had left-heart contrast following control injections and were excluded from further study. Eight of the remaining 10 animals had left-heart contrast following hydrogen-peroxide injections. No adverse effects on the electrocardiogram and left ventricular pressure were observed.

Mini-microbubbles:
A solid polysaccharide coating might protect a mini-microbubble of less than 10 microns from rapid dissolution so it could traverse the pulmonary bed (10,11).
Sixteen open-chested pigs were studied. Contrast-effects were monitored in the apical four-chamber views from an apical transducer position with a Toshiba SSH-10A phased array sector scanner.
A varying volume of a suspension with mini-microbubbles with a mean size of 10 microns in particles up to a size of 200 microns was injected in the internal jugular vein followed by a 5 cc saline flush. Intrapulmonary and intracardiac shunting were excluded by control injection of 5 ml of saline. In 12 out of 23 injections of mini-microbubbles left heart contrast was observed after a delay of more than 3 beats indicating transpulmonary transmission of mini-microbubbles.
No adverse effects were noticed.

The feasibility of transmission of echocardiographic contrast through the lungs has been demonstrated in these experiments. Liquids yielding contrast by physical (diethyl ether) or chemical (peroxide decomposition) means or sugar covered mini-microbubbles of gas have all been shown capable of producing left heart echocardiographic contrast. The problem is therefore toxicity. Few data are available at present, however. The ultimate method of noninvasive left heart echo contrast creation will probably be the one which has the least toxic effects.

Diethyl ether, a liquid which boils vigorously at body temperature is a very active source of echo-contrast but toxic when 2 ml or more are injected. Ziskin et al (7) did not observe toxic effects when small amounts were injected in animals. Small doses (0.3 ml) have been safely used in humans for many years for measuring the circulation time. These doses, however, seem insufficient to produce an effective left heart echo-contrast effect.
This may be also the case for hydrogen peroxide for which acceptable toxity has been demonstrated for right sided echo-contrast studies when small doses are used (1 ml of a 3% solution)(12). The use of "hard-shelled" mini- microbubbles appears to be the most promising approach.

Although toxicity studies in humans have not been performed, there are
several arguments to believe that they might be safe enough. No
adverse effects were seen during our animal studies, the poly-
saccharides used for the coating are used for intravenous injections,
and the tital amount of gas injected is small (approx.0.002 ml).
A great problem at present is to prevent degradation of the extremely
hygroscopic polysaccharide coating. Failure of achieving left sided
contrast in some of our experiments was probably due to the exposure
to the atmosphere and/or preparation of the mini-microbubble
injectate. Further study is obviously needed to optimize the use of
this promising new contrast agent for improving the success rate in
attaining left heart contrast with peripheral venous injection.

References

1. Meltzer RS, Tickner EG, Sahines TP, Popp RL: The source of
    ultrasound contrast effect. J Clin Ultrasound 8: 121, 1980.
2. Meltzer RS, Tickner EG, Popp RL: Why do the lungs clear ultra-
    sonic contrast ? Ultrasound in Med & Biol 6: 263, 1980.
3. Butler B, Hills B: The lungs as a filter for microbubbles. J Appl
    Physiol 47: 537, 1979.
4. Reale A, Pizzuto F, Gioffré PA, Nigri A, Romeo F, Martuscelli E,
    Mangieri E, Scibilia G: Contrast echocardiography: transmission
    of echoes to the left heart across the pulmonary vascular bed.
    Eur Heart J 1: 101, 1980.
5. Meltzer RS, Serruys PW, McGhie J, Verbaan N, Roelandt J: Pulmo-
    nary wedge injections yielding left sided echocardiographic
    contrast. Brit Heart J 44: 390, 1980.
6. Roelandt J, Meltzer RS, Serruys PW: Contrast echocardiography of
    the left ventricle. In: Rijsterborgh H (ed), Echocardiology,
    Martinus Nijhoff Publishers, the Hague/Boston/London, p 219,
    1981.
7. Ziskin MC, Bonakdarpour A, Weinstein DP, Lynch PR: Contrast
    agents for diagnostic ultrasound. Invest Radiol 7: 500, 1972.
8. Meltzer RS, Sartorius OEH, Lancée CT, Verdouw PD, Essed CE,
    Serruys PW, Roelandt J: Transmission of ultrasonic contrast
    through the lungs. Ultrasound in Med & Biol 7: 377, 1981.
9. Wang X, Wang J, Huang Y, Cai C: Contrast echocardiography with
    hydrogen peroxide. I: Experimental study. Chin Med J 92: 595,
    1979.
10. Bommer WJ, Mason DT, DeMaria AN: Studies in contrast echocardio-
    graphy: development of new agents with superior reproducibility
    and transmission through lungs. Circulation 59 and 60 (Suppl II):
    II-17, 1979.
11. Bommer WJ, Tickner EG, Rasor J, Grehl T, Mason DT, DeMaria AN:
    Development of a new echocardiographic contrast agent capable of
    pulmonary transmission and left heart opacification following
    peripheral venous injection. Circulation 62 (Suppl III): III-34,
    1980.
12. Wang X, Wang J, Chen H, Lu C: Contrast echocardiography with
    hydrogen peroxide. II: Clinical application. Chin Med J 92: 693,
    1979.

Limitations of M-Mode-Echocardiography in Patients with Unusual Locations of Hypertrophic Cardiomyopathy

E. Köhler, Med. Klinik B, University of Düsseldorf

Echocardiography in the past years seemed to be one of the most sensitive and specific methods for the diagnosis of hypertrophic obstructive cardiomyopathy (HOCM). The differential diagnosis against most other cardiac diseases which also show an enlarged left ventricular muscle mass can be evaluated with accuracy. Some diagnostic criteria of HOCM, however, like asymmetric septal hypertrophy (ASH), systolic anterior movement of parts of the mitral valve (SAM) or partial mesosystolic closure movement of the aortic valves are also seen in other heart diseases. But regarding this restriction, in most cases the diagnostic criteria of HOCM are so typical that the diagnosis can be made by 1- and 2-dimensional echocardiography also in those patients, in whom not all echocardiographic criterias of the disease are found.

In 1976 FALICOV a.RESNECOV (3,4) first reported the case of a patient suffering from HOCM with an intraventricular pressure gradient of 80 -100 mmHg and a midventricular obstruction downstream from the mitral valve. The M-Mode-recording in this patient only revealed an ASH without any "SAM"-phenomenon.

Studying all 177 patients with hypertrophic obstructive (HOCM) and hypertrophic nonobstructive cardiomyopathy (HNCM) in whom echocardiography was performed in our laboratory we also noticed discrepancies between the echocardiographic and the catheterisation data in some cases. In attempt to ascertain the value of M-Mode- and 2-dimensional echocardiography in hypertrophic cardiomyopathy we reviewed the data of our patients with HOCM, who revealed atypical echocardiographic and/ or angiocardiographic findings.

Case reports
Case 1: A 23 year old male was treated for some years because of systemic hypertension. Physical examination exhibited a low grade (2/6) systolic ejection murmur at the base of the heart. The M-Mode recording revealed a moderate thickening of the interventricular septum as well as of the left ventricular posterior wall. Neither at rest nor under provocation with amyl nitrite any anterior motion of parts of the mitral valve during systole could be observed. These echocardiographic findings were convenient with the anamnesis of systemic hypertension but they were not suspicious for HOCM. Because of the

systolic murmur of unknown origin, heart catheterisation was performed. The important finding was an intraventricular gradient of 100 mmHg during stimulation with isoprenaline or after extrasystolic beats respectively. The gradient only demonstrable at stimulation was not found across the left ventricular outflow tract but was located below the mitral valve between the midventricular and the apical region of the left ventricle. The left ventricular cineangiogram obtained in the 30° RAO and the 60° LAO position revealed an extremely narrowing of the left ventricular medial and apical parts with only an very small cavity at endsystole.

Case 2: This patient (male, 43 years) had typical clinical signs suspective for HOCM. During heart catheterisation an intraventricular gradient across the left ventricular outflow tract of 30 mmHg at rest and 60 mmHg after extrasystolic beats was found. Although there was no doubt about the diagnosis, different echocardiographic recordings obtained at different times showed confusing echocardiographic entities. The first recording, done in 1976, demonstrated a typical anterior movement of parts of the mitral valve (SAM) during systole and an only moderately thickened ventricular septum. Another recording in 1978 revealed only a distinct "SAM"-phenomenon. In 1981 no unequivocal "SAM" was demonstrable, although all other clinical findings still were suspective for HOCM. 2-dimensional echocardiography pointed out the typical bulging of a moderately thickened interventricular septum into the left ventricular outflow tract but also with this method no "SAM"-phenomenon was detectable.

Case 3: A 14 year old female also exhibited typical clinical features suspective for HOCM. During heart catheterisation a gradient under rest-conditions of about 60 mmHg was found across the left ventricular cavity. The cineangiogram revealed a distinct narrowing of the midventricular region of the left ventricle while the left ventricular outflow tract seemed to be of nearly normal width. The M-Mode recording in this patient failed the diagnosis of HOCM and showed only a moderate septal thickening with normal septal motions during systole.   unequivocal "SAM"-phenomenon was visible.

Case 4: A confusing series of echocardiograms was obtained from a patient with HOCM, who had an intraventricular pressure gradient of about 60 - 80 mmHg during his first catheterisation in 1976. The cineangiogram at that time revealed an extremely narrowing of the midventricular and apical parts of the left ventricle. The echocardiogram showed a markedly thickened interventricular septum of about 18 mm, but no "SAM". Aortic valve motion seemed to be quite normal. 3 years later the patient suffered from bacterial endocarditis of the aortic valve resulting in severe aortic insufficiency. At this time, the M-Mode-recording revealed a slightly enlarged left ventricle, high frequent diastolic vibrations of the anterior mitral valve leaflet, a premature closure of the mitral valve, and a slightly augmented left atrium. No "SAM", no septal thickening and no partial midsystolic closure movement of the aortic valves were found. Therfore this echocardiogram was in agreement with the diagnosis of severe aortic insufficiency but not suspicious for HOCM. This was in contrast to the auscultatory findings at that time. During catheterisation besides a marked aortic insufficiency an intraventricular pressure gradient of about 40 mmHg was found under resting conditions. The cineangiogram exhibited the typical anterior deviation of the left ventricular axis with a narrowing of the midventricular and the apical area.

Case 5: In a 39 year old male patient auscultation detected only a soft systolic murmur at the point of Erb. The ECG revealed slight abnormalities of the repolarisation phase and numerous multifocal ventricular premature beats. The apex cardiogram showed a prominent a-wave, the carotid pulse tacing was not typical for HOCM. The M-Mode-echocardiogram in this patient was suspective for HOCM because of a distinct "SAM"-phenomenon and a moderately thickened interventricular septum. In spite of this suspicious echocardiographic findings, the result of heart catheterisation was unexpected. The interventricular pressure gradient at rest was about 70 mmHg and at postextrasystolic beats over 150 mmHg. The cineangiogram revealed a nearly totally systolic midventricular occlusion.

Comments

Although echocardiographic entities like asymmetric septal thickening, systolic anterior movement of parts of the mitral valve or midsystolic closure of the aortic valves are not specific for hypertrophic obstructive cardiomyopathy (1,2,5), in most patients with an intraventricular gradient across the left ventricular outflow tract, the diagnosis can be made without difficulties, if adequate tracings are obtained. The retrospective analysis of the echocardiograms of 152 patients with typical clinical and angiographic fin-

dings for HOCM studied in our laboratory showed that the echocardiographic
recording in each case was evident or suspicious for HOCM at the first examination or at least at reassessment. This confirms that M-Mode-echocardiography is a highly sensitive and specific method for the evaluation of the typical form of hypertrophic obstructive cardiomyopathy. But diagnostic problems
become evident in patients, in whom the intraventricular gradient is located
in the midventricular or apical regions of the left ventricle, because of the
different pattern of hypertrophy. In these atypical cases of HOCM at the tip
of the mitral valve leaflets, the interventricular septum may be of normal
thickness and the systolic movement of the mitral as well as of the aortic
valves often show no abnormalities. Therefore in patients with clinical features suspective for hypertrophic cardiomyopathy, a quite normal M-Mode-
echocardiogram can not exclude the clinical diagnosis. In 25 patients with
HOCM, who revealed atypical angiographic features with midventricular or apical gradients, the diagnosis could be confirmed by M-Mode-echocardiography
only in 14 (=52%). This finding points out that M-Mode-echocardiography is
not an accurate method for the detection of atypical forms of hypertrophic
cardiomyopathies, because the hypertrophied areas of the left ventricle in
these patients are often not accessible to the M-Mode beam (6,7). Two- dimensional echocardiography revealed an unusual distribution of hypertrophy in
nearly all of these patients. Thickening of septum, left ventricular posterior and anterior wall was preponderately located midventricular or apical,
areas which can not be identified by conventional M-Mode-echocardiography
reliably. Two-dimensional echocardiography also has it's limitations. In
hypertrophied ventricles, the recognition of the endocardial surface may be
difficult. This results in an intraobserver variability. Furthermore, 2-di-
mensional echocardiography can not differentiate between patients with midventricular or apical HOCM on the one hand and those with hypertrophic
nonobstructive cardiomyopathy or other forms of left ventricular hypertrophy
on the other.
In conclusion our data indicate, that M-Mode-echocardiography is of limited
value in recognizing atypical locations of left ventricular hypertrophy. By
2-dimensional echocardiography midventricular and apical hypertrophy in most
cases is detectable reliably. But at this time, no echocardiographic characteristics are known to differentiate between the atypical obstructive and
nonobstructive form of hypertrophic cardiomyopathy.

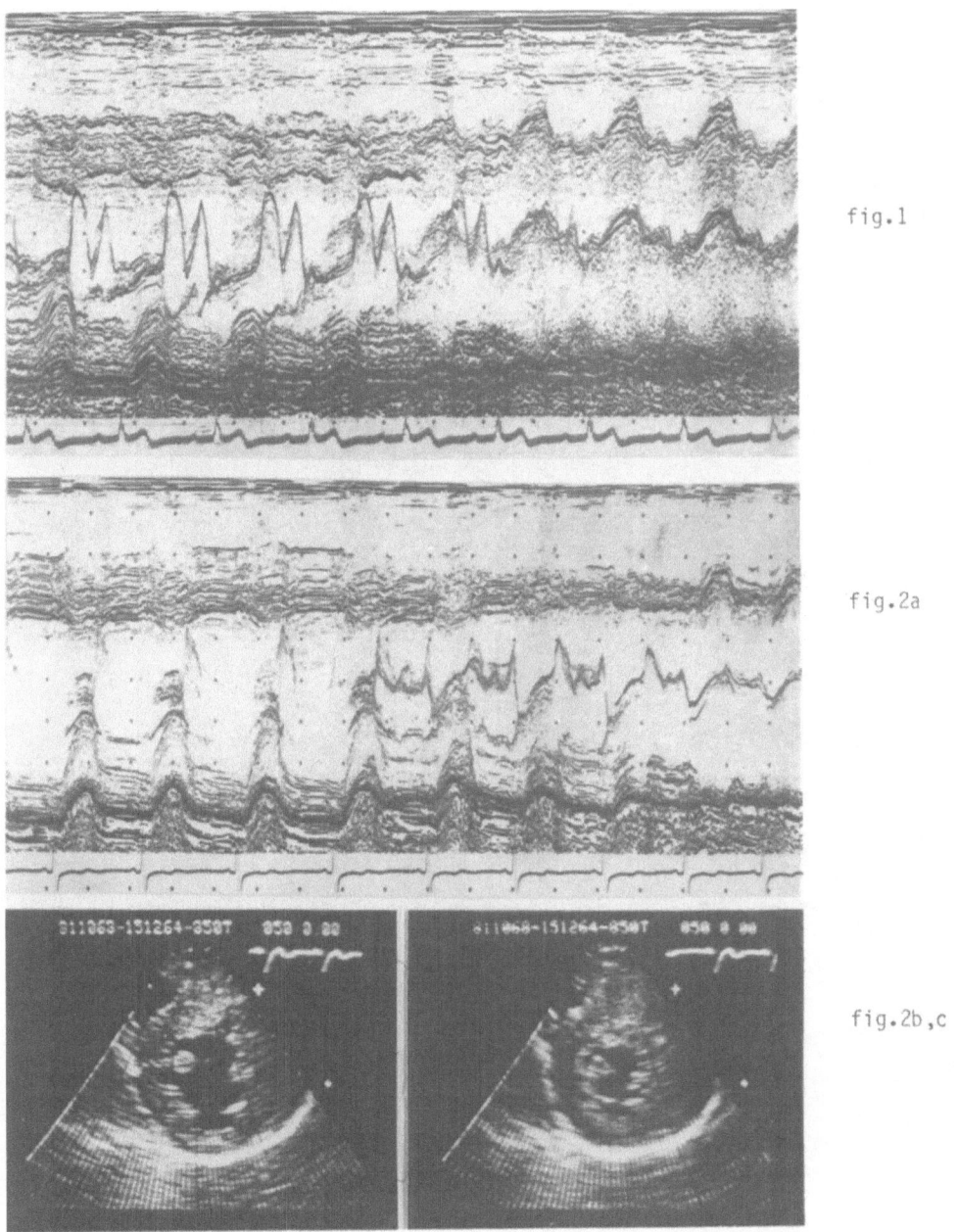

fig.1

fig.2a

fig.2b,c

fig. 1 a.2: M-Mode- and 2-dimensional echocardiograms at enddiastole (2a) and
at endsystole (2c) of 2 patients with apical HOCM

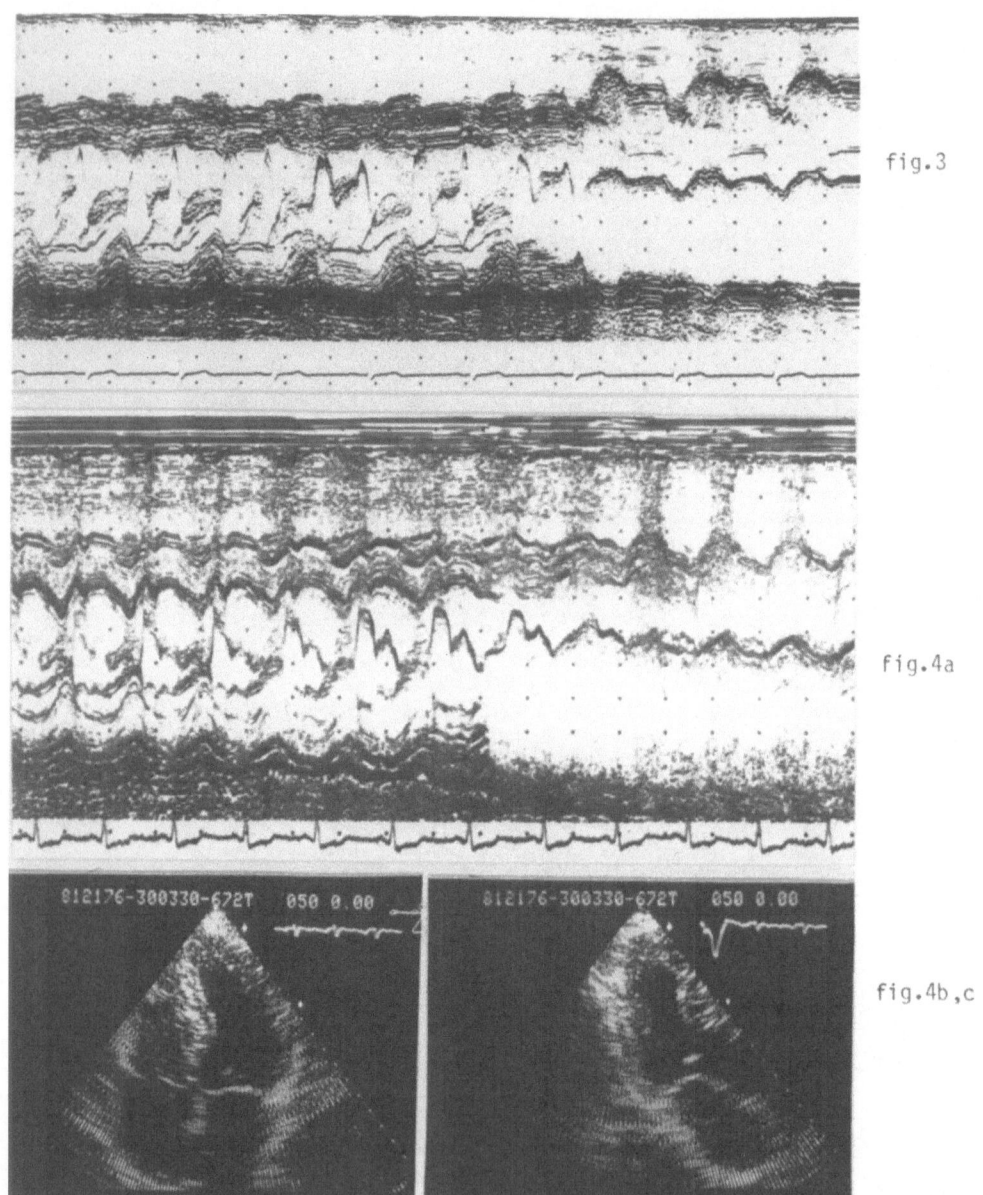

fig.3

fig.4a

fig.4b,c

fig.3 a. 4: M-Mode- and 2-dimensional echocardiograms of 2 patients with
medioventricular HOCM

References:

Doi,Y.,L.,W.J.McKenna,J.Gehrke,C.M.Oakley,J.F.Goodwin:
M Mode Echocardiography in Hypertrophic Cardiomyopathy:Diagnostic
Criteria and Prediction of Obstruction
Am. J. Cardiol. 45, 6 - 14 (1980)

Doi,Y.,L.,J.E.Deanfield,W.J. McKenna,H.J.Dargie,C.M.Oakley,J.F.Goodwin:
Echocardiographic Differentiation of Hypertensive Heart Disease and
Hypertrophic Cardiomyopathy
Br. Heart J. 44, 395 - 400 (1980)

Falicov,R.E.,L.Resnecov,S.Bharati,M.Lev:
Mid-Ventricular Obstruction: A Variant of Obstructive Cardiomyopathy
Am. J. Cardiol. 37, 432 - 437 (1976)

Falicov,R.E.,L.Resnecov:
Mid Ventricular Obstruction in Hypertrophic Obstructive Cardiomyopathy
Br. Heart J. 39, 701 - 705 (1977)

Cardin,J.M.,J.V.Talano,L.Stephanides,J.Fizzano,M.Lesch:
Systolic Anterior Motion in the Absence of Asymmetric Septal
Hypertrophy Circulation 63, 181 - 188 (1981)

Maron,B.J.,J.S.Gottdiener,R.O.Bonow,S.E.Epstein:
Hypertrophic Cardiomyopathy with Unusual Locations of Left Ventricular
Hypertrophy Undetectable by M-mode Echocardiography
Circulation 63, 409 - 418 (1981)

Maron,B.J.,J.S.Gottdiener,S.E.Epstein:
Patterns and Significance of Distribution of Left Ventricular
Hypertrophy in Hypertrophic Cardiomyopathy
Am. J. Cardiol. 48, 418 - 428 (1981)

DIGITAL PROCESSING OF 2-DIMENSIONAL CONTRAST ECHOCARDIOGRAMS

A.Wessel,R.Brennecke,P.Duhm,H.-J.Hahne,P.H.Heintzen
Department of Pediatric Cardiology and Biomedical Engineering
University of Kiel,Germany

The 2-dimensional ultrasonic imaging of the heart is an important diagnostic tool in cardiology. It provides information about anatomical structures and dynamic function of the heart. The peripheral injection of echo contrast material, such as glucose solution or saline,improves recognition of intracardiac defects. Using this contrast technique for determination of ventricular volume one disadvantage becomes obvious: contrast material and cardiac tissue show almost the same pattern in the ultrasonic image. Thus the borders of the cardiac chamber,which often are only poorly defined in the non-contrast echocardiogram,become unrecognizable in the contrast echocardiogram. The purpose of this study was to improve the analysis of contrast echocardiograms with special respect to border recognition by computerized processing techniques. In order to improve the border recognition in contrast echocardiograms we used modified digital image enhancement techniques primarily developed for digital video angiography.

Methods

A commercially available phased array sector scanner (ROCHE RT 400) was used to obtain 2-dimensional echocardiograms. Ultrasound frequency was 2.8 or 3.5 MHz and the signal processing section of the instrument was used without modification. The standard video signal generated by the digital scan converter (6 bit) of the instrument was recorded on video tape. For digitization the images could be selected from the video recordings by a digital frame grabber system with a resolution of 256x256x8 bit (1). The digitized image data were tranferred at a much slower, computer compatible rate to a standard digital disk (DEC RP04 , 80 Mbyte). The images were processed by FORTRAN-programs and results were tranferred back to the frame grabber for display. For some applications,a false colour display for enhanced visualization of contrast material and background structures was used as described below.

Glucose solution (5%) served as contrast material in all cases which is especially advantageous when performing contrast echocardiograms in infants and children,thus avoiding unfavourable salt load or allergic side effects. According to the weight of the child we injected 2 to 5 ml 5% glucose solution into a peripheral vein or via an angiocatheter into inferior vena cava or right atrium during heart catheter procedure. Opacification of the left ventricle was achieved by injecting the glucose solution into the left atrium or the left ventricle via catheter during routine catheterization.

ECG gated averaging of cardiac image data is used for noise reduction in nuclear imaging and video angiography. We applied this principle to ultrasonic real time sector image sequences for the same purpose. For gated averaging image data were selected only from heart cycles which did not differ more than 10% from the average duration. In order to detect errors in image registration (geometrical matching) due to respiratory motion and involuntary movement of the tranducer,we additionally used correlation techniques for the detection of mismatched images (4). Those images which not correlated well were excluded from further processing. Details of the averaging technique are shown in fig.1. The input image sequence is shown schematically as a block of data. With reference to the ECG,a small group of unprocessed images are selected around the same heart phase of several heart cycles. Thus,each heart phase is represented by a group of typically 10 to 20 images. In this example, for each pixel of each group,12 samples of the echo amplitude at this location can be extracted from the images of this group. We call this set of amplitude samples,which describe the brightness of a given pixel at a certain heart phase,a sample vector. The following data may be derived from the sample vector(5):

1. Mean value
2. Standard deviation of the samples.
3. Median value. Median filters are not subject to the blurring effects typical for averaging filters.

By applying one of these filters to all sample vectors new images are generated showing at each pixel the value of the mean,the standard deviation

42

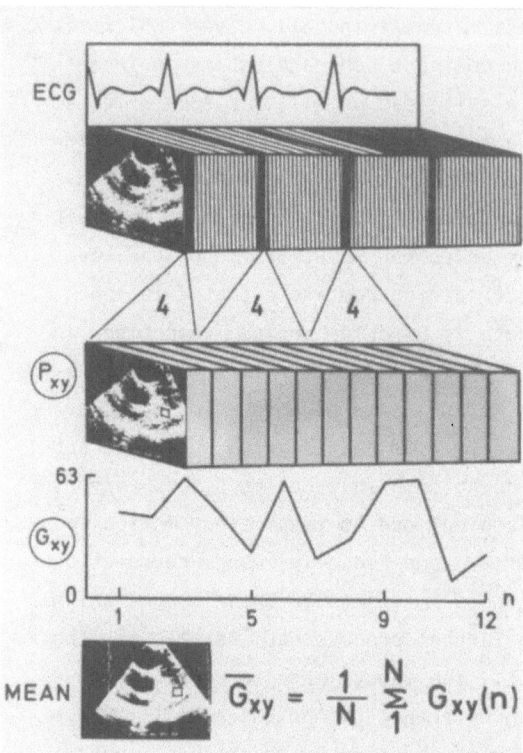

Fig.1: Principle of the computation of a mean image by ECG gated averaging.

or the median as computed for the corresponding sample vector. The selective display of regions which contain contrast material is especially important in quantitative studies such as determination of volume and function parameters. Subtraction of a contrast free background image from each contrast image has been recently implemented in angiography using digital electronic technology (1,2,3). In echocardiography however, the subtraction of a single background image from a single contrast image produces substantial subtraction artifacts due to large differences arising from granular structures in tissue regions of subtracted images. Therefore before subtraction the amount of spatial granularity of the sector images was reduced by ECG gated averaging as described above. A group of background and a group of contrast images were averaged separately. Then the two resulting averaged images were subtracted. Remaining subtraction artifacts could be reduced still further by taking into account the regional variation of echo amplitude fluctuations in the background image sequence. To perform this,

.the picture obtained by subtraction of the mean images was divided either by the standard deviation picture derived from the background images (SUB/SDB) or it was divided by the standard deviation image calculated from the background and contrast images (CCC). Because the formal similarity of this process with the determination of signal-to-noise ratio,we call these images SNR-images (subtraction signal-to-noise ratio image).

In the process of image subtraction,the background is suppressed which may reduce morphological information in some cases. In order to reintroduce this information into the display of subtraction images again,we developed a pseudocolour display technique(5).

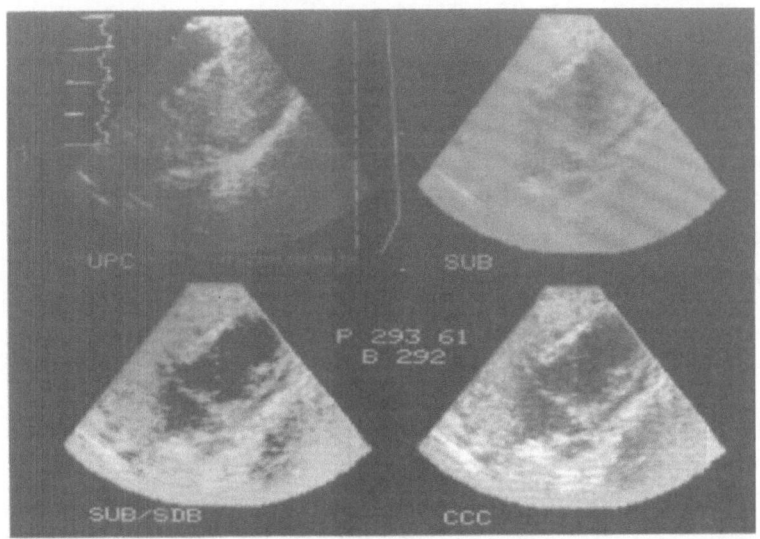

Fig.2: Apical 4-chamber view after injection of 5% glucose solution into the left atrium in a 14 years old boy with aortic stenosis. The contrast material opacifies the left atrium an the left ventricle.
Upper left: unprocessed picture (UPB)
Upper right: subtraction of background images from mean contrast image (SUB).
Lower left: result after processing by modified subtraction technique (SUB/SDB).
Lower right: image after processing after modified subtraction technique (CCC).

Results

The computerized image enhancement techniques were applied to more than 30 clinical contrast echocardiograms of the right and left ventricle from infants and children with congenital heart disease. Temporal filtering techniques producing mean or median contrast images showed only a smoother granular structure than the unprocessed picture but did not lead to an improved border delineation of the ventricular cavity. This could be achieved by subtraction techniques. Fig.2 shows a contrast echocardiogram of the left ventricle from a 14 years old boy with aortic stenosis, obtained after injection of glucose solution into the left atrium. In the non-contrast echo and in the unprocessed contrast image one cannot define the ventricular borders clearly. Simple subtraction of background images from the mean contrast image does not result in an adequate visibility of details such as ventricular wall and septum. Normalizing procedures of the subtraction image create the SNR-images with large contrasts (SUB/SDB and CCC). After this processing the ventricular cavity becomes sharply delineated. Fig.3 depicts the contrast echocardiogram of the right ventricle from a 6 years old girl with persistent ductus arteriosus. Creating a picture of the CCC type, the contrast is enhanced and the border delineation of the right ventricle is improved.

Discussion

Contrast echocardiography has proven to be helpful for detection of intracardiac defects,which are invisible in the non-contrast echocardiogram. Since, however, the echo contrast material often has a similar granular structure as the surrounding cardiac tissue it is difficult to define a cross section of the ventricular cavity for volume determination from the conventional unprocessed contrast echo. This fact is especially disadvantageous for depiction of the right ventricular cross section as this chamber is lying in the near field of the ultrasonic beam, which causes a poorly defined non-contrast image. This disadvantage may be diminished by applying digital image enhancement techniques to the contrast echocardiogram. Temporal filtering alone reduces imhomogenity of the contrast material distribution when several images from heart cycles are averaged.

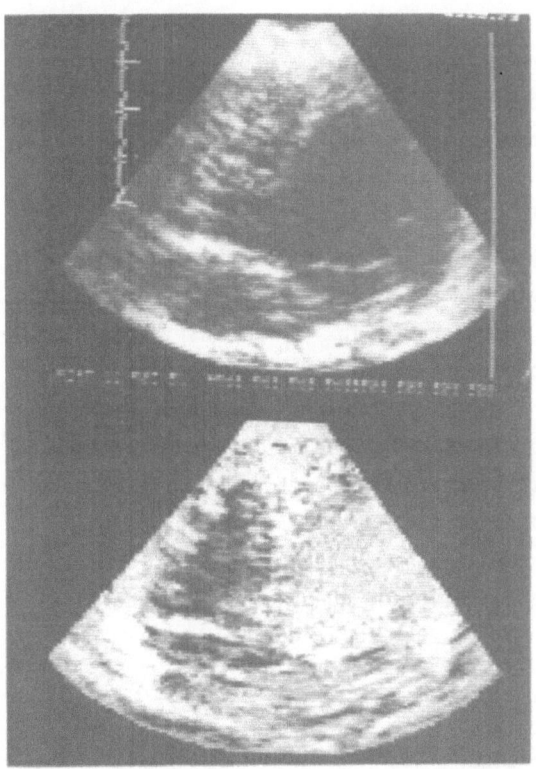

Fig.3: Apical 4-chamber view after injection of 5% glucose into the inferior vena cava, obtained from a 6 years old girl with persistent ductus arteriosus. Right atrium and ventricle are filled with contrast material. Unprocessed image in the upper part, in the lower part the same image after processing by modified subtraction technique (CCC).

Temporal filtering followed by simple subtraction is however,not sufficient for depicting ventricular borders from the contrast echocardiogram. Those processing procedures which lead to an increasing contrast between cardiac tissue and contrast material seem to be more suitable for improved border detection of cardiac chambers. We got the best contrast between tissue and contrast material after dividing the subtraction image by the standard deviation of the background image,thus producing the pictures called SNR-images. Using the CCC type procedure the contrast is softer than

created with the SUB/SDB technique and the picture seems to be less brilli-
ant. Nevertheless borders are well recognized. Further investigation will
be necessary to evaluate which of both processing techniques lead to the
more precise volume determination compared with other techniques for volume
determination, e.g. angiocardiography. Due to cardiac motion, the standard deviation may be overestimated in border regions of the ventricle. In
the normalization process, used to obtain the SNR-image this may lead to
suppression of border regions of the contrast material so that the area of
the ventricular cross section may be underestimated. Preliminary results
seem to suggest that the CCC type procedure could yield the most accurate
cross section of cardiac chambers.

The performance of the extraction techniques described must depend to some
extend on the echo signal processing characteristics of the ultrasonic
scanner used. Therefore standardization of the amplifier and the digital
scan converter section of these instruments seem to be necessary to achieve
wider clinical application of semiquantitative and quantitative echocardiographic image processing methods.

References

(1) Brennecke R, TK Brown, J Bürsch, PH Heintzen: Digital processing of
video- angiographic image series. Computers in Cardiology Long Beach,
California: IEEE Computer Society. 1976. p.255.

(2) Mistretta CA, RA Kruger, TL Houk et al.: Computerized fluoroscopy
techniques for non- invasive cardiovascular imaging. Proc. SPIE 152: 65.
1978.

(3) Ovitt TW, PC Christenson, HD Fisher: Intravenous angiography using
digital video subtraction. AJNR1:387,1980.

(4) Brennecke R, HJ Hahne, K Moldenhauer, JH Bürsch, PH Heintzen: Improved
real- time processing and storage techniques with applications to
intravenous contrast angiography. Computers in Cardiology p.191. Long
Beach, California: IEEE Computer Society. 1978.

(5) Brennecke R, Hahne HJ, Wessel A, Heintzen PH: Computerized enhancement
techniques for echocardiographic sector scans. Proc.Comp.Cardiol. IEEE
Comp. Soc., Long Beach, 1981

Acknowledgement

This work has been supported by a grant from the Deutsche
Forschungsgemeinschaft.

QUANTIFICATION OF CARDIAC FUNCTION BY COMPUTERIZED 2-DIMENSIONAL
ECHOCARDIOGRAPHY

S. Meerbaum, E. Carcia, K. Ong, and W. Zwehl
Cardiovascular Research Institute, Cedars-Sinai Medical Center,
Los Angeles, California, United States of America

INTRODUCTION

One of the promising developments in two-dimensional echocardiography (2DE) has been its use in quantitating global cardiac function
and mapping segmental ventricular contraction. Considering the very
large amount of spatial and temporal measurements to be processed, it is
not surprising that efforts are underway to computerize the acquisition
and analysis of 2DE images (1-5). This paper will indicate recent
progress at the Cedars-Sinai Medical Center (Los Angeles) in the
development and validation of real-time 2DE computerization.

Real-Time Computerization

A significant advance in methodology was introduced when Dr. E.
Garcia et al developed an interface which couples a standard medical
imaging computer system to the video output of current 2DE machines or
video tape recorders (6). This computer digitizes and stores the echo
images on magnetic disc in real-time at 30 frames per sec., thereby
overcoming several limitations of current 2DE. The speed of acquisition
is greatly increased over previous computer methods which digitized only
a single still frame at a time. The new system also displays several
different views of the heart simultaneously in a continuous closed-loop
fashion. Such simultaneous visualization of different cardiac images
is proving to be a highly desirable feature for assessment or comparison
of segmental wall motions. Since the echocardiogram is digitized, an
increasing amount of software is being provided for automatic quantitation of ventricular function. Computerization results in substantial
savings in time and labor, and avoids the inevitable subjectivity
associated with manual 2DE image processing.

Detailed computer algorithms have been developed. Thus, temporal
smoothing of the images replaces the contents of each pixel with a
weighted average of itself and pixels with same Cartesian coordinates

immediately before and after. Spatial smoothing uses a weighted average
of the pixel and eight surrounding ones within the same frame. Frame-
by frame automatic edge detection in 2DE images involves the computer
convolving a 3x3 Laplacian operator (second derivative) with the tempor-
ally and spatially smoothed images. A binary image is then created from
all the pixels that both exceed an echo amplitude threshold of the
smoothed image, and are within a preselected range of the Laplacian
images. The endocardial interface in a 2DE cross section is automatically tracked from the binary image by the computer searching from a
predefined center of the ventricular lumen until an intensity threshold
is encountered at its interface. This starts the process of automatically tracing and endocardium all around the ventricle (Fig. 1).

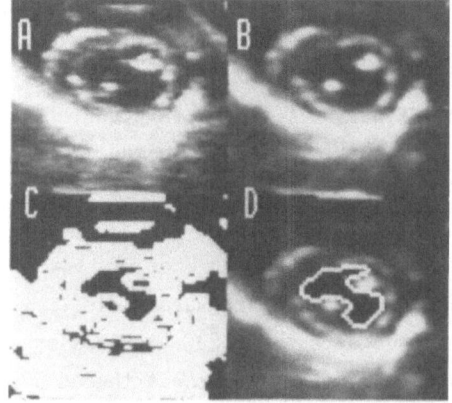

FIGURE 1. Progression of computerized processing of 2DE image: selected
video frame of a dog's digitized papillary short axis cross section (A),
space-time smoothed image (B), binary image (C) and automated edge
delineation (D).

With the endocardial outline extracted, the images are suitable for
computerized frame-by-frame quantitation of global and regional ventricular function. Thus, validated reconstruction from 2DE apical and
short-axis cross-sectional views of the left ventricle can be used to
derive ventricular volumes and global ejection fraction (7-13). Ana-
lytical methods, using fixed or floating referencing, provide standard
subdivision of the cross-sectional images into segments, which can then
be analyzed frame-by-frame for regional wall motions (14,15). The computer system displays the results of computations in the form of charts,
showing alterations in cross-sectional areas or reconstructed ventricular
volumes throughout the cardiac cycle. The percent systolic fractional
area change or global ejection fraction are indicated, and derivatives

can also be plotted (Fig. 2). A segment-by-segment bar graph displayed
by the computer presents a map of regional contraction and wall thickness.

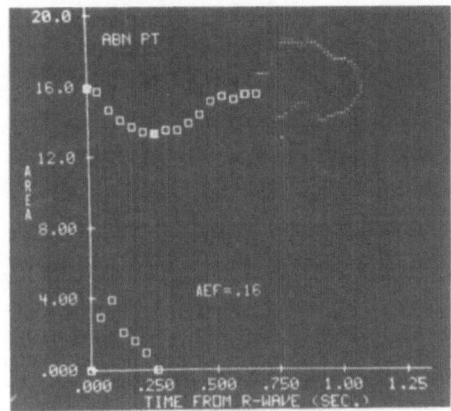

FIGURE 2. Papillary level 2DE short-axis section in a patient with acute
myocardial infarction. Real-time computer system display shows change
in section intraluminal area throughout a cardiac cycle, a computed
systolic fractional area ejection fraction, frame-to-frame endocardial
outlines, and area derivative.

The 2DE images obtained in our closed-chest dog preparations are
generally excellent, allowing full utilization of the above real-time 2DE
computerized system. A sample application in an experimental study of
myocardial ischemia is shown in Figure 3, allowing computerization of
measurements previously performed by hand drawn 2DE methods (16,17).
Current clinical 2DE image quality is known to be variable. While very
good images are obtained in most normals and some patient subsets, only
a limited number of patients with coronary artery disease are presently
suitable for the 2DE real-time quantitative computerization. It remains
necessary to enhance the clinical 2DE cardiac images, particularly to
minimize echo dropouts and improve endocardial definition. Nevertheless,
the multiple cineloop display of digitized images provided by the
computer system have been employed by us and found advantageous in
several clinical 2DE studies which did not permit automated edge
detection. Thus, a two-view display allows an investigator to set up
one dynamic view of a control and next to it an intervention facilitating
comparison study (18). Conventional 2DE methods would entail repeated
rewinding and successive playback of required portions of the study,
and the evaluation would not be as comprehensive a s when images are
viewed side by side.

50

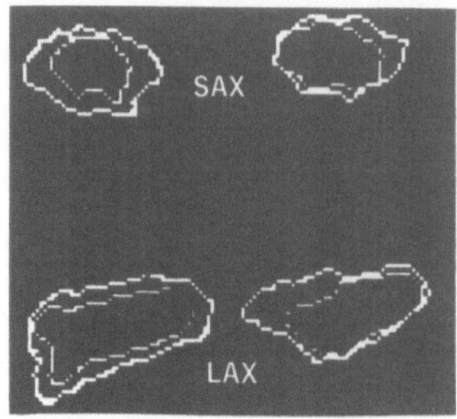

FIGURE 3. Superimposed end diastolic and end-systolic computer delineated endocardium in a 2DE short-axis (top) and long-axis (bottom)
cross sectional view of a dog's left ventricle. Control state on left
and occlusion of theproximal left anterior descending coronary artery
(on right). Note distinct regional akinesis in segments subserved by
the occluded coronary artery.

Validations of the 2DE Computer System

The 2DE computer system was validated by us in two experimental
studies. First in canine left ventricular slabs and subsequently in
closed-chest dogs employing contrast cineventriculography as a commonly
accepted "standard". A preliminary evaluation has also been performed
in a series of Cath Lab patients.

A. In Vitro Validations

In this study of left ventricular slabs (19) computer algorithms for automated edge detection in 2DE images were validated against
measurements of slab dimensions. The computer technique was compared
with the conventional hand drawn 2DE methodology, and interobserver
reproducibility was also determined. The previously described computer
instrumentation included the Nova minicomputer with 128K word program
and 256K word image memories, an 80 M Byte disk storage, and 512x512
pixel video display, with 256 gray levels. The 2DE images were
digitized in a 64x64 matrix and acquisition rate was 30 frames/sec. A
region of interest was located under software control. Digital space-
time smoothing reduced noise and effects of dropouts. Figure 4 compares
the computer processed image with the actual canine slab. Automatic
edge detection of endocardium was as described above.

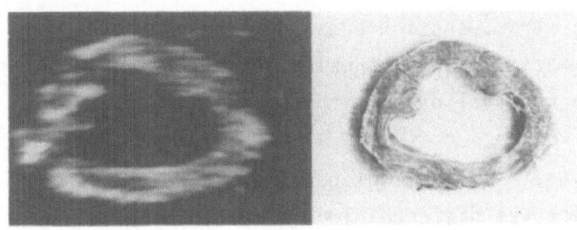

FIGURE 4. Xerox of canine slab (left) compared to computer digitized and smoothed 2DE image of the same slab section (right).

The study was performed in 29 10mm wide canine left ventricular slabs. 2DE imaging of slabs was carried out in a water bath. Cross-sectional intraluminal areas and segmental areas were computed from (1) directly documented slab dimensions, (2) hand drawn 2DE slab section images, and (3) computer processed slab 2DE images.

Slab intraluminal area varied from 3.3 to 18.3 cm^2. Comparing the intraluminal areas obtained with computerized 2DE, hand drawn 2DE and direct slab measurements, correlation coefficients were .95 to .96 and standard error of estimate ranged from 1.0 to 1.32 cm^2 (Fig. 5).

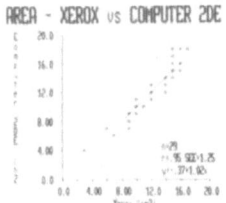
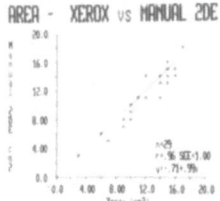
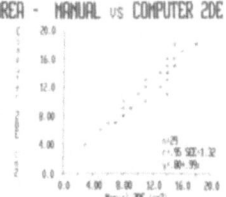

FIGURE 5. Linear re-ression graphs indicating excellent correlation between real-time computerized 2DE delineated area of canine slabs with (1) direct area measurement (xerox) and (2) the area manually outlined from 2DE images.

Similar comparisons of hand drawn 2DE vs computerized 2DE derived segmental areas (12 per slab) yielded correlations (r = .79 - .95 with SEE = .07 - .27 cm^2). Thus, this study in ventricular slabs indicated the validity of computer processing of 2DE images.

B. In Vivo Experimental Validation

This study in closed-chest dogs (20) examined the automated left ventricular endocardial delineation in characteristic two-dimensional echo images of the beating heart. Cross-section areas derived by the computer from 2DE images were compared against manually drawn 2DE, and computer reconstructed LV volumes were validated with contrast ventriculography.

In 13 normal closed-chest dogs, 4-5 excellent quality short-axis cross-sectional images were obtained at different levels of the left ventricle, as well as one long-axis view. All images were stored on 1/2 inch video tape. Representative cardiac cycles were digitized in real-time from video to disk using a 64x64 matrix format at 30 frames/sec.

The first step in the conventional manual method of 2DE image processing consisted of a dynamic review of endocardial left ventricular wall motion to identify the end-diastolic (largest) and end-systolic (smallest) short-axis cross-sectional area. Stop frame images were drawn directly from the video screen, with the outlined borders re-checked and verified by repeated viewing of the wall dynamics. Ventricular length in end-diastole and end-systole was read from 2DE long-axis sections.

The computer method involved (1) space time smoothing of frame-by-frame images throughout the cardiac cycle, (2) closed-loop movie format display to identify end-diastole and end-systole by cross-sectional area, (3) dynamic range expansion, and (4) Laplacian threshold operator to identify endocardium. Left ventricular volume computation (with either manual or computer 2DE approach) used a modified Simpson reconstruction with ventricle length and the 4-5 short-axis cross-sectional areas. The cineangio LV volume analysis employed a simple area-length type analysis.

Comparison of 2DE end-diastolic and end-systolic short-axis cross sectional areas automatically derived by computerized edge detection indicated a high correlation coefficient vs. manually drawn outlines (.98 and .89) and a small SEE (1.4 and 1.5 cm^2). Similarly, ventricular volumes derived by the two modalities of 2DE correlated well (r = .92 and .91), with small SEE (10.8 and 7.5 cc). Compared to contrast ventriculography, the computerized 2DE derivation of both end diastolic and end systolic left ventricular volumes correlated very well (r = .93 with SEE = 11.4 cc, and .96 with SEE = 5.1 cc) (Fig. 6).

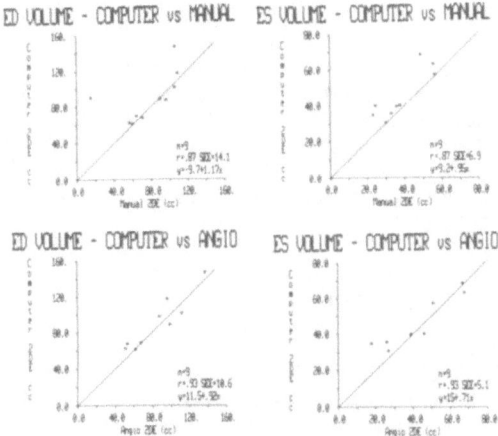

FIGURE 6. End diastolic (left) and end systolic (right) volumes of
canine left ventricles derived and reconstructed by manually drawn
2DE and computerized 2DE techniques. Linear regression plots show
very good correlation of the two methodologies, and excellent
validation of computerized 2DE against contrast cineangiography.

Computerized edge detection of the superior 2DE images obtained in
dogs allowed accurate analysis of left ventricular cross sectional areas
and volume reconstruction. In addition, the 2DE computer should offer
important advantages of objectivity and speed.

COMMENT

It must be emphasized that computerized quantitative analysis of
global and regional cardiac function requires satisfactory 2DE definition of the endocardial (and epicardial) interface. The superior 2DE
images obtained in the dog demonstrated reproducibility and validity of
the 2DE computer system. While clinical 2DE studies have presented a
much lower yield of images suitable for quantitative measurement by
either computerized or hand drawn methods of analysis, a recent examination of a patient subset from the catheterization laboratory with
satisfactory 2DE images indicates similar suitability of the automatic
edge detection technique and good condition with cineangiography (21).
Further development of computerized image processing promises wider
application of the new system in clinical echocardiography.

ACKNOWLEDGEMENTS

We wish to acknowledge the effort of the following co-workers:
Eliot Corday, M.D., Stephen Corday, M.D., Ronald Levy, M.D., Roberto
Haendchen, M.D., William Childs, and Matthew Bennet of Medical Data
System, Ann Arbor, Michigan

54

REFERENCES

1. Price RR, Erickson JJ, Jones TB, Fleisher AF, Partain CL, James AE
    Jr: A digital signal and image processing system for ultrasono-
    graphy. Proceedings of the 25th Annual Meeting of the AIUM,
    American Institute of Ultrasound in Medicine. Oklahoma City,
    Sept 1980, p 202
2. Skorton PJ, McNary CA, Child JS, Shah PM: Computerized image
    processing in cross-sectional echocardiography. Am J Cardiol
    45:403, 1980
3. Matsumoto M, Matsuo H, Kitabatake A, Inove M. Hamanaka Y, Tamura S,
    Tanaka K, Hiroshi A: Three-dimensional echocardiograms and two-
    dimensional echocardiographic images at desired planes by a
    computerized system. Ultrasound Med Biol 3:163, 1977
4. Garrison JB, Weiss JL, Maughan WL, Tuck OM, Guier WN, Fortuin NJ:
    Quantifying regional wall motion and thickening in two-dimensional
    echocardiography with a computer-aided contouring system. IN:
    Computers in Cardiology. Long Beach, September, 1977, pp 25-35,
    IEES Computer Society.
5. Kuwuhara M, Shigeru E, Kitagawa H, Ishimi K: Automatic analysis of
    two-dimensional echocardiograms. Med Info 80, p 210-213, IFIP,
    North-Holland, 1980
6. Garcia E, Gueret P, Bennett M, Corday E, Zwehl W, Meerbaum S, Corday
    S, Swan HJC, Berman D: Real-time computerization of two-dimensional
    echocardiography. Am Heart J 101:783, 1981
7. Wyatt HL, Heng MK, Meerbaum S, Hestenes JD, Cobo JM, Davidson RM,
    Corday E: Cross-sectional echocardiography. I. Analysis of
    mathematic models for quantifying mass of the left ventricle in
    dogs. Circulation 60:1104, 1979
8. Wyatt HL, Heng MK, Meerbaum S, Gueret P, Hestenes JD, Dula E,
    Corday E: Cross-sectional echocardiography. II. Analysis of
    mathematic models for quantifying mass of the left ventricle
    in dogs. Circulation 60:1104, 1979
9. Gueret P, Meerbaum S, Wyatt HL, Uchiyama T, Lang TW, Corday E:
    Two-dimensional echocardiographic quantitation of left ventricular
    volumes and ejection fraction: Importance of accounting for
    dyssynergy in short-axis reconstruction models. Circulation 62:
    1308, 1980
10. Folland ED, Parisi AF, Moynihan PF, Jones RJ, Feldman CL, Tow DE:
    Assessment of left ventricular ejection fraction and volumes by
    real-time two-dimensional ejection fraction and volumes by real-
    time two dimensional echocardiography. A comparison of cineangio-
    graphic and radionuclide technique. Circulation 60:760, 1979
11. Schiller NB, Acquatella H, Ports TA, Drew D, Goerke J, Boswell R,
    Carlsson E, Parmley WW: Left ventricular volume from paired biplane
    two-dimensional echocardiography. Circulation 60:547, 1979
12. Carr KW, Engler RL, Forsythe JR, Johnson AD, Gosink B: Measurement
    of left ventricular ejection fraction by mechanical cross-sectional
    echocardiography. Circulation 59:1196, 1979
13. Wyatt HL, Meerbaum S, Heng MK, Gueret P, Corday E: Cross-sectional
    echocardiography. III. Analysis of mathematic models for
    quantifying volume of symmetric and asymmetric left ventricle.
    Am Heart J 100:821, 1980
14. Parisi AF, Moynihan PF, Folland ED, Feldman CL: Quantitative
    detection of regional left ventricular contraction abnormalities
    by two dimensional echocardiography - Analysis of methods.
    Circulation 64:4, 752-760, 1981

15. Gueret P, Meerbaum S, Broffman J, Uchiyama T, Corday E: Differential effects of nitroprusside on ischemic and nonischemic myocardium demonstrated by two-dimensional echocardiography. Am J Cardiol 48:59-68, 1981

16. Wyatt HL, Meerbaum S, Heng MK, Rit J, Gueret P, Corday E: Experimental evaluation of the extent of myocardial dyssnergy and infarct size by two-dimensional echocardiography. Circulation 63:607, 1981

17. Meerbaum S, Wyatt HL, Heng MK, Lang TW, Farcot J, Davidson R, Corday E: Quantification of ischemic dysfunctioning myocardium in dogs (abstr). Circulation 55 and 60 (suppl III): III-89, 1977

18. Zwehl W, Childs W, Levy R, Meerbaum S, Berman D, Corday E: Comparison between computer-aided two-dimensional echocardiography and nuclear ventriculography during bicycle exercise testing. Dtsch. Ges. Kreislauffosd., Z Kardiol. Suppl, 1982

19. Garcia E, Levy R, Zwehl W, Corday SR, Haendchen R, Childs W, Meerbaum S, Corday E: Validation of automated computer analysis of left ventricular two-dimensional echocardiography (abstract). Circulation 64:1981

20. Zwehl W, Haendchen R, Garcia E, Levy R, Wyatt HL, Corday S, Meerbaum S: Validation of automated left ventricular edge detection images processed by computerized two-dimensional echocardiography. Circulation 64:IV 67, 1981

21. Levy R, Garcia E, Zwehl W, Murphy F, Corday SR, Childs W, Meerbaum S, Corday E: Objective echocardiographic quantitation of left ventricular volumes by use of automated computerized edge-detection analysis in canines and humans (abstract). Am J Cardiol (in press, February, 1982)

AUTOMATIC AND INTERACTIVE IMAGE PROCESSING OF 2-D ECHOCARDIOGRAMMS FOR
ANALYSIS OF LEFT VENTRICULAR FUNCTION.

E. GRUBE, B. BACKS, M. ZYWIETZ
MEDICAL HOSPITAL, UNIVERSITY OF BONN, DEPARTEMENT OF CARDIOLOGY
5300 BONN, WEST-GERMANY.

Due to the noisy appearance and low reflected signal energy from boundaries
characteristic for 2-D echocardiographic images, specific reflection properties and accuracies of automatic and manual border extraction are greatly reduced. Therefore digital processing of two dimensional echocardiogramms
in our institution is focused on three basic areas:
1. The first being the enhancement of the two dimensional images to create
   optimal displays for both clinical and research use.
2. The second area is the development of algorithms for the automatic detection of ventricular boders.
3. The third area is the automatic extraction of quantitative features from
   two dimensional echocardiogramms.
Through several image enhancement techniques the evaluation of computer
generated displays is greatly facilitated and the user may thus explore
the effects of various filters, transformations, summations and other interactive processing steps (Fig. 1-3).

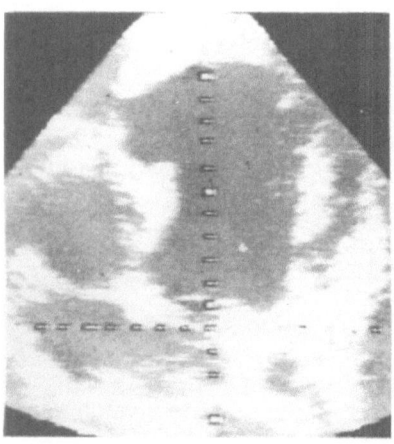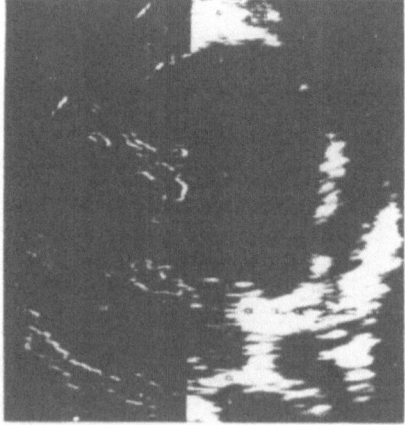

FIGURE 1a) Original 2-D echocardiogramm(4-chamber view) 1b) Processed image
(gradient and contrast enhanced).

By automated and manual techniques the recognition patterns of 2-D echocardiogramms and angiogramms can be compared particularly by definition
and extractions of endocardial borders. If the endocardial and/or the epicardial interfaces are appropriate judged on the basis of manual identification of these boundaries one should be able to analyze segmental wall
motion and ventricular function parameters by an automatic processing system.

In the following study we tested the hypothesis that the application
of digital computer image processing systems to digitized 2-D echocardiogramms should be more accurate and faster in the judgement of left ventricular
function parameters and determination of segmental wall motion abnormalities
as compared to the manual input of unprocessed echocardiogramms.

METHODS:

A total of 36 patients were studied by 2-D echocardiography and angiocardiography for the evaluation of the cardiac status in various disease
states. 15 patients had coronary artery disease with a history of a previous
myocardial infarction and corresponding segmental or global wall motion
abnormalities. 9 patients had no abnormal contraction patterns or abnormal
left ventricular function. 12 patients had valvular heart disease (2 aortic
stenosis, 4 aortic insufficiency, 3 mitral insufficiency, 3 mitral stenosis)

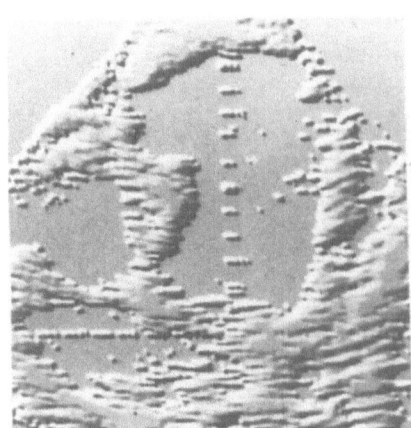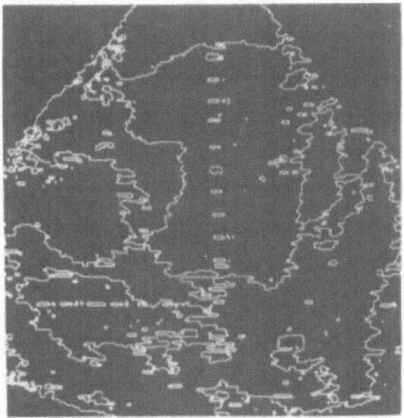

FIGURE 2a) Pseudoplastic 2-D image and 2b) contour extracted 2-D image
of an anterior-apical aneurysm viewed in the 4-chamber projection.

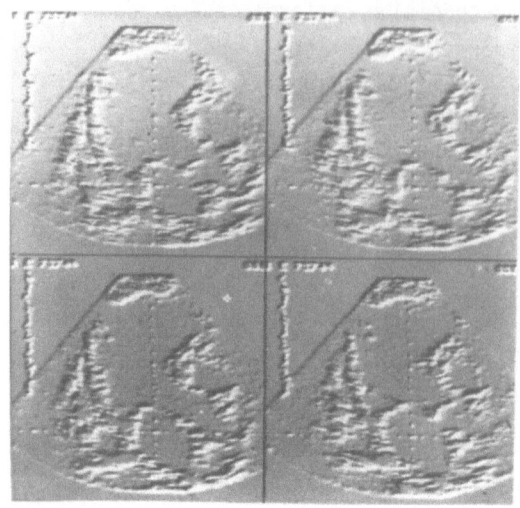

FIGURE 3) Serial display of 2-D pseudoplastic images in an apical 2-chamber view in a patient with an antero-apical aneurysm.

2-D studies were performed using standard views (LX,SX,4-CH,2-CH) with a simultaneous TM-echo recording. Angiogramms were performed in the 30° RAO and 60° LAO projections. 2-D echocardiographic studies and angiogramms were stored on a video tape for later evaluation.

The extraction of the endocardium was done in two steps: 1) First it was identified by image processing techniques using averaging and different filters as well as grey level discrimination (Fig. 1a-3), 2) secondly the endocardium was traced by an experienced observer. Then the manual and automated inputs were compared by direct superimposition of the two silhouettes qualitatively and by comparing the 2-D distances and TM distances quantitatively.

Following edge definition, several wall motion analysis programms were applied. In the LAO-, RAO-, 2-CH- and 4-CH-views we used a floating axis system with superposition of the long axis (Fig.6-7), in the short axis view we used a fix axis system .

Endsystolic-, and enddiastolic volumes as well as ejection fraction were computed using Simpson's rule in single and biplane views. Segmental wall motion was analyzed by determining theshortening of 48 radii or by computing the regional EF based on an area change method.

Image processing was done at the University of Bonn using a Medical Image Processing System "CA 2000". An overview of the image processing scheme and the CA 2000 is shown in Fig. 4-5)

FIGURE 4) Overview of the image processing scheme

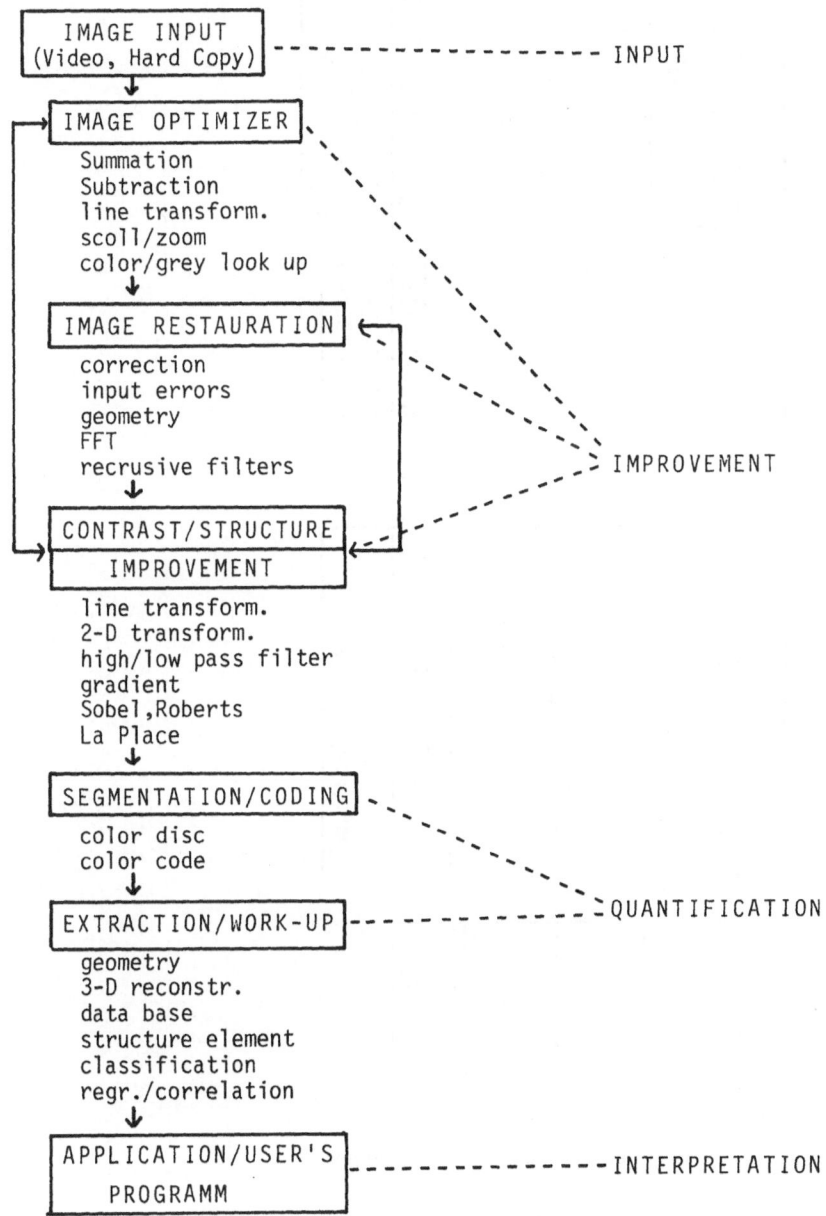

60

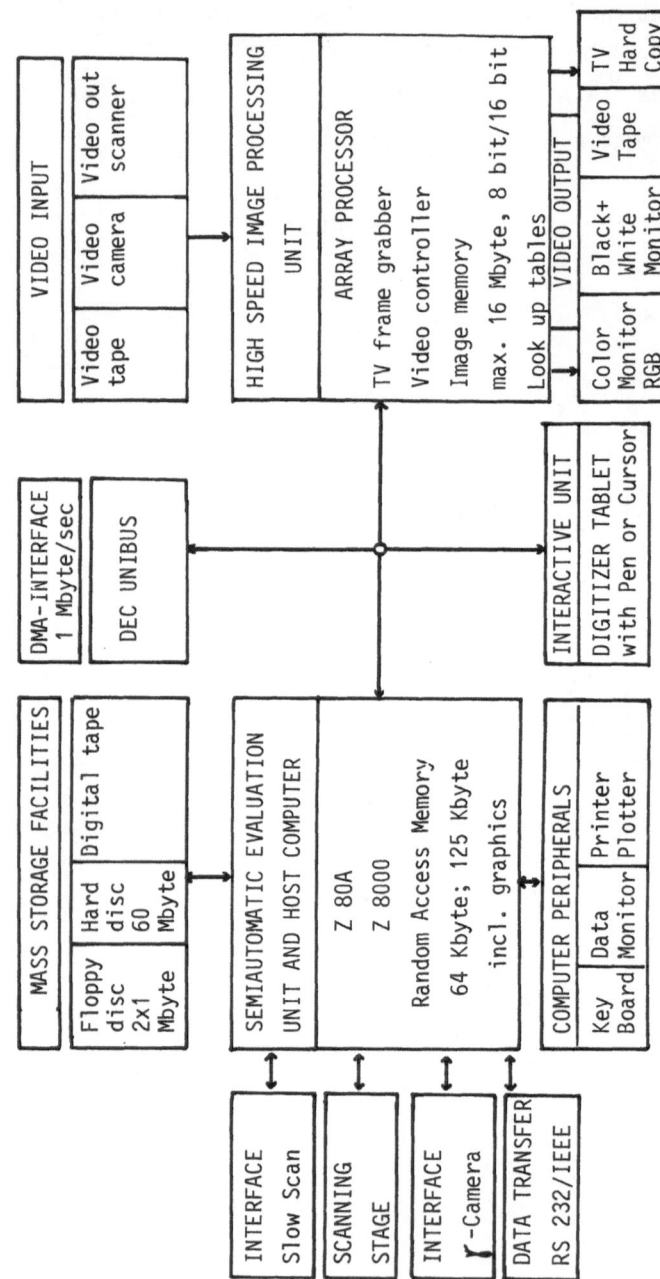

FIGURE 5) Medical Image Processing System "CA 2000"

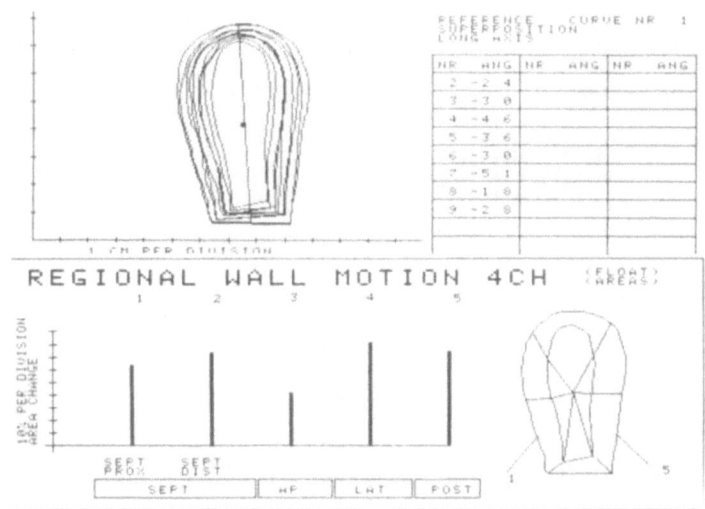

FIGURE 6) Endocardial outlines throughout one cardiac cycle with the angle of superimposition and regional wall motion analysis by the area change method with the determination of the regional EF in an apical 4-CH view.

2-D pictures were digitized using an optical densitometer with a 512 by 512 matrix with 8 bit corresponding to 256 grey levels. Multiimage averaging grey level evaluation, image segmentation and color coding were performed by a high speed image processing unit. Wall motion and volumetric studies of the left ventricle were performed by a Z 80A or Z 8000 host computer.

RESULTS AND DISCUSSION

Evaluation and comparison of 2-D and angiographic boundaries detected and traced by the computer and by the researcher were excellent. Accordingly the evaluation of left ventricular volumes and wall motion was equally good. Enddiastolic volumes, endsystolic volumes and ejection fraction determined by manual border input (man) and computer input (comp) correlated well. EDV_{man}/EDV_{comp} r= .89; ESV_{man}/ESV_{comp} r= .94; EF_{man}/EF_{comp} r= .91.

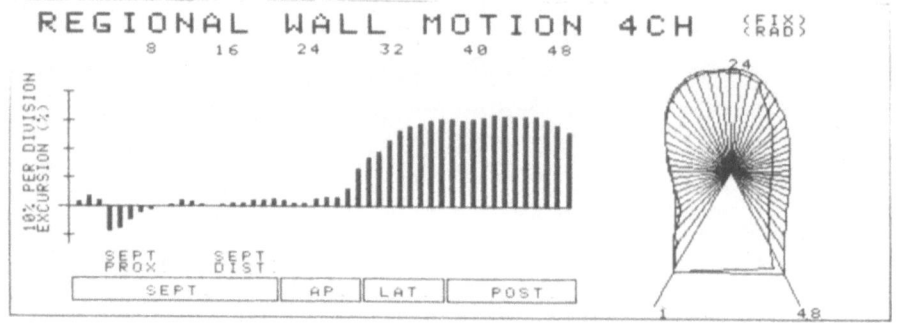

REGIONAL WALL MOTION 4CH {FIX}{RAD}

RADIAL SHORTENING (%)

REGION:	1	2	3	4	5	6	7	8	9	10	11	12
	2.	4.	2.	-8.	-7.	-4.	-2.	-1.	.	1.	2.	2.
REGION:	13	14	15	16	17	18	19	20	21	22	23	24
	1.	.	1.	1.	1.	2.	2.	3.	2.	1.	1.	3.
REGION:	25	26	27	28	29	30	31	32	33	34	35	36
	3.	3.	6.	13.	17.	19.	23.	27.	28.	29.	30.	31.
REGION:	37	38	39	40	41	42	43	44	45	46	47	48
	31.	30.	31.	31.	32.	32.	32.	32.	32.	31.	29.	26.

FIGURE 7) Determination of regional wall motion by the radii method in a patient with an apical/septal infarct. (Echo 4-chamber view).

The slope of the line of regression was closer to the line of identity in the computer generated volumes of processed images.

There was a 100% agreement in the analysis and location of segmental wall motion both using area or radii analysis between the manual and computer borderinput.

A quantitative comparison between M-mode measurements and processed and unprocessed 2-D echocardiographic measurements disclosed a superior correlation between TM-echo/processed images (r= .90) than between TM-echo/unprocessed images (r= .83)

From these preliminary studies we conclude that some of the disadvantages of two dimensional images such as speckled appearance, low reflected energy, granular structures, poor border definition and an unfavorable signal to noise ratio can be overcome by image processing techniques.

The results were reproducible and the quatitative measurement demonstrated an even closer correlation to TM echo measurements.

With the addition of digital scan converters to two dimensional instruments
direct digital access to ultrasonic data is possible and image processing
techniques (image averaging, grey level histogramm evaluation, image selection and segmentation, color coding) for boundary detection may be used.
Our studies showed that the use of processed images and algorithms from
2 dimensional video images are fast and reliable compared to conventional
off-line evaluation of unprocessed echocardiogramms by an experienced
observer.

These techniques can be used to establish pictorial data base systems and
three dimensional left ventricular reconstructions as well as to further
characterize biological tissue.

In our view only further improvement of grey level resolution, direct
acquisition, digitization and computer interfacing of ultrasonic data will
increase the accuracy and reproducibility of 2-dimensional echocardiographic evaluations for objective, quantitative determination of cardiac
structure and function.

We would like to express our gratitude to Mr. L.Heider and Mr. G.Hillje
KONTRON- Image Analysis GmbH.

ECHOCARDIOGRAPHIC DETECTION OF WALL MOTION ABNORMALITIES BEFORE
AND AFTER STREPTOKINASE THERAPY IN PATIENTS WITH ACUTE MYOCARDIAL
INFARCTION.
P. SCHWEIZER, R. ERBEL, W. MERX

1. INTRODUCTION

Several clinical and experimental studies have demonstrated,
that two-dimensional echocardiography can rapidly detect and
localize contraction abnormalities due to acute myocardial infarction. The extent of regional disturbance correlated remarkably well with angiographic asynergy and it showed also positive correlation to the size of morphologically proven transmural infarction (1,2).

Furthermore, follow-up evaluation of patients during the
acute stage of infarction detected prognostically important
alterations in cardiac topography. In animal experiments distinct-
time-courses of regional function due to different interventions
could be observed non-invasively (3-5).

The current study in patients with acute myocardial infarction
was undertaken to determine whether the extent of regional contraction abnormality being serially followed up with two-dimensional echocardiography may be influenced with early successful
intracoronary thrombolytic recanlization of the occluded vessel.

2. PROCEDURE

2.1. Material and methods

2.1.1. Patients. 42 patients with acute transmural myocardial
infarction fulfilled the criteria for intracoronary streptokinase
therapy as well as the criteria for repeated registration of high
quality two-dimensional echocardiograms. There were 28 patients
with anterior wall infarction and 14 patients with inferior infarction. The patient collective was further divided in two
subgroups according to the different time interval between be-

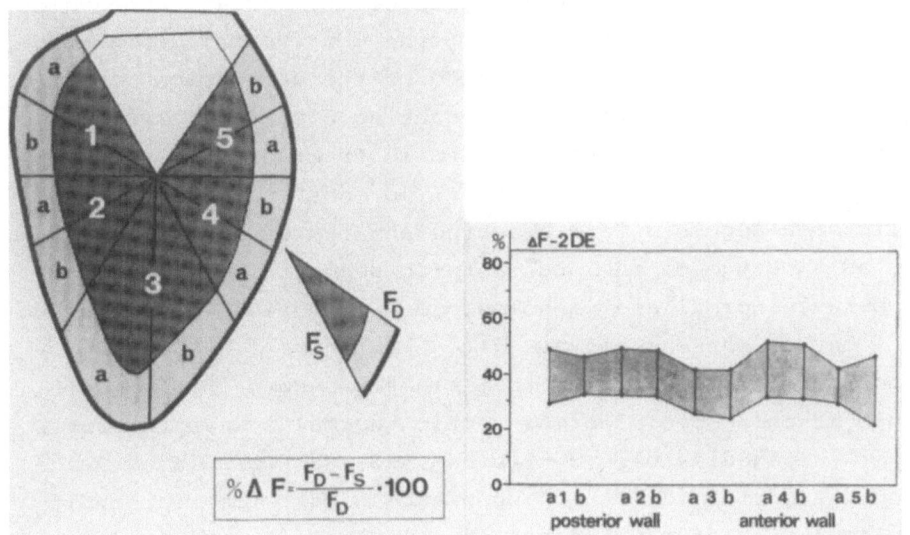

Figure 1: Left: Area based method for quantification of segmental wall motion abnormalities. 1o segmental areas are defined by radii emanating from the endsystolic center of gravity. Right: The normal contraction range represented by the tolerance limits (lower limits)and the mean values (upper limits) was echocardiographically established in 32 patients.

ginning of the symptoms of infarction and the recanalization of the occluded vessel. In group A (16 pts) the occluded vessel was open within 4 hours from the beginning of symptoms (mean interval $X = 2oo \pm 28$ min.), whereas in patient group B intracoronary thrombolysis was successful only later than 4 hours or remained ineffective.

2.1.2. Echocardiographic evaluation. Two-dimensional echocardiographic studies were performed using a VARIAN-34oo R phased array sector scanner. At the time of the first study optimum transducer position on the chest wall (apical window) was marked to maintain the same cross section in the individual from day to day. Studies were performed immediately before invasive therapeutic intervention was performed, on the second and third day of hospitalization and 3 to 4 weeks afterwards. Registrations were recorded on a 3/4 inch video cassette recorder for subsequent analysis.

2.1.3. Data analysis. Apical two-chamber cross section was

selected for the quantitative analysis of the serial echocardiographic studies. The inner border of the left ventricle in both
enddiastole and endsystole was traced on the television monitor.

Regional wall motion was assessed using a computer system.
The center of gravity of the endsystolic frame of the left
ventricle was used as inner fix point. 1o endsystolic and 1o enddiastolic area segments were measured and the differences expressed as % change of the enddiastolic segment area (% Δ F).
Limits between normal and pathological wall motion were obtained
with 32 control persons and are given in figure 1.

Furthermore, the length of the akinetic segment of the left
ventricle in this special cross-section normalized to the total
length of the enddiastolic outline (% AKS) was calculated. Data
analysis was performed without knowledge of the time interval
between occlusion of the infarct vessel (beginning of symptoms)
and recanalization.

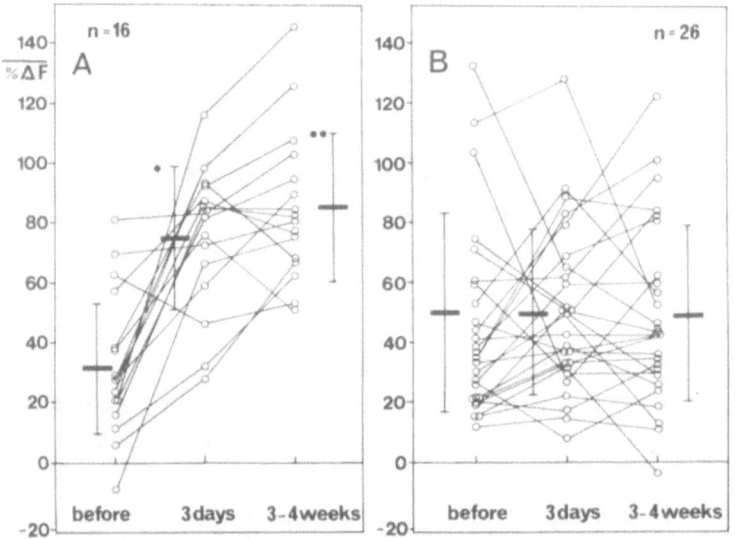

Figure 2: Temporal changes of segmental area ejection fractions
within the ischemic zone. Patients are grouped according to the
time interval between beginning of the symptoms and recanalization of the infarct vessel (group A: earlier than 4 hours).

3. Results

During the initial study period pronounced regional contrac-

tion abnormalities in correspondance to the infarct vessel could
be observed in all patients. The temporal changes within the
ischemic zone are illustrated in figure 2. The %Δ F of those segments beeing pathological during the follow-up period were
summed up and are given for each control period.

In patients group A with early recanalization of the infarct
vessel the function of the ischemic segments improved from % Δ F
32,9 $\pm$ 22 % to 75 $\pm$ 23 % (p < 0,o5) on the third day after the
acute event and showed a distinct further improvement 3-4 weeks
later (84$\pm$25,p < 0,o1) . In B there were no significant temporal
variations concerning the whole study group despite individual
changes from period to period.

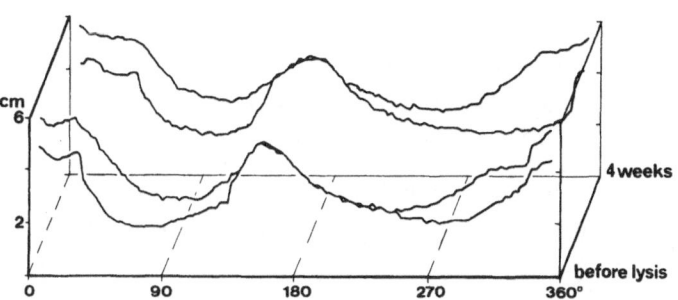

Figure 3: Example of the temporal behaviour of regional contraction in a patient with early recanalization of the infarct vessel
(time interval 3 hours). Each plot shows the percentage radial
shortening in systole and diastole against the angle o-360°.
Large akinetic zone of the anterior wall, which improves 4 weeks
later.

Figure 3 and 4 give examples of the temporal changes of contraction pattern being observed in a patient with anterior wall
infarction and short interval between the beginning of symptoms
and reopening of the infarct vessel.

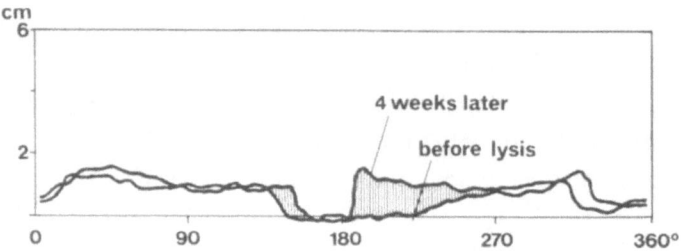

Figure 4: Same example as in figure 3. Plots of the difference between the percentage radial snortening in systole as well as in diastolic clearly demonstrating the reduction of the akinetic segment 4 weeks later.

The different temporal behaviour of regional dysfunction between study group A and B could also be demonstrated with the determination of the length of akinetic segment:

	before	2nd day	3rd day	3-4 weeks
A:AKS	22 ± 9	15 ± 13	$13,5 \pm 11$	13 ± 12 % (p < o,o1)
B:AKS	29 ± 12	27 ± 8	27 ± 8	$26,5 \pm 9$ % n.s.

4. COMMENT

Two-dimensional echocardiography offers the ability to evaluate serially regional left ventricular function in patients with acute myocardial infarction (3,6).

In contrast to other investigators the apical long axis cross section was selected for analysis, because to our experience it is easier to obtain even in critically ill patients. The section plane can be reproduced using the cardiac valves and chambers as landmarks.

Pronounced segmental wall motion abnormalities been localized in correspondence to the occluded vessel were observed, in all patients during the acute stage of ischemia. Dependent of the time interval between occlusion and recanalization of the infarct vessel, two patient groups were distinguished. The comparison of the results of both groups clearly showed a significant reduction in the area of contraction abnormality during the follow-up in those patients undergoing very early reperfusion. These results are consistent with previously reported cineangiographic data (7,8).

Those findings share some limitation, because no direct estimation of myocardial vitality is possible from quantitation of regional left ventricular function. Segmental wall motion abnormalities can be assosciated with both, myocardial ischemia and infarction.

REFERENCES

1. Weiss JL, BH Bulkley, GM Hutchins, SG Mason: Two-dimensional echocardiographic recognition of myocardial injury in man: comparison with postmortem studies. Circulation 63: 4o1, 1981

2. Schweizer P, R Erbel, W Merx, W Krebs, F vErckelenz, H Lambertz, S Effert:Wall motion abnormalities in acute myocardial infarction. Correlation between two-dimensional echocardiography and cineangiography. Europ Heart J 2 (Abstr): 1o8, 1981

3. Eaton LW, JL Weiss, BH Bulkley, JB Garrison, ML Weisfeldt: Regional cardiac dilatation after acute myocardial infarction. Recognition by two-dimensional echocardiography. New Engl J Med 3oo: 57, 1979

4. Wyatt HL, S Meerbaum, MK Heng, J Rit, P Gueret, E Corday: Experimental evaluation of the extent of myocardial dyssynergy and infarct size by two-dimensional echocardiography. Circulation 63: 597, 1981

5. Meltzer RS, CN Woythaler, AJ Buda, GC Griffin, WD Harrison, RP Martin, DC Harrison, RL Popp: Two dimensional echocardiographic quantification of infarct size alteration by pharmacologic agents.

6. Visser CA, KI Lie, G Kan, R Meltzer, D Durrer: Detection and quantification of acute, isolated myocardial infarction by two dimensional echocardiography. Am J Cardiol 47: 1o2o, 1981

7. Rentrop P, H Blanke, KR Karsch, W Rutsch, M Schartl, W. Merx,
    R Dörr, D Mathey, K Kuch: Changes in left ventricular function
    after intracoronary streptokinase infusion in clinically evol-
    ving myocardial infarction. Am Heart J 1o2: 1188, 1981

8. Mathey DG, G Rodewald, P Rentrop, K Leitz, W. Merx,
    BJ Messmer, W Rutsch, ES Bücherl: Intracoronary strepto-
    kinase thrombolytic recanalization and subsequent surgical
    bypass of remaining atherosclerotic stenosis in acute myo-
    cardial infarction: Complementary combined approach effecting
    reduced infarct size, preventing reinfarction, and improving
    left ventricular function. Am Heart J 1o2: 1194, 1981

ECHOCARDIOGRAPHIC MAP OF THE LEFT VENTRICLE.   A METHOD
TO LOCALIZE MYOCARDIAL INFARCTION

T. TOUCHE, P. VERVIN, D. MARTIN, R. PRASQUIER

Description of 2D echographic left ventricular segmental
wall motion is hampered by lack of accepted standards and by
the difficulty to convey in a written record the complex anatomical features of areas of asynergy as assessed by multiple
views imaging.

A simple pictorial method, derived from anatomical study
of the left ventricle, is therefore proposed to improve the
precision of the reporting procedure.

I.   METHODS

1.   SEGMENTAL ANATOMY OF THE LEFT VENTRICLE (Fig. 1)

The left ventricle is divided into 4 walls through longitudinal lines: anterior wall (from the septum to the medial
edge of anterior papillary muscle), lateral wall (including
anterior papillary muscle and limited by lateral edge of
posterior papillary muscle), inferior wall (including posterior papillary muscle and limited by the septum) and septum.
Each wall is subdivided in a basal, midventricular (or papillary) and apical level. Basal and midventricular levels
of septum and lateral wall are further subdivided into superior and inferior halves. The left ventricle is therefore
divided into 16 segments.

Planimetry of these 16 segments in 4 normal human hearts
showed that the surface ratio between the largest and the
smallest was always less than 2: these segments have therefore a roughly similar size.

72

ANATOMIC SEGMENTATION OF THE LEFT VENTRICLE

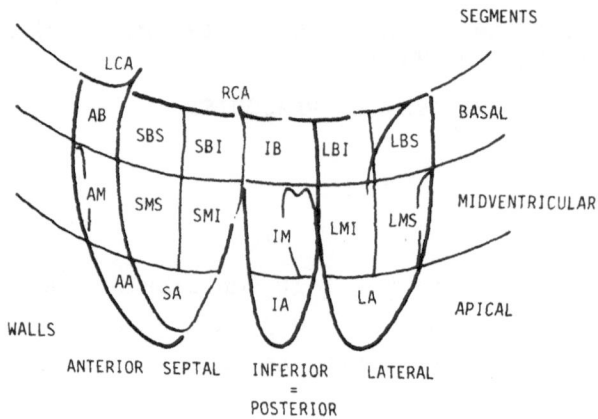

Figure 1. First letter refers to wall: A anterior, S septum, I inferior,
L lateral. Second letter refers to level: B basal, M midventricular,
A apical. Third letter refers to further subdivision: S superior,
I inferior. LCA: left coronary artery RCA: right coronary artery.

2. <u>LEFT VENTRICULAR ECHOGRAPHIC MAPPING IN PATIENTS</u> (Fig. 2)

This scheme of segmental division was used in 100 consecutive patients with old (more than 3 weeks) myocardial infarction. Standard parasternal and apical views were supple-
mented whenever possible or necessary by intermediary or
oblique views, in order to obtain a better delineation of
area of asynergy.

Results were reported on a schematic drawing of the
different left ventricular sections, using a 3 colour code
qualitative assessment of myocardial thickening: no systolic
thickening, some systolic thickening or inadequate visualization. The different regions of individual sections were then
retraced with the same colour code on a myocardial map where
relative positions of standard left ventricular sections had
been predetermined. Whenever recorded sections were atypical,
the results could be reported on the ventricular map according

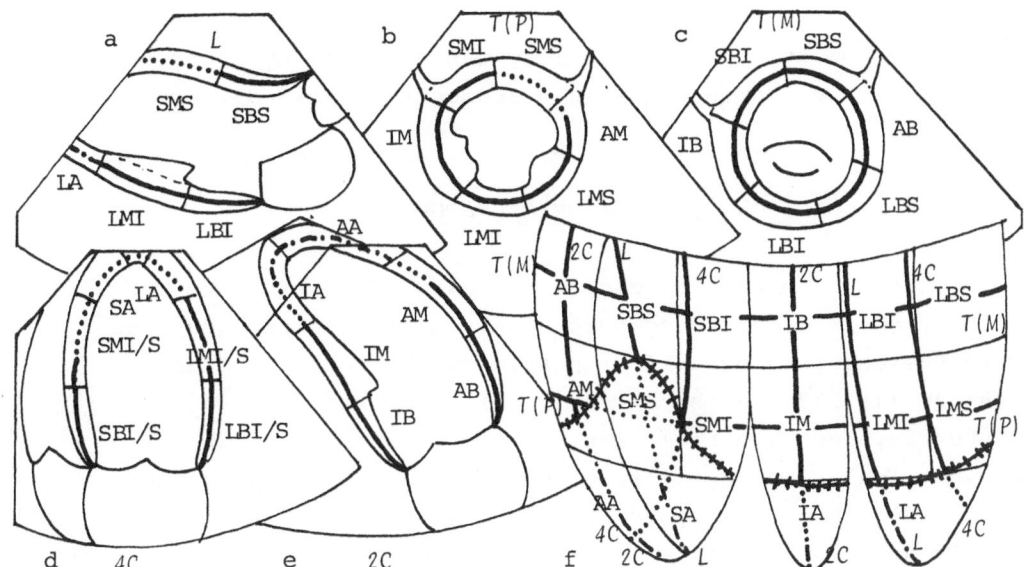

Figure 2: Echographic mapping of an anterior MI. a, b, c, d, e: findings
in standard views   f: drawing on the ventricular map.
..........no systolic thickening
——————— presence of systolic thickening
—.—.—.—.— inadequate visualization
++++++++++ limits of infarcted area

to their relative topography.

Limits of the akinetic regions as derived from each section
were then joined together on the myocardial map: this allowed
for a three dimensional geometrical display of the involved
ventricular area.

Many ventricular segments are displayed by more than one
section. Whenever a discrepancy occurred for the regional
assessment in the different sections, recordings were reanalysed.

The echocardiogram is then reported as the drawing of the
ventricular map with the areas of asynergy and as the analysis
of individual segments, each segment being defined as partially
abnormal (when less than three quarters of its area were abnormal), totally abnormal, normal or not visualized, when no
visualized outline intersects the central portion of the
segment.

3. REPRODUCIBILITY

Interobserver reproducibility was assessed by separate
readings of 50 examinations (800 segments) by two different
observers.

4. COMPARISON WITH ANATOMICAL STUDIES

Three anatomical studies of myocardial infarctions were
reanalysed in order to compare usual infarction topographies
with the echocardiographic reportings. In these studies,
Lenègre (1) 212 hearts, Sayen (2, 3) 44 hearts, Savage (4)
24 hearts, left ventricle was divided into 3 levels (basal,
midventricular and apical); although each level was further
subdivided into 8 segments and not 6 (and 4 for the apical
level) as in our echocardiographic report, this did not prevent
from a comparative analysis.

This comparison was performed on isolated anterior and
posterior infarctions. Similarly to Sayen, who describes
"central" areas with fixed vascular supply, we selected for
the topographical analysis of myocardial infarctions "key
segments" that were easily recorded and usually involved in
the infarction process. Apical septal (SA) and basal inferior
(IB) segments were selected as key segments for respectively
anterior and posterior myocardial infarction.

II. RESULTS

1. PERCENTAGE OF SEGMENTAL VISUALIZATION

Adequate visualization in more than 70% of the patients
could be obtained in every segment excepted the superior half
of the lateral wall and of the anterior wall.

2. REPRODUCIBILITY

There was complete agreement in 698 (87%) segments, only

7 (1%) complete disagreements between the two observers (normal
vs abnormal) and 95 (12%) partial disagreements over either
quality of the recording or degree of segmental involvement.

Disagreement was significantly lower (5% vs 16%,p<.001)
for segments that were visualized in two echographic sections
by both observers (n=220) than for segments that could be
interpreted in only one section (n=580).

3. TOPOGRAPHICAL EXTENSION AND COMPARISON WITH ANATOMICAL
    SERIES

3.1. Percentage of segmental involvement
Very frequently involved segments (>40%) include apical
segments, midventricular septal and inferior segment, and
basal inferior segment. Unusually involved segments (<10%)
include basal anterior, superobasal lateral and superomid-
ventricular lateral segments.

Results from Lenègre were closely similar(1).

3.2. Localization and extension of anterior and posterior
infarction
Isolated anterior infarction was in our series defined
by the involvement of the anterior key segment without
involvement of posterior key segment. In Fig. 3a are shown
two frequent different localizations: anteroseptoapical and
large anterior.

There were 51 isolated anterior infarctions. SA and AA
were constantly involved and SMS, IA and LA were frequently so.
Other less usually abnormal segments were SMI, AM, SBS, SBI,
IM, AB, LMI, LMS, LBS with a decreasing frequency. Some of
these segments are usually only partially abnormal. (Fig. 3b)

Pathological studies were reexamined, the SA segment being
assimilated to Sayen's segment 4 and Savage's segment A2, and
the IB segment being assimilated to Sayen's segment 24 and
Savage's segment B7. Results of this comparison are presented
in figures 3c and 3d; although infarct extension is much larger
in the anatomical series, topography of the infarcted area is
similar.

76

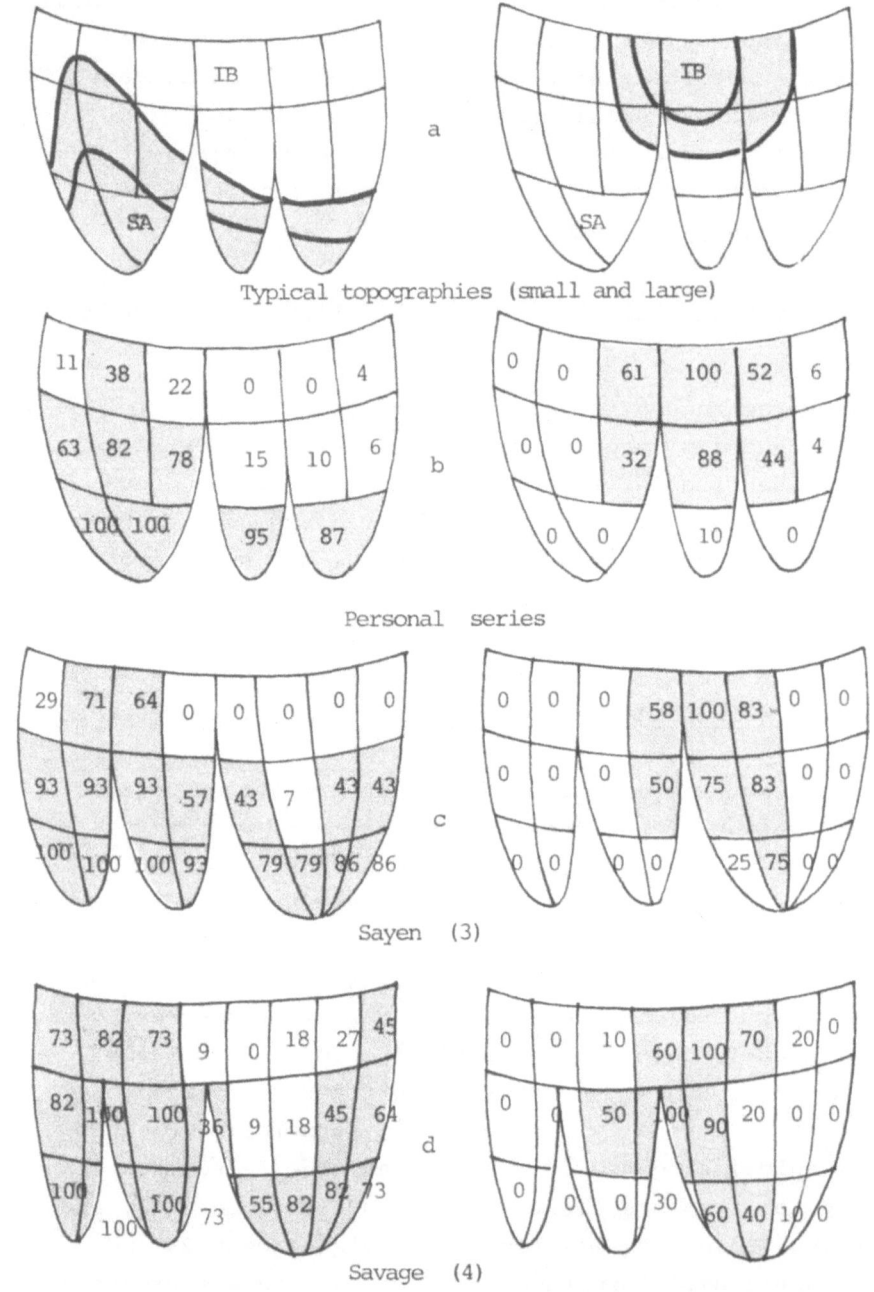

Typical topographies (small and large)

Personal series

Sayen (3)

Savage (4)

Fig. 3 Anterior MI   Fig. 4 Posterior MI

Typical myocardial infarctions. Numbers correspond to percentage
of segmental involvement.

Isolated posterior infarctions were defined by IB without SA involvement. In figure 4a are shown two typical localizations, posterior and posterolateral.

There were 28 isolated posterior infarctions; extension occurred, usually partially, to segments IM, SBI, LBI, LMI and SMI (fig. 4b). There is a definite similarity to anatomical results.

3.3. Exceptions to usual topography

They were distinctly unusual; besides 10 patients with associated anterior and posterior infarctions, and 3 non-interpretable echocardiograms, there were 2 posterior infarctions without IB visualization, 5 lateral infarctions and 1 normal study.

In Sayen's study (3), 5 anterior or posterior transmural infarctions and in Savage's study (4), only 1 anterior infarction did not involve the key segment.

III. DISCUSSION

The present study was undertaken in order to determine the reliability of a method of specific echocardiographic description and pictorial display of segmental wall asynergy. Myocardial thickening was studied because it is a more specific index of myocardial function than wall displacement (5) and is also less dependant upon the choice of a reference system (6,7). Quantitative echographic analysis of wall thickening is however feasible in a small minority of patients and of segments because of inadequate image quality and resolution limitations. In our experience, echographic qualitative assessment of absence of myocardial thickening is accurate and reproducible, whereas distinction between normal motion versus hypokinesis is not (8).The comparison to pathological findings of myocardial infarctions limited anyway the study to the analysis of complete absence of local thickening. The inclusion of some older large pathological studies (1, 3, 4) allowed to correlate echocardiographic findings with a wider spectrum of myocardial

infarctions small and large, than would presumably be available
from prospective anatomical studies in our CCU's era.

Our reproducibility findings were satisfactory; the very
good results obtained for segments that could be adequately
visualized in different sections underscore the value of
multiple views imaging of the heart. Topography of asynergy
was similar to the pathological findings: the strikingly
uniform pattern of most myocardial infarctions around some
key areas which are almost always involved is well known by
the echocardiographers.

The entire mapping procedure is fast and easy to perform;
it is well suited to serial studies. It leads to a more careful and more homogeneous analysis of segmental motion and the
pictorial display is readily accepted by the clinician; moreover it can include "atypical" sections increasing the diagnostic value of tomographic scanning analysis of ventricular
area: assessment of wall motion in atypical sections should
however only be attempted by someone who can relate these
sections one to each other, usually limiting it to the physician who performed the examination.

This ventricular mapping is not intended as an accurate
quantitative tool for segmental wall motion analysis; this
would await for position locating systems (9), improvements
in image quality and computer enhancement programs. We feel
it is less arbitrary than the usually employed indices of
asynergy based upon comparison with angiography and fixed
limited number of ventricular segments (8, 10, 11) where un-
certainties can occur from distorsion of ventricular geometry
by aneurysmal distension and from frequent partial involvement
of large segments, when the need arises for a "all or none"
answer as to the presence or absence of asynergy.

We found after the completion of our study a very similar
approach by Edwards and col (12), who describes a segmental
echographic analysis of ventricular motion based upon autopsic
study, with division of the left ventricle into 14 segments.
The major discrepancy between the two classifications is the
choice in Edward's study of the postero medial papillary

muscle as the dividing point between the ventricular septum and inferior free wall: this leads to a septal area of 40% of the total LV circumference at the basal and midventricular level which is higher than in our experience (30%).

Correlative autopsic and echocardiographic studies (13) should lead to an improvement in the topographical descriptive capabilities of 2D echocardiography.

BIBLIOGRAPHY

1. LENEGRE J. Anatomie pathologique des cardiopathies par athérosclérose coronarienne. Ed. Lenègre et Soulié. Maladies de l'appareil cardiovasculaire I, 1024 Flammarion publ. Paris 1968.
2. SAYEN JJ, SHELDON WF. The heart muscle and the electrocardiogram in coronary disease. Difficulties of description and illustration of ventricular muscle lesions with a method for their graphic representation in a myocardial map. Am Heart J. 38 688, 1949.
3. SAYEN JJ, SHELDON WF, WOLFERTH CC. A new classification of ventricular myocardial damage derived from the clinicopathologic findings in 100 patients. Circulation 12:321, 1955.
4. SAVAGE RM, WAGNER GS, IDEKER RE, PODOLSKY SA, HACKER DB. Correlation of post mortem anatomic findings with electrocardiographic changes in patients with myocardial infarction. Retrospective study of patients with typical anterior and posterior infarcts. Circulation 55:279, 1977.
5. LIEBERMAN AN, WEISS JL, JUDGUTT BI, BECKER LC, BUCKLEY BH, GARRISON JG, HUTCHINS GM, KALLMAN CA, WEISFELDT ML. Two dimensional echocardiography and infarct size: relationship of regional wall motion and thickening to the extent of myocardial infarction in the dog. Circulation 63:730, 1981.
6. MOYNIHAN PF, PARISI AF, FELDMAN CL. Quantitative detection of regional left ventricular contraction abnormalities by two dimensional echocardiography. Analysis of Methods. Circulation 63: 752, 1981.
7. PARISI AF, MOYNIHAN PF, FOLLAND ED, FELDMAN CL. Quantitative detection of regional left ventricular contraction abnormalities by two dimensional echocardiography. Accuracy in coronary artery disease. Circulation 63: 761, 1981.
8. PRASQUIER R, BARTHELEMY M, VERVIN P, HANOUN CH, TOUCHE T, AUMONT MC, GOURGON R. Echocardiographie bidimensionnelle dans l'infarctus aigu du myocarde. Arch. Mal. Coeur 72: 1069, 1979.
9. BKINKLEY JF, MORITZ WE, BAKER DW. Ultrasonic three dimensional imaging and volume from a series of arbitrary sector scans. Ultrasound Med. Biol. 4: 317, 1978.
10. KISSLO JA, ROBERTSON D, GILBERT BW, VON RAMM O, BEHAR VS. A comparison of real time two dimensional echocardiography and cineangiography in detecting left ventricular asynergy. Circulation 55: 134, 1977.
11. HEGER JJ, WEYMAN AE, WANN LS, DILLON JC, FEIGENBAUM H. Cross sectional echocardiography in acute myocardial infarction:detection and localization of regional left ventricular asynergy.Circulation 60: 531, 1979.

12. EDWARDS WD, TAJIK AJ, SEWARD JB. Standardized nomenclature and anatomic basis for regional topographic analysis of the heart. Mayo Clinic Proc. 56: 479, 1981.
13. WEISS JL, BUCKLEY BH, GARRISON JG, HUTCHINS GM, KALLMAN CA, WEISFELDT ML. Two dimensional echocardiography and infarct size: relationship of regional wall motion and thickening to the extent of myocardial infarction in the dog. Circulation 63: 739, 1981.

Diagnostic value of 2-dimensional echocardiography in the
early detection of acute myocardial infarction

Schartl, M., Disselhoff, W., Rutsch, W., Schmutzler, H.

Dept. of Cardiology, Free University Berlin,
Klinikum Charlottenburg

Introduction

In acute myocardial infarction the mortality within the first
4 hours accounts for 60 % of the total mortality. This may
be reduced by means of intense hemodynamical monitoring and
possibly by rapid therapeutical intervention like intracoronary thrombolysis. This ist what makes an early diagnosis of
evolving myocardial infarction important.
The diagnsotic tools within the first 4 hours are clinical
symptoms and the ECG, but not blood parameters like CPK
which usually is not found to be elevated within this time.
The 2-dimensional echocardiography is a new method in
detection of regional wall motion abnormalities. It is now
used in the diagnostic of acute myocardial infarction (1,2,
5,6,7). Several of the reports given did not meet the
criteria for establishing the sensitivity of this method (1,
2,6,7). In other cases the 2-d echocardiogram was performed
later then 4 hours after the onset of chest pain (5). We
therefore compared in a prospective study the diagnostic
value of the 2-d echocardiography with that of the ECG in
the early detection of acute myocardial infarction.

Material and Methods

89 patients (16 female and 73 male, mean age 53 ± 12 years)
admitted to the coronary care unit with the suspected
diagnosis of acute myocardial infarction because of chest
pain less than 4 hours ago were included into the study.
2-d echocardiography was performed after a mean time of
178 ± 62 min following the onset of angina. Patients were

excluded from the study if more than 4 hours had elapsed from the onset of pain or if tney had a history of previous infarction. The final decision if a patient actually did suffer from acute myocardial infarction was made later basing upon all available data (ECG, CPK, coronary angiogram) except for the echo findings. 56 patients did have a transmural myocardial infarction (anterior infarction 18, anteroseptal infarction 8, anterolateral infarction 3, inferior infarction 20 and inferolateral infarction 7). In 4 patients the infarction was not transmural (inferior infarction 3, anterior infarction 1). The remaining 29 patients did not have a myocardial infarction but in the following test 7 of them were shown to have a coronary arteries disease. One patient had an aneurysm of the aorta descendens.

In all cases 12 lead ECGs and blood samples for creatine phosphocinase analysis were taken on admission and every following day. Cross sectional echocardiographic studies were also performed with the patient in the left lateral position using a 90° mechanical sector scanner. Recordings were made in five views: parasternal long axis, parasternal short axis (mitral valve), parasternal short axis (papillary muscle), apical four chamber view and apical two chamber view. On the basis of these five views the left ventricle was divided into 9 segments: septal basal (ventral, dorsal), septal apical (ventral, dorsal), apical, diaphragmatic, posterobasal, anterobasal, anteroapical, infero lateral and superior lateral. The recordings were analysed from an observer who had no knowledge of the ECG findings. The right ventricle was analysed if possible. According to a semiquantitative score each segment was labelled o = normal, 1 = hypokinetic, 2 = akinetic or 3 = dyskinetic. The total score for all 9 segments was then summed up and taken as an indicator of the degree of regional wall motion abnormality. In 53 cases coronary angiogram and ventriculogram additionally within the first 5 hours after the onset of pain were performed.

Results

CPK and ECG

Except for one case CPK was found normal in all patients
with acute myocardial infarction within the first 4 hours
after the onset of angina.

The results of the ECG during the first 4 hours after the
onset of pain were classified as follwos: true positive if
the ECG was diagnostic (ST-segment and/or QRS complex
changes) or if it indicated possible myocardial infarction
(ST-segment changes) in patients with acute myocardial
infarction; false positive when a positive or possible
positive ECG occured in patients without acute myocardial
infarction; false negative if the ECG was negative in an
acute myocardial infarction patient; true negative when a
negative ECG was found in a patient without acute myocardial
infarction. For the ECG by itself we found a specificity of
72 %, a sensitivity of 93 %, a positive predictive value of
88 % and a negative predictive value of 83 %. 3 patients with
posterior infarction and 1 patient with LBBB were judged
false negative. False positive ECG was found in 8 cases
with ST-elevation in the anterior leads (6) and in 1 case
with posterior lead ST-elevation. 1 patient was suffering
from Prinzmetal angina and the time lag between ECG
registration and echocardiography accounted for the
discrepancy.

Cross sectional echocardiography

The visability of several segments of all patients (n = 89)
was: septal basal 92 %, septal apical 92 %, apical 82 %,
diaphragmatic 78 %, posterobasal 87 %, anterobasal 77 %,
anterolateral 89 %, superior lateral 87 %, superior lateral
85 %. Complete examination could be done in 65 cases (74 %).
The echocardiographic findings were classified as follows:
true positive ore false positive if the 2-d echocardiography
demonstrated any regional wall motion disorder in patients
with or without acute myocardial infarction; true negative

or false negative if no regional wall motion abnormality
could be detected in patients without or with acute
myocardial infarction or if sufficient quality of echo
recording could not be achieved. Echocardiographic detection
of wall motion disorder in evolving myocardial infarction
was found to be specific 86 %, sensitivity was 87 %,
positive predictive value 93 % and negative predictive value
76 %. In 4 cases hypokinesia of the posterior wall and in
1 case akinesia of the apical segment were thought to be
seen without any other evidence of coronary heart disease
in these patients. False negative results were due to
insufficient imaging quality in 3 cases, failure to
visualize non transmural infarctions in 2 cases (inferior
myocardial infarction) and transmural infarctions in 3 cases
(posterior 2, anterior 1).

Localisation of acute myocardial infarction
46 patients with known coronary angiograms and complete
echocardiographic examination were selected for a more
detailed analysis ot the localisation and extent of
myocardial infarction.
In 15 patients with inferior myocardial infarction (ST-elevation in II, III, aVF) the posterobasal segment was found
to be involved 15 times, the diaphragmal segment 4 times,
the septal basal-dorsal segment 5 times, the superior lateral
segment 3 times. Additional motion disturbance of the right
ventricle could be found in 4 cases of these 15 patients.
9 patients hat a proximal occlusion and 2 a proximal subtotal stenosis of the right coronary artery. Twice the
occlusion site was the middle third, once the distal third
of the right coronary artery and once the left circumflex
artery was found to be proximally occluded.
In 7 patients with inferolateral infarction (II, III, aVF,
V_{5+6}) the akinetic segment 7 times was posterolateral,
5 times diaphragmal, 6 times superior lateral, 2 times
inferolateral and 5 times septal basal-dorsal. Occlusion

of the right coronary artery was seen 3 times, ramus margi-
nalis sinister 1 time and left circumflex 3 times (twice
the proximal and once the middle third). 15 patients with
anterior myocardial infarction (I, II, aVL, V_{2-6}) showed
involvement of the anterolateral, septal apical-ventral and
of the apical segment in all cases. In 6 cases the anterobasal segment, in 8 the inferolateral, were involved. The
left anterior descending artery (LAD) was occluded proximally in 12 cases and in 1 case showed subtotal stenosis.
In 2 cases the middle third of the LAD was the site of
occlusion.

In 8 patients with anteroseptal infarction (ST elevation
V_{1-4}) the following segments showed motion disorder: apical,
septal-ventral 6 times, anterolateral 4 times, anterobasal
2 times, apical 7 times and inferolateral 2 times. The LAD
was occluded 4 times in the proximal and in the middle third
respectively.

In one patient with anterolateral infarction (V_{3-6}) the LAD
was found to be occluded proximally. The anterolateral,
anterobasal, inferolateral and apical segments were involved.
These data make it clearthat an infarction can simply be
localized in the posterior or anterior wall by ECG as well
as by 2-d echocardiography. But 2-d echocardiography can
differentiate the segments involved more exactly which the
ECG ist not able to do. Therefore a correlation cannot be
found neither between the number of altered ECG leads and
the number of segments involved (r = 0,48) nor between the
number of altered ECG leads and the score of wall motion
disorder (r = 0,43). This means that the exact extent of
infarcted tissue could be estimated only by 2-d echocardiography and not by ECG. In anterior wall infarction the ECG
as well as 2-d echo allow to predict that the LAD will be
affected but do not give more detailed information. In
posterior infarction the left circumflex artery or right
coronary artery possibly are occluded. This cannot be
differentiated very well neither by ECG nor by 2-d echo.

Hemodynamics

The score of wall motion disorder as determined by 2-d echo
does not relate to the left ventricular enddiastolic
pressure (r = 0,26) nor to the cardiac index (r = 0,42).
Those patients however with posterior infarction also
affecting the right ventricle did have a markedly higher
right atrial pressure than those with posterior infarction
without affection of the right ventricle.
4 out of 46 patients with acute myocardial infarction died
within the first 7 days, but echocardiographic findings did
not suggest a risk constellation for these 4 patients.

Discussion

Our results show that in most cases the ECG is a reliable
and sufficient method to detect acute myocardial infarction.
The rather often false positive ECG diagnosis in our patients
probably results from the doctor wish not to make any
mistakes who therefore in doubtful cases prefers to assume
an acute myocardial infarction rather than to overlook it.
In the cases for example 2-d echocardiography can be helpful
in the diagnostic because we never made a wrong diagnosis
when ECG and echo were combined. But it might be possible
to overlook a non transmural infarction. Nearly in all cases
of acute myocardial infarction the ECG was diagnostic except,
for exampel, for the patient with LBBB in which the
demonstration of a asynergy was very important to make the
correct diagnosis. But in this case wie also knew that there
was no history of previous infarction. Although the
sensitivity and specificity for 2-d echo findings were
equally high as for the ECG findings in our group we should
not forget that 2-d echo does not allow a differentiation
between ischemic tissue andacute or chronic infarction.
Therefore 2-d echocardiography only can supply additional
proof in the diagnostic of acute myocardial infarction.

The ECG allows only a simple information about the localization and the extent of myocardial infarction. This can be done with more differentiation by 2-d echocardiography but with an only moderate prediction of the involved coronary vessel. The better description of the extent of myocardial infarction however does not seem to be of great advantage since the score of wall motion abnormality does not correlate to hemodynamic parameters nor does it allow a prognostic index by which high risk patients might be identified in the early diagnostic of acute myocardial infarction. The main advantage of the 2-d echocardiography in acute myocardial infarction probably are the possibility to register changes after therapeutical intervention (3) and the detection of complications such as pericardial effusion, rupture of the ventricular septum or left ventricular thrombi (4).

References

1. Regional cardiac dilatation after acute myocardial infarction. Eaton, L.W., J.L. Weiss, B.H. Bulkley, J.B. Garrison, M.L. Weisfeldt
N E J M 300 (1979) 57

2. Cross-sectional echocardiography in acute myocardial infarction: detection and localisation of regional left ventricular asynergy. Herger, J.J., A.E. Weyman, L.S. Wann, J.C. Dillon, H. Feigenbaum
Circulation 60 (1979) 531

3. Two-dimensional echocardiographic quantification of infarct size alteration by pharmacologic agents. Meltzner, R.S., J.N. Woythaler, A.J. Buda, J.C. Griffin, W.D. Harrison, R.P. Martin, D.C. Harrison, R.L. Popp
Amer. J. Cardiol. 44 (1979) 257

4. Two-dimensional echocardiographic identification of surgically correctable complications of acute myocardial infarction. Mintz, G.S., M.F. Victor, M.N. Kotler, W.R.Parry, B.L. Segal
Circulation 64 (1981) 91

5. Early detection of acute myocardial ischemia and infarction by cross-sectional echocardiography. Monaghan, M.J., K. Daly, G. Jackson, D.E. Jewitt. Echocardiology, ed H. Rijsterborgh, Martinus Nijhoff Publishers (1981) 93

6. Estimation of myocardial involvement in patients with acute myocardial infarction by two-dimensional echocardiography. Nixon, J.V., K.A. Narahara, T.C. Smitherman Circulation 62 (1980) 1248

7. Detection and quantification of acute isolated myocardial infarction by two-dimensional echocardiography. Visser, C.A., K.I. Lie, G. Kan, R. Meltzer, D. Durrer Amer. J. Cardiol. 47 (1981) 1020

SENSITIVITY OF ONE- AND TWO-DIMENSIONAL ECHOCARDIOGRAPHY IN
DETECTING INFARCTED SCAR TISSUE

K. V. OLSHAUSEN, H. C. MEHMEL, W. KÜBLER

1. INTRODUCTION

The healing process of an acute myocardial infarction
involves the deposition of collagen and the formation of scar
tissue which alter the acoustic properties and the wall thickness of the affected ventricular wall segment. Although M-mode
echocardiography is limited in scanning the left ventricular
cavitiy, several studies claimed a high degree of success in
detecting infarcted scar tissue (2, 8). 2D-echocardiography
has been shown to be superior to M-mode in analyzing left
ventricular wall motion abnormalities (4, 5). This study was
underteken to compare the sensitivity of one- and two-dimensional echocardiography for scar tissue in patients after
myocardial infarction.

2. PATIENTS AND METHODS

65 consecutive patients with clinically and later angiographically proven remote (more than four weeks) first myocardial infarction were studied by one- and two-dimensional echocardiography. The studies were performed using a PICKER ECHO-
VIEW 80C one-dimensional and 60° mechanical scanning probe.
The two-dimensional echocardiograms were recorded using a
SANYO VTC-7100 video cassette recorder enabling re-examination
in real-time and slow motion.

All accessible windows were utilized. These included in
the one-dimensional technique:
a) The parasternal standard position as well as the lower
   intercostal windows if feasible.
b) The subcostal/subxiphoid window.

c) The lateral scan a few centimeters left of the parasternal
   border.

In the two-dimensional technique the following views were
recorded (fig. 1):

a) Long axis view

b) Two short axis views: At the mitral valve and at the
   papillary muscles.

c) The apical four chamber view.

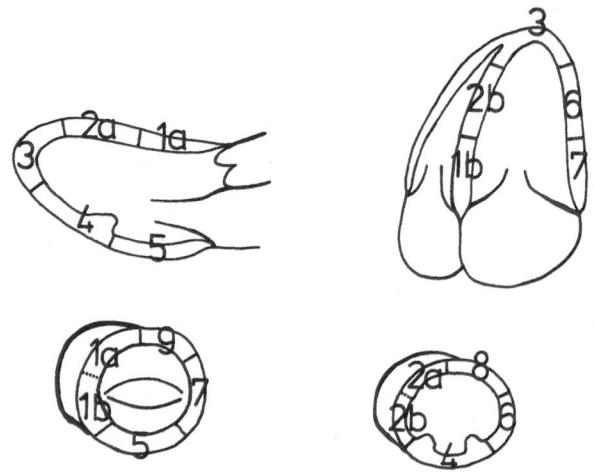

Figure 1: Segmental division of long-axis, short axis and
          apical four chamber cross sectional views.
          1a Anterior basal septal   5 Posterobasal
          1b Medial basal septal   6 Inferior lateral
          2a Anterior apical septal   7 Superior lateral
          2b Medial apical septal   8 Anterolateral
          3 Apical   9 Anterobasal
          4 Diaphragmatic

The apical short axis view was omitted because technically
satisfactory recordings were not reliably obtained. Owing to
inadequate recordings 9 patients (14%) had to be excluded
from the study. If, in the one-dimensional recording, the
lateral or subcostal view was not feasible the patient was
nevertheless kept in the study in order to compare 1D- to
2D-echocardiography.

Thus the study included 56 patients (48 males, 8 females, mean age 55±12 (mean ± SD) years, range 28 to 65 years). 31 patients had an anterior wall infarction (AWI), 25 patients a posterior wall infarction (PWI).

According to (3, 8) the following M-mode criteria for scar tissue were applied:

a) The septal or posterior wall myocardium measured less than 7 mm thick in mid diastole.

b) One area of myocardium was more echo-producing than either its opposing wall or an adjacent area of the same wall. An example of changing density within an anterior myocardial infarction is shown in figure 2.

c) One area of myocardium was 30% thinner than an adjacent area within a sector scan.

d) Reduced systolic thickening of septum or posterior wall of less than 30%.

For the detection of scar tissue at least two criteria had to be present.

The 4 two-dimensional left ventricular views were divided into 9 segments, with the basal and apical septal segment further subdivided into anterior and medial (7). These 11 wall segments were then analyzed for scar tissue without prior knowledge of the ECG findings, peak CK values or M-mode findings. Criteria for scar tissue in 2D-echo were similar to 1D-criteria:

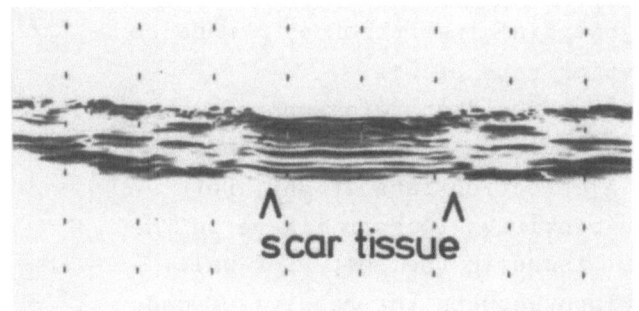

Figure 2: Changing density within a sliced anterior wall infarction in a water bath.

a) A thinner wall than the adjacent tissue.
b) A more echo-producing wall than the adjacent tissue.
c) A reduced or absent ventricular wall motion.
At least two criteria were necessary in order to identify
scar tissue.

CK values were determined every 8 hours after infarction.
The highest CK value of each patient was selected as a rough
estimate of infarct size.

3. RESULTS

The standard parasternal M-mode view was available in all
selected patients whereas the true lateral scan was feasible
in only 38% (21/56 patients) and the subcostal view in 79%
(44/56 patients).

The amount of scar tissue detected by M-mode echo is shown
in table 1:

Table 1: Scar tissue detected by M-mode echocardiography

	AWI (n=31)		PWI (n=25)	
	n	%	n	%
Standard position and lower intercostal views	13	42	8	32
Standard and lateral views	16	52	8	32
Standard and subcostal views	17	55	14	56
Total (all windows)	20	65	14	56

Altogether scar tissue could be seen in 34 patients out of
56 patients with remote myocardial infarction by M-mode echocardiography, i.e. a detection rate of 61%.

The scar tissue detected by 2D-echocardiography is shown
in table 2. In 48 out of 56 patients scar tissue could be
detected by 2D-echo, i.e. a detection rate of 86%. Both
techniques seem to be more sensitive to scar tissue in the
anterior wall than to scar tissue in the posterior wall.

Figure 3 shows a comparison between the results of one-
and two-dimensional echocardiography. The location of all
hypokinetic, akinetic and dyskinetic segments detected by

Table 2: Scar tissue detected by 2D-echocardiography

	AWI (n=31)		PWI (n=25)	
	n	%	n	%
Long axis view	21	68	21	84
Short axis view (mitral valve)	8	26	9	36
Short axis view (papil. muscles)	16	52	19	76
Apical 4 chamber view	10	32	10	40
Total (all views)	27	87	21	84

2D-echo is illustrated in fig. 3. The findings were subdivided according to the location of the infarction and whether M-mode echo was successful in finding scar tissue. For the AWI it can be seen that scar tissue in the anterior basal septal or anterior apical septal segment usually is found by M-mode echo. Lesions in segment 8 (anterolateral) or 9 (anterobasal) without involvement of the septal segments are difficult to detect by M-mode echo. Similar findings apply to PWI: All lesions in segment 5 (posterobasal) are found by 1D-echo, whereas lesions in segment 4 (diaphragmatic) are not always recognized as scar tissue by M-mode echocardiography. The reason for this is that the posterobasal segment as the direct opposite wall of the septum is easier to register from the standard position than the diaphragmatic segment and that the caudally swept echo beam does not hit the diaphragmatic segment perpendicularly.

One would expect that the ability of 1D-echo to detect scar tissue to be influenced by the size of infarction. Therefore the highest CK value as a rough estimate of the infarct size and the number of positive and negative M-mode registrations were compared (table 3). The figures of this table indicate that the detection of scar tissue is influenced by the infarct size.

In 6 patients with peak CK values above 1500 IU scar tissue could not be detected by 1D-echo: 4 patients suffered from AWI. The scar tissue was located in the apical segment. 2 patients suffered from a PWI: in both cases the scar tissue was

94

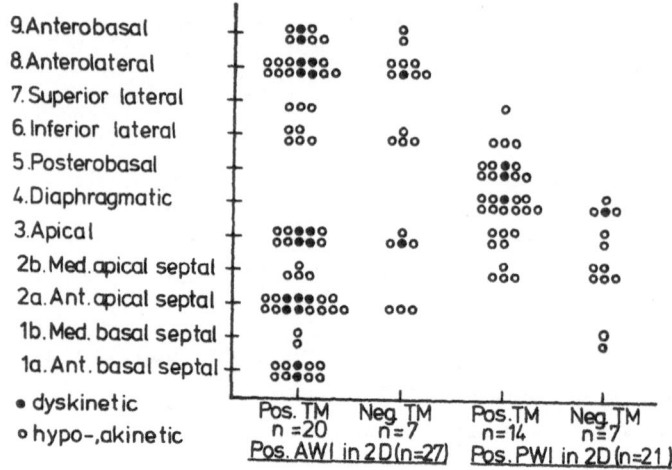

Figure 3: Comparison between the results of one- and two-
dimensional echocardiography. Dyskinetic segments
and aneurysms in 2D ● , hypokinetic and akinetic
segments ○ . Further details in the text.

located in the diaphragmatic segment close to the apical
segment and spreading into the medial apical septal segment.
In these cases the right coronary artery was dominant.

In 8 patients scar tissue could not be detected by 2D-echo
yielding a rate of detection of 86%. 7 of these patients had
a peak CK value below 1000 IU indicating a relatively small
infarct size. According to the results of the cardiac
catheterization 4 missed lesions were located in the apical,
2 in the anterior apical septal, 3 in the diaphragmatic and
1 in the inferior lateral area. Technical difficulties and
rather small infarct size are the main reasons for missing
these infarcted areas. Neither the standard parasternal view,
nor the apical short axis view nor the apical four chamber
view (near field of the transducer) yields a reliable and
comprehensive picture of the apical and adjacent segments
in all cases. These limitations particularly apply to a 60°
mechanical sector probe where the registrations have to be
superimposed in large ventricles to receive a complete

Table 3: Peak CK value and detection of scar tissue (M-mode)

Maximum CK	1500 IU	1500 IU	all
Positive M-mode	13	21	34
Negative M-mode	16	6	22
Total	29	27	56

$$\chi^2 = 6.4 \quad p < 0.05 \quad \text{(two-tailed-test)}$$

registration of the left heart. Our data are consistent with the findings of (6), but they differ slightly from the results reported by (1).

4. CONCLUSIONS

Even with all accessible windows the sensitivity of M-mode echocardiography in detecting scar tissue is only fair (61%). Considering 14% of the examinations were technically inadequate the sensitivity is even lower. Only positive registrations can be regarded as diagnostic. The additional M-mode views (subcostal and lateral) give an additional sensitivity of about 25%, but they are not always feasible. Particularly the lateral scan is difficult to obtain.

Negative M-mode registrations do not exclude a significant scar tissue: In AWI these are usually located at the anterolateral or apical segment, in PWI at the diaphragmatic or medial apical septal segment. The sensitivity for scar tissue is higher in AWI than in PWI, and it is correlated to the peak CK value at the time of infarction.

The sensitivity of 2D-echocardiography in detecting scar tissue is high (86%) and better than in 1D-echo. Difficulties can still occur in imaging scars in the apical and the adjacent regions in the case of small infarctions.

5.   REFERENCES

1. Bubenheimer P, Moser H, Roskamm H.: Sensitivity of echocardiography in localizing infarcted scars: A comparative
   evaluation of two-dimensional and time motion echocardiography. Eur. Heart J. 2(Suppl. A), 110, 1981

2. Corya BC, Rasmussen S, Feigenbaum H, Black MJ, Knoebel SB:
   Echocardiographic detection of scar tissue in patients
   with coronary artery disease. (abstr.) Am. J. Cardiol.
   37: 129, 1976

3. Corya BC, Rasmussen S, Feigenbaum H, Knoebel SB, Black
   MJ: Systolic thickening and thinning of the septum and
   posterior wall in patients with coronary artery disease,
   congestive cardiomyopathy, and atrial septal defect.
   Circulation 55: 109, 1977

4. Heng MK, Lang TW, Toshimitsu T, Meerbaum S, Wyatt HL,
   Lee SS, Davidson R, Corday E: Quantification of myocar-
   dial ischemic damage by 2-dimensional echocardiography.
   Circulation (Suppl. III) 56: 125, 1977

5. Kisslo JA, Robertson D, Gilbert BW, von Ramm O, Behar VS:
   A comparison of real-time, two-dimensional echocardiography
   and cineangiography in detecting left ventricular asynergy.
   Circulation 55: 134, 1977

6. Kronik G, Mösslacher H, Schmoliner R: Differentialdiagnose
   zwischen diffusen Myokarderkrankungen und koronarer Herz-
   erkrankung mit Hilfe der zweidimensionalen Echokardiographie. Herz/Kreislauf 13, 113, 1981

7. Monaghan MJ, Daly K, Jackson G, Jewitt DE: Early detection
   of acute myocardial ischemia and infarction by cross-
   sectional echocardiography. In: Echocardiology ed:
   Rijsterborgh H. pg. 93, Martinus Nijhoff Publishers,
   The Hague/Boston/London

8. Rasmussen S, Corya BC, Feigenbaum H, Knoebel SB:
   Detection of myocardial scar tissue by M-mode echocardiography. Circulation 57: 230, 1978

Two dimensional Echo Imaging and Pulsed Doppler Blood Flow Detection: A comprehensive approach to cardiovascular diagnosis

Donald W. Baker

Center for Bio Engineering
University of Washington, Seattle, WA USA

The integration of two Dimensional imaging with Pulsed Doppler is much more than a simple convienence. Certainly it provides a possible mechanism for the determination of volumetric blood flow rates or the calibration of velocity. Researchers in increasing numbers are showing how to use the 2D image to determine local anatomy and Doppler transducer beam orientation with respect to the blood flow vector. Quantitation of both image and flow parameters is important as well as intrinsic to improved cardiovascular diagnosis. The real significance of combining image and blood flow data may lay within the potential of multiformat programable instrumentation and a holistic system approach to diagnosis.[1] These promise to make possible significant advances in diagnostic sensitivity and accuracy in the future.

The current alternative to this systems approach is the assembly of a number of highly specialized dedicated instruments where the output from each one contribute only small portions of the overall diagnostic data base. Usually these dedicated instruments will come from different sources and have no practical or planned interrelationship thus detracting from the overall efficiency of the diagnostic procedure. Occassions probably arise when the highly dedicated instruments will be cost effective, however, the modern cardiovascular diagnostic center may not be one of these.

The design and evolution of a clinically effective instrument is influenced by many considerations including medical, technical, educational, economic, and human factors. Since all viable clinical instruments must ultimately pass through a commercialization process another set of factors influence the eventual characteristics a device may have. World market considerations such as disease prevalence and distribution, educational backgound and experience, local economic conditions, distribution and support capabilities all weigh on a final design. Manufacturing and selling costs become significant considerations as well as the danger of rapid obsolences from both the manufacturing as well as clinical point of view. The idea of combining imaging with blood flow capabilitaies in a single "Duplex" instrument is influenced by all these factors, some much more than others.[2,3] The most important is medical.

One approach to evaluating the effectiveness of using ultrasound as a diagnostic modalities is to ask the question, "What is it we are attempting to do with ultrasound techniques in diagnosis?" A possible answer that serves best to support combined Echo-Doppler thinking is, "We are attempting to characterize the current physical "STATE" of the disease process in all its manifestations." This characterization is based on the study of how ultrasonic energy interacts with stationary and moving structures.

BIOLOGICAL STATE CONCEPTS

Before one can discuss ultrasonic interactions we must define the concept of normal or disease "STATE" as it might be used in medical diagnosis.

By "STATE" we mean the set or list of physical parameters and derived functions which can be used to characterize or describe the current physical status of the biological process. The medical categories that form the basis for the "STATE" set of parameters include:

- Anatomy
- Blood Flow
- Blood Pressure
- Tissue properties.

The physical dimensions or parameters with which the specific characteristics of each of the medical categories can be defined in terms of include:

Anatomy   size - shape - length - area - volume - velocity
Flow   velocity - acceleration - volume rate - time and space-profiles
          - gradients - temperal and spatial flow disturbance patterns
Pressure magnitude - gradients
Tissue   density - image texture - scattering - reflection.

The fundamental ultrasound measurement upon which all dimensional or distance information is derived is the echo roundtrip transit time along the sound beam. If the sound beam axis is scanned either in a linear or sector fashion within a plane one has the basis for area calculations. If the image scan plane is swept in a direction normal to itself one has the basis for three dimensional volume determinations. From volume measurements can come derivations of mass if density can be determined.

Pulsed Doppler instruments provide basic information about structure or blood velocity along the sound beam axis by detecting the Doppler shift of the echos. In special cases continuous wave Dopplers can be used to overcome the nyquist sampling limitation of phase coherent Pulsed dopplers. From velocity information one can derive acceleration and displacement parameters. The true vector velocity of the flow requires knowledge of the angle between the sound beam axis and flow vector. This can be determined within a plane using two dimensional imaging. Determination of the true velocity vector orientation requires three nonplaner Doppler transducers and vector triangulation schemes. When a pulsed Doppler is used with Echo ranging and two dimensional imaging, maps or profiles of velocity or acceleration in two and three dimensional space can be made. Multigate pulsed Dopplers used with M-mode Echo and two-dimensional imaging devices allow rapid assesment of spatial velocity distributions from cardiac and peripheral structures. Real time two dimensional blood flow imaging is an interesting concept with significant clinical application, however only rudimentary feasiblity has been demonstrated to date.

DISEASE STATE

Disease in "STATE" thinking is defined as an expanding sequence of "STATE" changes which lead to the failure of one or more critical functions. For example in a given normal subject the mitral valve has a set of physical parameters i.e., size, location, tithering, leaflet thickness, compliance, and velocities which can describe its normal state or character.

With the onset of certain disease process these parameters begin to change, in many cases in a detectable and measurable way. Leaflet thickness and compliance plus tithering changes, leading to orfice area reduction, are examples of change with rheumatic stenotic valvular disease. So it is said that these physical parameter changes constitute a "STATE" change. In every case of disease such parameter changes are characteristic and intrinsic to the process.

DIAGNOSIS

Diagnosis in "STATE" thinking becomes the process of identifying changes in the value or character and relationship of the state parameters. The earlier and more specific this can be done in the process the more sensitive and accurate the diagnosis might be. Because of the rather stochastic variability of the biological parameters there is never a clear deliniation between the so called normal "STATE" set and the disease altered set. This fact will probably limit the ultimate sensitivity of any given method. This variability is a kind of Biological noise limit beyond which simple approaches cannot venture.

The sequence of diagnosis and treatment in "STATE" thinking can be described in general form from the following steps.

- Generation of the "STATE" pattern
- Comparison and differentiation of the present "STATE" set from the previous or so called "normal" state set of physical parameters and dimensions
- Evaluation of "STATE" changes as a guide in the management of interventions which are planned to shift physical parameters back to the individuals normal "STATE" values.

The characteristics of the optimal instrument configuration can be derived from the "STATE" diagnosis approach. Several examples of disease "STATE" progression can be used to point out the instrument requirements. These examples will attempt to show that the clinicians impression of the current disease "STATE" will depend on when in the time course the diagnosis is attempted and upon what instruments are actually used.

CORONARY ARTERY DISEASE

A simplified description of the progression of myocardial disease might proceed in the following sequence, from Figure 1.

- Impaired myocardial blood flow
- changes in myocardial tissue properties
- regional or global contractile and mechanical property changes
- electrical excitation altered
- regional wall thickness and motion change
- ventricular chamber size and shape changes
- alteration of ventricular flow patterns
- reduction in ejection rate and cardiac output

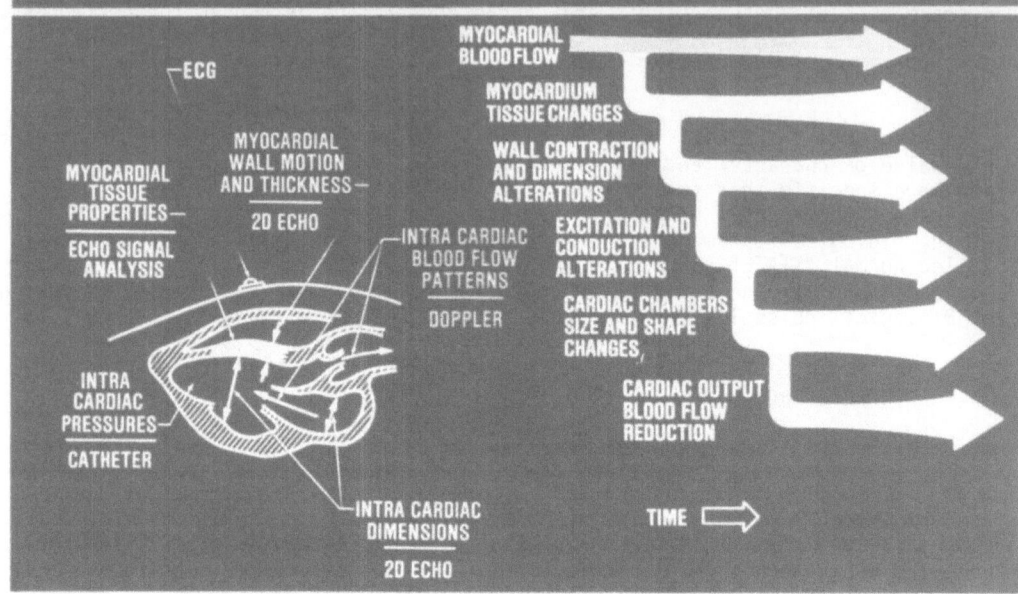

Figure 1.   Myocardial disease stemming from a reduction of coronary arterial
             blood flow leads to a progression of physical "STATE" parameter
             changes. Early and specific detection of the "disease state"
             depends on what instruments are used and when the investigation
             is done. Wall motion abnormalities are the earliest easily
             detected signs using imaging devices.

These can be summarized into three primary groups as follows:

- blood flow changes
- tissue changes
- anatomical or structural changes.

Our ability to make the diagnosis will depend on the type and capability of
the instrument used at each stage of the disease progress. For example an
ultrasonic flow meter able to detect and evaluate coronary and myocardial blood
flows might provide the earliest and most sensitive diagnosis. If tissue
changes follow myocardial blood flow impairment then some type of ultrasonic
tissue analysis would be the most sensitive at this stage. Myocardial contraction patterns, wall thickness and timing probably follow tissue changes from
blood flow reductions. For most clinicians this stage is the first opportunity
they will have to detect the presence of coronary artery disease using either M-
mode or 2D imaging displays. If the disease advances farther, before diagnosis
is attempted or made, even more gross changes might be detected in ventricular
size and shape using 2D imaging. Ultimately at some point blood flow changes
will occur to reduce ventricular flow ejection, acceleration and finally cardiac
output.

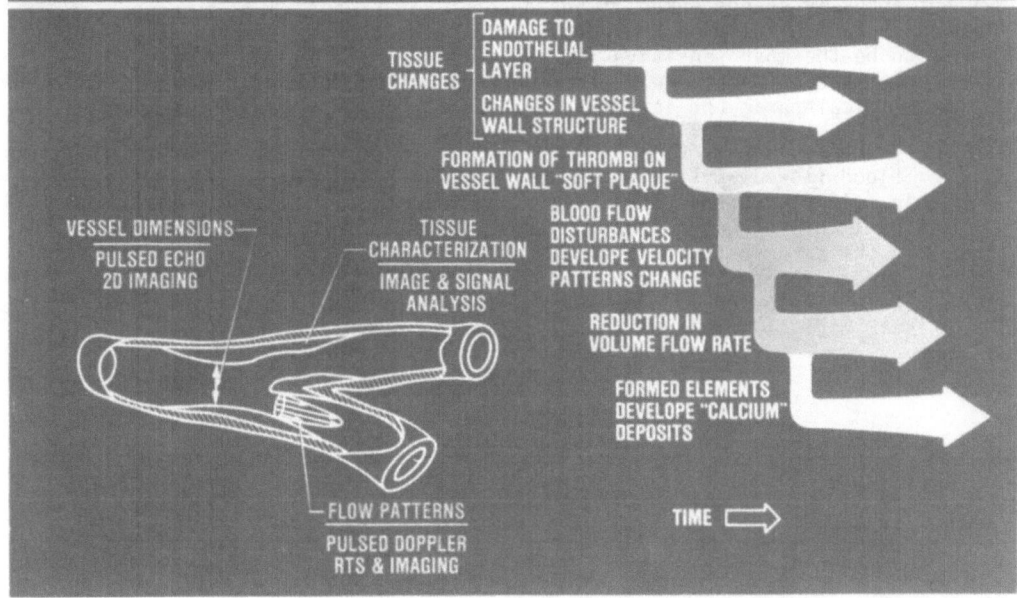

Figure 2.   Carotid arterial disease has its own special set of "disease
STATE" parameters which evolve with time. Blood flow disturbances are the earliest and most easily detected indications
of an altered vessel lumen.

The progression of coronary artery disease is diagrammed in schematic form
in Figure 1. The arrows represent the time sequence for each broad category of
disease "STATE" change i.e., blood flows, tissue alterations, and anatomical
changes. The width of the arrow represents the relative ease with which a particular change can be evaluated. For example we are currently unable to detect
coronary flow or tissue changes with current instruments. Anatomical size and
shape along with motion changes are readily detected with 2D imaging and M-mode
instruments. Gross blood flow changes occur later in the disease progression
and can in many cases be evaluated with Pulsed Doppler and 2D imaging or with
continuous wave devices applied on the ascending aorta.

CAROTID ARTERIAL DISEASE

The development and progression of arterial occlusive disease follows a
quite different sequence than coronary artery disease and leads to a different
combination of critical "state" parameters. The role of blood flow evaluation
takes on a new significance compared to anatomical imaging. Blood vessel wall
tissue parameters change but are difficult to assess. Figure 2 shows the
"Disease STATE" progression in general terms. Peripheral vascular disease
appears to begin with a change in the vessel wall and intima which are primarily
of tissue, origin. These may be the earlist physical manifestiations of
arterial occlusive disease that could be detected with ultrasound, however, no
practical clinical techniques or instruments exist to function at this level.

The changes in vessel wall lead to a sequence of various plaque developments ranging from fatty streaks to acoustically transparent soft plaques and finally calcified formed element plaques. Most of these lead to an alterations in vessel crossectional geometry and possible total occlusion. Ulcerated plaques may not actually change lumen dimensions but can produce flow distrubances. Research and clinical experience have demonstrated that blood flow distrubances appear to be the most sensitive indication of disease in the carotid bifurction. The broader arrows in Figure 2 denote the primary role of blood flow as a significant clinical parameter in this disease process.

For carotid, artery disease the combination of 2D tissue imaging and pulsed Doppler blood flow analysis is the most sensitive and accurate diagnostic tool available. If tissue characterization could be developed along with higher resolution imaging the threshold of sensitivity could be pushed even lower. Generally the same instrument concepts that were used for detection of coronary artery disease can be used here, except for higher ultrasound frequencies for higher image resolution and the emphasis on the pulsed Doppler and Spectral analysis to optimize and take advantage of the very sensitive flow indicator of disease.

AORTIC INSUFFICIENCY

This cardiac valvular problem leads to still another "disease state" progression situation which has its own most sensitive indicators and optimal instrument requirements. Figure 3 depicts the progress of this problem beginning with valve tissue or tithering alterations. Aortic valve dimensions and motion might change at an early stage, but may not be visualized by 2D real time imaging. In this case a regurgitant jet of blood flow may be present in the left ventricular outflow track. This jet may or may not cause flutter in the anterior mitral valve leaflet, the only other indicator of this defect. As the disease "STATE" progresses large back flows may be detected in the ascending aorta. Eventually with increasing regurgitation ventricular chamber dimensions may enlarge to the point of being detectable by M-mode and 2D real time imaging. If the only instrument available is an M-mode or 2D device, then there is a real and significant chance to miss the early stages of this valvular problem.

COMPREHENSIVE APPROACH TO CARDIOVASCULAR DIAGNOSIS

It should be possible in general to evaluate and describe most all cardiovascular disease processes interms of "Disease STATE" parameters within the three broad groups of:

- Anatomy - structure

- Blood flow defects

- Tissue characteristics

These can be further defined into a set of physical parameters derived by using 2D imaging with pulsed Doppler flow detection and with tissue signature analysis. In a given situation the instrument format, echo or Doppler, and the operating frequencies will, along with appropriate signal analyse and displays, provide the most sensitive and accurate clinical diagnosis.

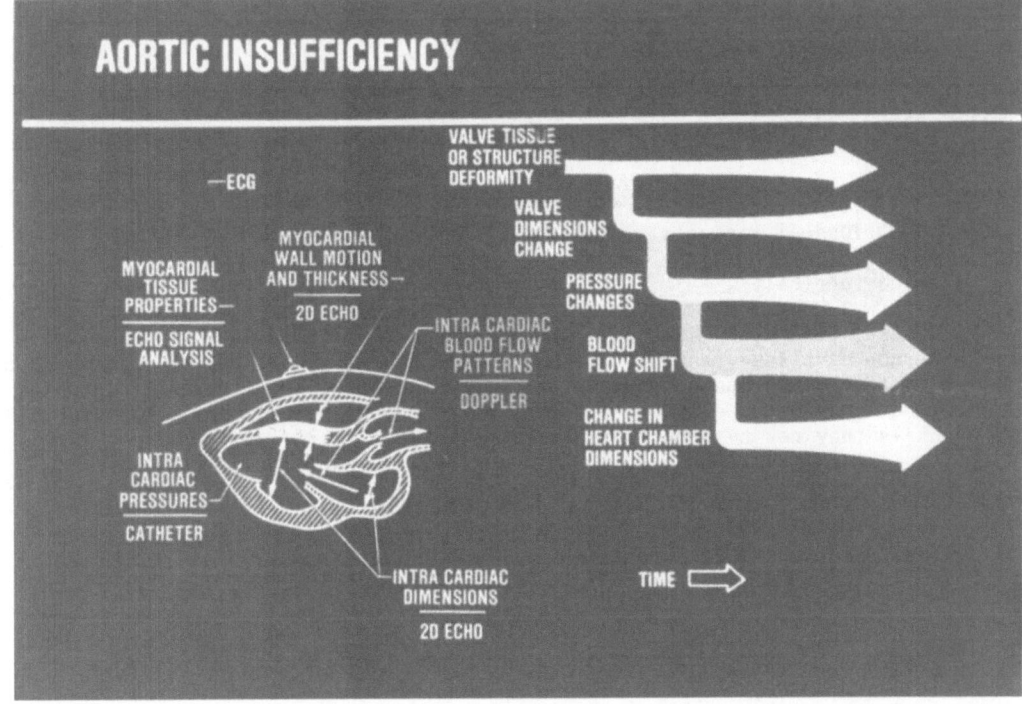

Figure 3.   Aortic insufficiency is most readily detected at an early stage using pulsed Doppler with real time imaging. Anatomical changes occur later in this disease process.

The optimization of the instrument configuration to match the disease profile at a given time and situation is required to provide the optimal diagnosis based on the ultrasonic findings. This leads to the requirement that instruments be highly adaptable to the clinical and physical circumstances. Human factors come to play in terms of instrument control and displays to insure maximum information flow from the patient subject to the user interpreter.

SUMMARY

The same underlying diagnostic and instrument concepts apply to most all cardiovascular diagnostic situations. The principal factors that affect instrument characteristics and operating frequency are relative size and depth of the organ or structure of interest.

The sensitivity, specificity and/or accuracy of a diagnostic procedure depends on optimizing the instrument performance in terms of those "Disease STATE" parameters which can be most readily differentiated from the "Normal STATE" parameters.

The most effective instruments will be those which can be adapted to deal

104

optimaly with the primary "STATE" set of;

o   Anatomical Dimensions
o   Blood Flows
o   Tissue characteristics

wheather it is;

o   Adult or Pediatric Cardiac
o   Peripheral Vascular
o   Abdominal
o   Obstetrical.

   "Disease STATE" progression in any of these clinical catagories usually moves through a tissue, anatomy and blood flow phase. The temperal sequence and degree of "STATE" change depends on the particular disease. The ability to detect and analyze these changes depends on the instrument capabilities and on how easily they can be brought to bear on the problem.

REFERENCES

1.   Baker, D.W., A comprehensive approach to cardiac measurements. Developments in Cardiovascular Medicine, Vol. 1, Echocardiology, pp. 15-27, Martinus Nijhoff, the Hague 1979

2.   Baker, D.W., Applications of Pulsed Doppler Techniques. Radiologic clinics of North America, pp. 79-103, Vol. 18, No. 1, April 1980

3.   Phillips, D.J. et.al., Detection of Peripheral Vascular Disease using the Duplex Scanner III.   Ultrasound in Medicine and Biology, pp. 205-218, Vol. 6, No. 3-A, 1980

USEFULNESS OF DOPPLER ECHOCARDIOGRAPHY IN THE DIAGNOSIS OF VALVULAR
HEART DISEASE

KENT RICHARDS AND SCOTT CANNON. UNIVERSITY OF TEXAS HEALTH SCIENCE
CENTER AT SAN ANTONIO, SAN ANTONIO, TEXAS 78284

BASIC CONCEPTS

The concepts necessary to intelligently apply Doppler echocardiography
to clinical cardiology are simple but must be thoroughly understood.

Doppler Equation

A cylinder of ultrasound is broadcast from a transducer through the
chest wall into the heart. As the sound encounters structures of
differing acoustic density, a small portion is reflected back into the
transducer. According to the Doppler Principle (Figure 1), the change
in frequency of reflected sound is directly proportional to the velocity
of the blood volume sampled (V), the frequency of the transmitted ultrasound (carrier frequency, F_c), and the cosine of the angle between the
transmitted sound and the velocity field encountered (COS θ); this
product must be multiplied by two and divided by the speed of ultrasound
in tissue ($C_T = 1.5 \times 10^{-5}$ cm/sec):

$$F_D = (F_C)(2/C_T)(COS\ \theta)(V)$$

Rearranging the equation:

$$V = \frac{(F_D)(C_T)}{2(F_C)(COS\ \theta)} = K\ \frac{(F_D)}{(COS\ \theta)}$$

$$K\ (a\ constant) = \frac{(C_T)}{2(F_C)}$$

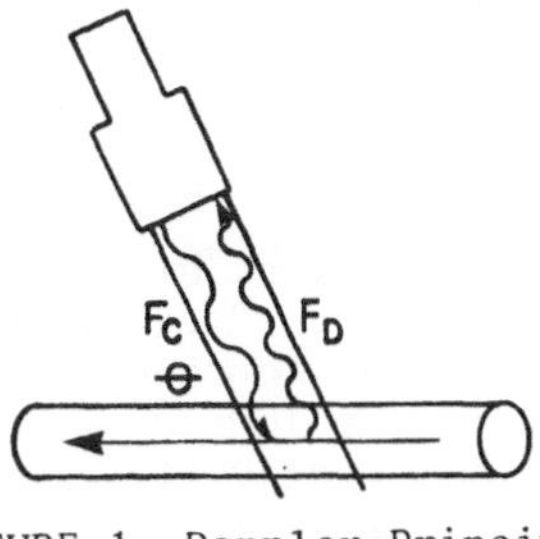

FIGURE 1. Doppler Principle

Thus, both the Doppler frequency shift and the cosine θ must be known
if velocity is to be calculated.

Signal Information Content

The reflected Doppler ultrasound signals contain three types of
information necessary to characterize intracardiac blood velocity:
time (T), Doppler frequency (F_D), and signal amplitude (decibels, dB).
Simply speaking, the amplitude of a Doppler signal at a given time and
frequency, is proportional to the number of blood cells moving at that
velocity and time. A three-dimensional display must be utilized to
graph this information. Two formats are currently used (Figure 2). In
the gray-scale display, time is in the X-axis, frequency in the Y-axis
and amplitude in the Z or gray-scale axis (weak signals are light;

106

strong signals are dark). In the hidden-line plot, line graphs are
generated for every 10 msec of data: time is in the X-axis, frequency
in the Y-axis, and amplitude as deviation of each line above its zero
level. Both displays allow resolution of velocity direction relative
to the transducer. The gray-scale display provides best temporal
resolution. The hidden-line display allows best resolution of frequency
and amplitude. Both formats are clinically useful.

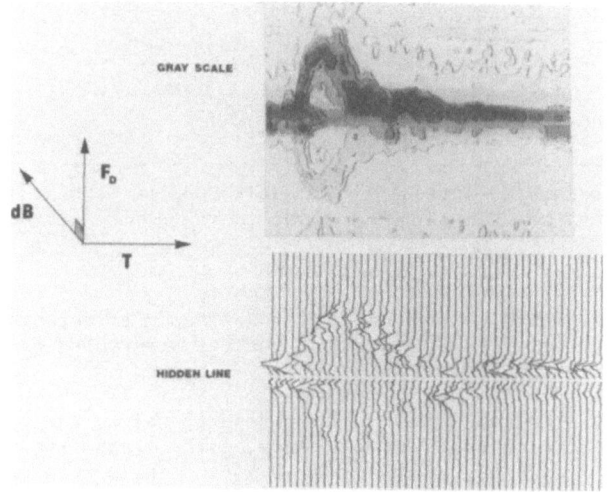

FIGURE 2. Doppler spectral signals from ascending
aorta graphed using gray scale or hidden line format

Velocity Patterns Induced by Stenosis

Flow in a normal straight blood vessel (Figure 3) is laminar and the
velocity profile across the vessel is blunt. This implies that velocity
near the wall is similar to velocity in midstream. Doppler signals
obtained by sampling a volume containing blood from the near wall to
midstream, would have frequencies near the same value; they would be
described as narrow-band. As blood enters an area of stenosis, velocity
increases; the Doppler frequency obtained by sampling within the stenosis
is elevated. A jet formed within the stenosis, extends beyond the
narrowing and causes a parajet flow disturbance. A blood volume sampled
beyond or along side such a jet, would contain multidirectional components at different velocities. Doppler signals would contain many
different frequencies at a given time and would be described as broad-
band. Both characteristics of blood flow distal to a stenosis - increased
velocity and flow disturbance - are useful in identifying and quantifying
valvular heart disease.

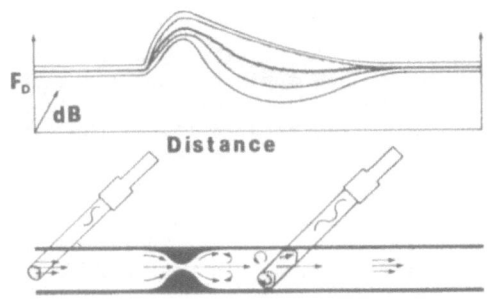

FIGURE 3. Blood velocity vectors (arrows) & Doppler signals corresponding
to anatomical sites proximal to, within, & distal to a stenosis in a
straight tube are illustrated.

Range-Gating

The velocity patterns within an entire heart are very complex; the
regions which must be sampled to identify and quantitate disease are
small and localized. The ultrasound beam transmitted into the heart is
a cylinder; ultrasound is reflected from all tissues within that cylinder
and thus the returned signal contains information from all sites pene-
trated (Figure 4). Range-gating, which allows the operator to select a
sample volume along that cylinder, is accomplished by pulsing the
transmitted signal. A brief burst of ultrasound is transmitted and the
transmitter is turned off. The receiver operates only at a time that
will allow reception of reflected sound from the chosen depth. The
combination of transducer orientation and range-gating allows selective
sampling of specific locations within the heart. M-mode and 2D records
of sample volume position relative to cardiac anatomy allow documentation
of the site sampled.

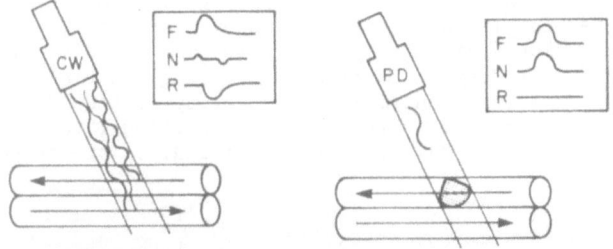

FIGURE 4. Doppler signals of forward (F), net (N), & reverse (R) channels
are shown from two oppositely directed velocity fields. With continuous
wave (CW) Doppler, range-gating is absent; summation of forward & reverse
signals produces a net signal near zero. With pulsed-Doppler (PD), range-
gating allows correct registration of the selected field.

Calculation of Parameters from Doppler Signals

Parameters indicative of cardiac function may be calculated from
either velocity data or from raw Doppler frequency data.

Velocity Data

Blood velocity determination requires measurement of two variables: Doppler frequency shift, and angle between the incident sound beam and the velocity field. Volume flow (Q) can be calculated if mean velocity ($\overline{V}$) and vessel cross-sectional area (A) at the site of Doppler sample volume, are known:

$$Q = A\overline{V}$$

If flow is bidirectional, forward flow (Q_F) and reverse flow (Q_R) may be estimated by measuring mean velocity ($\overline{V}_F$ & $\overline{V}_R$), duration of flow (T_F & T_R) and vessel cross-sectional area (A_F & A_R) in each direction:

$$QF = (\overline{V}_F)(T_F)(A_F)$$

$$QR = (\overline{V}_R)(T_R)(A_R)$$

The fraction of flow reversing, or regurgitant fraction (RF), is the ratio of Q_R/Q_F. If cross-sectional areas are the same during forward and reverse flow, the equation simplifies to:

$$RF = (\overline{V}_R)(T_R)/(\overline{V}_F)(T_F)$$

The pressure gradient (ΔP) across a stenosis can be calculated if all the energy components (E) responsible for the gradient, can be measured:

$$\Delta P = E_{convective} + E_{inertial} + E_{viscous}$$

In cardiac valve stenosis, convective forces are most important; the simplified Bernoulli Equation has been used to calculate pressure gradient:

$$\Delta P = K(V)^2$$

Flow Disturbance Data

In addition to increased velocity, vascular stenosis induces flow disturbance or frank turbulence in flow distal to the stenosis. This is manifest in the Doppler signal as spectral broadening. Figure 5 contrasts narrow-band versus broad-band Doppler signals from the ascending aorta. The signals can be contrasted by comparing the area of the frequency-time envelopes at a given energy level. Likewise, the variance of amplitude with respect to frequency at a given time allows differentiation of normal from abnormal. If severity of flow disturbance or volume distribution of flow disturbance are proportional to severity of stenosis, their measurement may provide useful indices of the severity of stenosis.

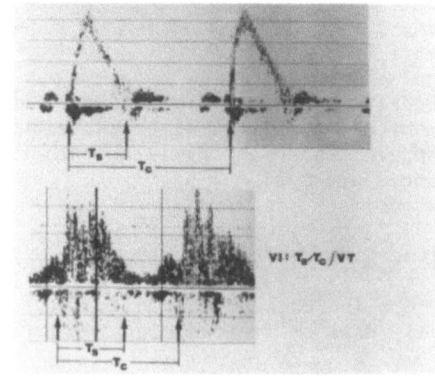

FIGURE 5. Doppler gray-scale spectral records of a normal (top) and aortic stenosis (bottom) patient illustrate prolongation of systolic flow disturbance time/cycle length time (Ts/Tc) and enlargement of systolic time-frequency envelope area (cross-hatched) characteristic of flow disturbance produced distal to a stenotic aortic valve.

APPLICATION TO SPECIFIC LESIONS

Aortic Stenosis

Detection of aortic stenosis (AS) and determination of its severity in adults can be accomplished using two separate Doppler echocardiographic techniques.

Pulsed Doppler Echocardiography (PDE) has been used to assess parameters which reflect flow disturbance induced in the ascending aorta distal to or surrounding the jet. The transducer is positioned at the suprasternal notch and the ultrasound beam adjusted to visualize the aortic arch in its long axis (Figure 6). The sample volume is positioned in the center of the ascending aorta 2 cm above the aortic valve. Normal individuals have narrow-band Doppler signals; those with aortic stenosis have broad-band signals. The duration of flow disturbance induced by systole is prolonged in AS. The combination of spectral broadening and prolongation of the duration of the flow disturbance makes the velocity-time envelope area a useful indicator of the presence of AS.

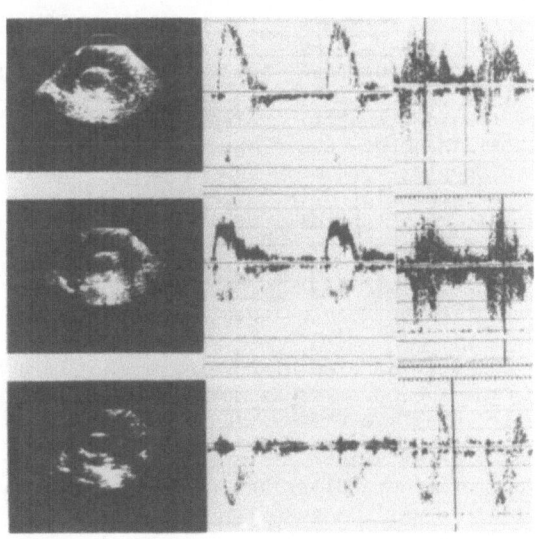

FIGURE 6. Doppler sample volume position in ascending (top), transverse (middle) and descending (bottom) aorta illustrate characteristic gray-scale spectral records in normal (middle column) and AS patients (right column). Spectral broadening present in ascending aorta because of AS reverts to narrow-band flow in the descending aorta.

In a series of 31 patients examined with a 3 MHz duplex pulsed Doppler with real-time, gray-scale spectrum analysis, all 17 patients with AS and 14 with no AS were correctly identified using the velocity-time envelope area alone (1). In a separate series of 24 patients with AS and mild or absent aortic regurgitation, Doppler examination was performed in the same manner (1a). Doppler signals were analyzed using a minicomputer which calculated sequential Fourier transforms, generated a 3-dimensional hidden-line display and extracted the following parameters which were regressed against $\overline{AP}$ determined at cardiac catheterization (abbreviations: SD = Standard Deviation, Freq = frequency):

PARAMETER	R =
Systolic Time-Freq Envelope Area (A)	.80
Spectral Width (Peak-Mean) at Peak Freq (Fp→m)	.79
SD of Average Systolic Freq (SD Av Freq)	.75
SD along Peak Freq Line (SD Pk Freq)	.74
SD at Mid-quarter of Systole (SD Mid ¼ Freq)	.82

Multivariant linear regression equations were calculated for the data and correlated with ΔP:

$\Delta P =$	R =
$23.8 + .029(A) + .0071(Fp{\to}m)$	.85
$17.6 + .020(A) + .021(SD\ Av\ Freq) + .0063(Fp{\to}m)$	.86
$20.2 + .022(A) + .0075(SD\ Pk\ Freq) + .0067(Fp{\to}m)$	.85
$21.1 + .022(A) + .012(SD\ Mid\ ¼\ Freq) + .0063(Fp{\to}m)$	.85

The data demonstrate that parameters which reflect flow disturbance can be generated from PDE signals obtained distal to stenotic aortic valves and that these parameters correlate with the pressure gradient present across these valves.

Continuous Wave Doppler Echocardiography (CWDE) has been used to measure peak temporal, peak spatial velocity (V_{max}) in the ascending aorta. The transducer was placed at either the suprasternal notch, or the first or second right intercostal space and the ultrasound beam directed toward the aortic valve. The transducer was manipulated until the highest frequency audio output was obtained. Using a 2 MHz continuous wave Doppler with mean and maximal frequency shift estimators, peak velocity was calculated in 14 patients with catheterization-proven valvular AS. Peak systolic pressure gradient across the aortic valve was calculated using the formula:

$$\Delta P = 4\ (V_{max})^2$$

The correlation between calculated and recorded pressure gradient was 0.85 (2,3).

Both analysis of flow disturbance parameters by PDE and measurement of V_{max} by CWDE show promise as methods of estimating severity of AS noninvasively in native valves.

Aortic Regurgitation

Doppler echocardiography is useful in detecting aortic regurgitation (AR) as well as quantifying its severity.

Detection of AR in native or prosthetic valves can be achieved with greatest sensitivity and specificity by utilizing duplex pulsed Doppler echocardiography (PDE). The transducer is placed at the cardiac apex and a 2- or 4- chamber view which includes the high left ventricular outflow tract (LVOT) is obtained. The sample volume is positioned to record systolic flow out the LVOT and high enough to avoid inflow from the mitral valve; the region below the aortic valve is carefully scanned to detect localized diastolic regurgitant jets (4,5,6). Care must be taken to avoid diastolic artifacts which might mask or mimic the pandiastolic, broad-band spectral pattern of AR. Figure 7 contrasts gray-scale spectral tracings in a normal (left upper), and a patient with AR (right upper). Artifacts characteristic of valve leaflets or wall motion (left lower) and mitral valve flow (right lower) are illustrated.

In a series of 49 patients studied with PDE, Ward (7) correctly identified 86% of 49 patients with catheterization-proven AR; 7% false positive results were noted. In a series of 35 patients with 49 catheterization-proven lesions, we (1a) used 3 MHz duplex pulsed Doppler with gray-scale spectral display to detect left-sided valvular heart disease. Satisfactory examination of LVOT was accomplished in 29 patients. The area within the lowest energy diastolic velocity-time envelope was measured in each patient in KHz X seconds. In the 13 patients who had no AR, the diastolic envelope ranged from .13-.49 ($\overline{.31}$) KHz X Sec; the value for 16 patients with trace to 3+ AR was .12-2.58 ($\overline{1.43}$) KHz X Sec. One of the 16 patients who had angiographic evidence of AR had a spectral area which overlapped with the normals; this false negative patient had only minimal AR at catheterization. No false positive results were noted. There was easy exclusion of AR in 6 patients who had isolated mitral stenosis despite the presence of atrial fibrillation in three. These data support the clinical usefulness of PDE characterization of LVOT blood velocity in the diagnosis of AR.

FIGURE 7. Gray-scale Doppler spectral records from LVOT demonstrate normal pattern (top left), AR pattern (top right), pattern due to valve leaflet or wall artifacts (bottom left), and pattern due to mitral valve inflow due to mitral stenosis (bottom right).

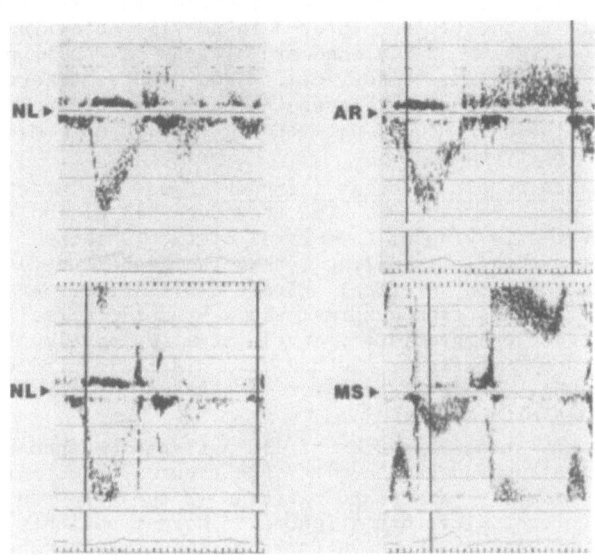

Quantification of AR is best accomplished by determining regurgitant fraction (RF). This can best be accomplished in the descending rather than ascending aorta because of more uniform velocity profiles in the former. Boughner (8) used a 2.2 MHz continuous-wave Doppler to non-invasively estimate regurgitant fraction in 15 patients with catheterization-proven AR. Doppler signals were obtained from the junction of the transverse and descending portion of the aorta. Peak velocity envelopes were plotted for each patient. The regurgitant fraction was calculated from the ratio of diastolic velocity-time area (A_d) divided by systolic velocity-time area (A_s):

$$RF_D = \frac{A_d}{A_s}$$

There was good correlation (r=.91) between catheterization and Doppler (RF_D) regurgitant fractions.

   An alternative approach to quantification of severity of AR
utilizes mapping of the area of diastolic flow disturbance within the
left ventricle. Theoretically, the volume of left ventricular blood in
which flow is disturbed by the regurgitant jet, is determined by the
severity of AR. Using two-dimensional echocardiography to verify sample
volume position, Bommer et al (8a) outlined the borders of the diastolic
flow disturbance in the left ventricle. A correlation between the
extent of the flow disturbance and the severity of AR was noted. Such
measurements remain time consuming and require considerable experience;
perhaps the advent of multigate two-dimensional flow-imaging will
improve sensitivity and speed to this approach of quantitating severity
of AR.

Mitral Stenosis

   The diagnosis of mitral stenosis (MS) can be easily made in most
patients with M-mode or 2-dimensional echocardiography. Though accurate
methods exist by which mitral valve area can be determined by 2-
dimensional echo, difficulty in estimating the effective hemodynamic
orifice is frequently encountered in heavily calcified or severely
deformed valves. Doppler echocardiography may be of particular usefulness in these cases. Likewise, it should be remembered that Doppler
parameters correlate most accurately with transvalvular pressure gradient
and thus provide a second parameter useful in determining need for
surgical intervention.

   Pulsed Doppler echocardiography is useful in detecting the
presence or absence of MS. The transducer is placed at the cardiac apex
and a short-axis view of the mitral orifice obtained. The sample volume
is adjusted to allow sampling within the highest-velocity portion of the
jet produced by the orifice. Figure 8 illustrates gray-scale Doppler
spectral tracings from a normal and a stenotic mitral valve. The area
of the lowest energy diastolic velocity-time envelope was measured in 17
normal and 6 MS patients who had mean diastolic gradients ($\overline{\Delta P}$) =
8-22 $\overline{14}$ mmHg. There was complete separation of normals from
individuals with MS (1a).

   In an extensive series of 156 patients who had both cardiac
catheterization and good quality PDE records of mitral orifice velocity,
Thuillez et al (9) described patterns in the zero-crosser signals which
allowed correct differentiation of 44 normal patients from 112 with MS.
Further analysis of the wave forms allowed correct determination of mild,
moderate and severe pressure gradient in all but 4 of 112 patients. The
Doppler analysis was not hampered by the presence of mitral regurgitation
in 39 and aortic valve disease in 32 patients.

   Continuous-wave Doppler has been shown useful in accurately
estimating pressure gradient across stenotic mitral valves. In a series
of 10 patients in whom simultaneous catheterization and Doppler exams
were performed, there was excellent correlation between actual transvalvular pressure gradient and that calculated using Doppler-determined
maximum velocity and the Bernoulli Equation (10). Consideration of
calculated $\overline{\Delta P}$ and atrioventricular pressure half-time (both derived from
Doppler) allowed more accurate assessment of severity of MS (11).

FIGURE 8.   Gray-scale
Doppler records from mitral
valve orifice in normal and
MS patients illustrate
increased frequency in mid-
diastole characteristic of
MS.   Increase in spectral
time-frequency envelope area
is seen in MS.

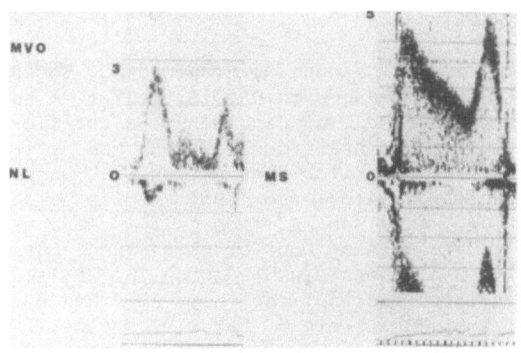

Mitral Regurgitation

Detection of mitral regurgitation (MR) and determination of its
severity is accomplished primarily with use of range-gated PDE.

Detection of MR is accomplished by placing the transducer at the
cardiac apex and obtaining a 2- or 4-chamber view of the mitral leaflets
at the level of the valve orifice.   The sample volume is positioned on
the left atrial side of the mitral orifice and the region behind the
leaflets scanned to detect localized, wide-band pansystolic spectral
tracing.   Figure 9 contrasts gray-scale spectral records in a normal
versus a patient with MR.   Measurement of the lowest energy systolic
time-velocity envelope area allowed complete separation of 17 normal
patients from 10 with MR proven at catheterization (1a).   The differential diagnosis of MR from congenital (12) or acquired (13) ventricular
septal defect can be easily and accurately accomplished with PDE.

Quantification of the severity of MR is also possible using duplex
PDE.   The severity of regurgitation is determined by defining the depth
and width of the regurgitant jet within the left atrium.   A high correlation was noted between Doppler and catheterization-determined
severity of MR (r =.88) (14).

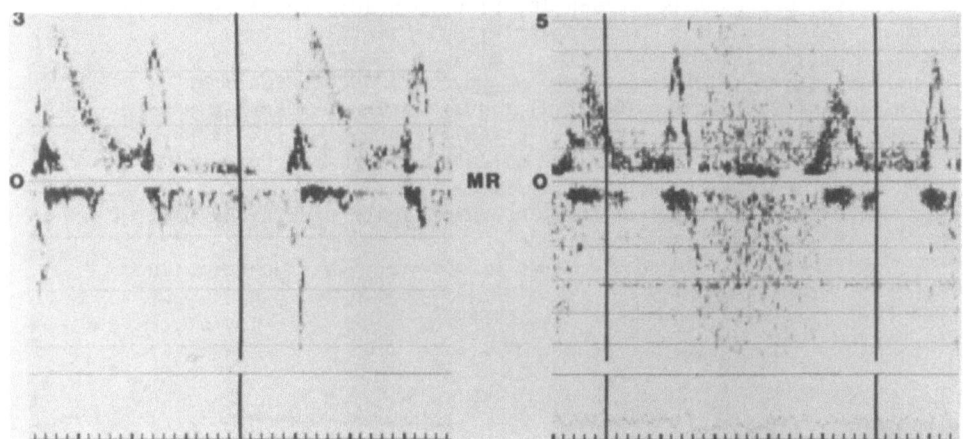

FIGURE 9.   Doppler gray-scale spectral records from normal and MR
patients obtained on the left atrial side of the mitral valve
illustrate broad-band systolic flow disturbance characteristic of MR.

114

REFERENCES

1. Richards KL, Cannon SR, Crawford MH, Sorensen SG: Diagnosis of valvular disease with Doppler real-time spectral analysis. American College of Cardiology Scientific Sessions, 1982.
2. Hatle L: Noninvasive assessment and differentiation of left ventricular outflow obstruction with Doppler ultrasound. Circulation 64:381-386, 1981.
3. Hatle L, Angelsen BA, Tromsdal A: Noninvasive assessment of aortic valve stenosis by Doppler ultrasound. Br Heart J 43:284, 1980.
4. Baker DW, Rubenstein SA, Lorch GS: Pulsed Doppler echocardiography: Principles and applications. Am J Med 63:69-80, 1977.
5. Lorch G, Rubenstein S, Baker D, Dooley T, Dodge H: Doppler echocardiography - Use of a graphical display system. Circulation 56:576-585, 1977.
6. Johnson SL, Baker DW, Lute RA, Dodge HT: Doppler echocardiography: The localization of cardiac murmurs. Circulation 48:810, 1973.
7. Ward JM, Baker DW, Rubenstein SA, Johnson SL: Detection of aortic insufficiency by pulse Doppler echocardiography. J Clin Ultrasound 5:5-10, 1977.
8. Boughner DR: Assessment of aortic insufficiency by transcutaneous Doppler ultrasound. Circulation 52:874-879, 1975.
9. Thuillez C, Theroux P, Bourassa MG, Blanchard D, Peronneau P, et al: Pulsed Doppler echocardiographic study of mitral stenosis. Circulation 61:381-387, 1980.
10. Hatle L, Brubakk A, Tromsdal A, Angelsen B: Noninvasive assessment of pressure drop in mitral stenosis by Doppler ultrasound. Br Heart J 40:131-140, 1978.
11. Hatle L, Angelsen B, Tromsdal A: Noninvasive assessment of atrioventricular pressure half-time by Doppler ultrasound. Circulation 60:1096-1104, 1979.
12. Stevenson JG, Kawabori I, Guntheroth WG: Differentiation of ventricular septal defects from mitral regurgitation by pulsed Doppler echocardiography. Circulation 56:14-18, 1977.
13. Richards KL, Hoekenga DE, Leach JK, Blaustein JC: Doppler-cardiographic diagnosis of interventricular septal rupture. Chest 76:101-103, 1979.
14. Abbasi AS, Allen MW, DeCristofaro D, Ungar I: Detection and estimation of the degree of mitral regurgitation by range-gated pulsed doppler echocardiography. Circulation 61:143-147, 1980.
1a. Richards K, Cannon S, Crawford M. Sorensen S: Pulsed Doppler echocardiographic assessment of aortic stenosis. Proc Cardiovascular Applications of Echocardiographic Doppler Systems, May 11, 1982, Paris, France.
8a. Bommer WJ, Mapes R, Miller L, Mason DT, DeMaria AN: Quantitation of aortic regurgitation with two-dimensional Doppler echocardiography. Am J Cardiol 47:412, 1981.

CLINICAL VALUE AND LIMITATIONS OF PULSED DOPPLER ECHOCARDIO-
GRAPHY IN PEDIATRIC CARDIOLOGY

D.A. REDEL

1. INTRODUCTION

Echocardiography provides valuable non-invasive methods for
the examination of the cardiovascular system. Especially two-
dimensional echocardiography (2D) is very illustrative of morphology and dynamics of the cardiac chambers, the valves and the
great vessels and is evolving as a reliable method for diagnosing
heart disease in children. Some details, i.e. the anatomy of the
atrioventricular valves can be clarified even better with the
aid of 2D than by angiocardiography.

But standard echocardiographic technics do not provide direct
information about blood flow. They can only visualize certain
secondary phenomena as diastolic flutter of the anterior mitral
leaflet or the interventricular septum in aortic regurgitation
or midsystolic closing of the aortic valves in subaortic stenosis.

2. PROCEDURE

2.1. Theoretical remarks

As ultrasound waves are reflected from cardiac structures and
the corpuscles of the streaming blood their frequency is shifted
in proportion to the velocity of the reflecting object (Doppler
effect).

Special devices have been developed that allow the extraction
of the frequency shift from the composite ultrasound echo (1, 2)
If ultrasound energy is emitted in a pulsed mode (pulsed Doppler
technics) there is the advantage of range-gated velocity detection
within a sample volume of the dimensions of 2 x 4 mm. Such a
system yields simultaneously the M-mode display of the region
under investigation and can be relatively simply combined with
a two-dimensional echocardiograph.

Its disadvantage is the inability of processing shifted frequencies beyond a certain limit, this is dependent on the depth of penetration.

Continuous wave Doppler systems do not possess these velocity limitations but they lack the range-gated properties that allow a localisation of flow phenomena along the ultrasonic beam axis.

Another crucial point is the spectral analysis of the Doppler shifted frequencies. A simple device is obtained by zero-crossing detection and graphical display of the frequencies as a time intervall histogram (TIH). Blood flow characteristics as spectral broadening, timing and direction of flow velocities can thus be recorded. But this inexpansive device lacks a satisfactory frequency resolution of the spectrum and is very liable to gain artefacts. A more sophisticated approach is fast Fourier transformation (FFT) of the Doppler spectrum. This allows a quantitative analysis of the frequency shift, artefacts are eliminated.

2.2. Material and methods

We report abour our experiences with a two-dimensional pulsed Doppler system (2DD) with TIH frequency display (atl Mk V) in the cardiologic examination of more than 4.000 patients over a period of two years.

In such a system Doppler flow analysis can be used as a focussed, two-dimensional orientated stethoscope to detect and localize blood flow disturbances. Thus 2D findings can be further elucidated.

In some cardiac defects flow characteristics correlate well with physiological or pathological pressure gradients between heart chambers and/or vessels.

The identification of cardiovascular structures in simple and complex heart disease is another usefull application of 2DD.

3. RESULTS

3.1. <u>Cardiac defects with shunt</u> are common in children with congenital heart disease and may occur isolated or in combination with other cardiac abnormalities.

3.1.1. <u>Ventricular septal defects</u> (VSD) can be visualized by 2D if their diameter amounts more than 3 mm (3, 4). Volume and direction of shunting is determined by the pressure difference between both ventricles. Pressure difference depends on the size of the defect, resistance of the pulmonary vessels or development of a right ventricular (RV) outflow tract gradient. A small VSD may cause a large left-to-right shunt if RV pressure is low, a large VSD may have only minimal shunting if RV pressure is high because of outflow tract obstruction or elevated pulmonary resistance. In any case morphological 2D findings together with flow characteristics across the defect and within the pulmonary artery describe the hemodynamic situation of a VSD (fig. 1).

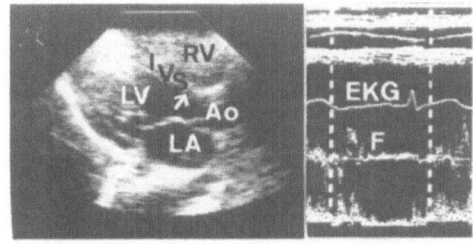

FIGURE 1. Small membraneous VSD (parasternal long axis), sample volume (arrow) samples late systolic flow across the defect (F at the right). Flow disturbance indicate normal RV pressure. IVS- interventricular septum, LV-left ventricle Ao-aortic root, LA-left atrium

3.1.2. <u>Atrial septal defects</u> (ASD) of the ostium secundum and ostium primum type can be visualized easily by 2D in infants (5). In older children direct proof can be difficult. Demonstrating the typical pretricuspid shunt pattern across the interatrial septum is very helpful in establishing the diagnosis and can distinguish ASD from other causes of pretricuspid left-to-right shunt (fig. 2). The flow pattern corresponds exactly with the simultaneously measured pressure difference between the atria in ASD. A short period of right-to-left shunting in late diastole and early systole allows ultrasonic contrast medium to enter the left atrium thus proving an interatrial communication by M-mode echocardiography (6).

118

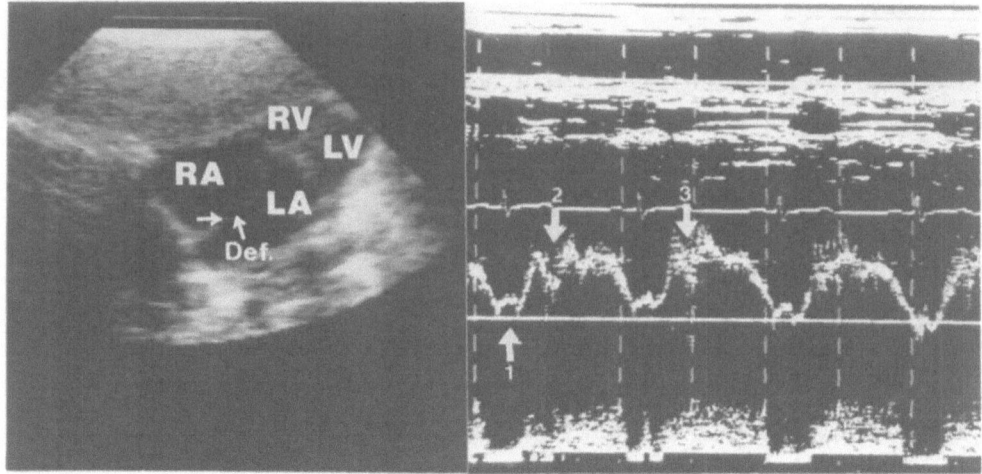

FIGURE 2. Atrial septal defect of the ostium secundum type
(Def.) (subcostal four chamber view). Sample volume (arrow)
lies within the ASD. TIH (on the right) shows the typical
flow pattern of pretricuspid shunting. First arrow in TIH
marks the short period of right-to-left shunt in late diastole
and early systole, second and third arrows mark the systolic-
diastolic left-to-right shunt.

3.1.3. <u>Patent ductus arteriosus</u> (PDA) may become a life-
threatening cardiovascular problem in preterm babies. Its
direct visualization by 2D is not as reliable as stated by
other autors (7). Pulmonary veins or branches of the pulmonary
artery can be easily mistaken for a PDA. Structure identification by 2DD is very helpful in establishing the diagnosis and
determining shunt direction (fig. 3). In neonates with ductus-
dependent heart disease under prostaglandin E therapy adequacy
of ductal blood flow can be demonstrated.

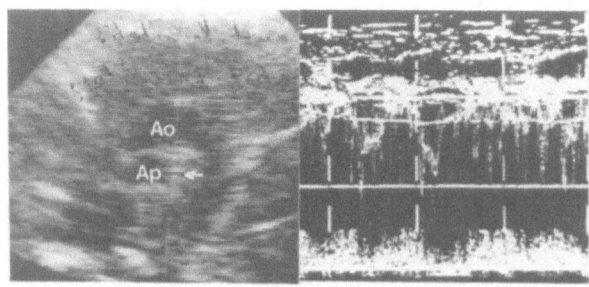

FIGURE 3. Direct visuali-
zation of PDA (arrow)
(suprasternal position).
Aortic arch (Ao), ascen-
ding and descending aorta
and right pulmonary ar-
tery are shown (Ap).
Position of the sample
volume in the PDA. Con-
tinuous flow across the
PDA indicating left-to-
right shunt.

3.2. Stenoses and regurgitations of valves

3.2.1. Pulmonic stenosis (PS) is the most common valve stenosis in children. Reliable echocardiographic criteria for its diagnosis have not been worked out. Flow disturbances in the pulmonary artery and its branches is a typical Doppler finding in PS (8). With the use of 2DD it is possible to localize the level of obstruction below, at or above the valve.

3.2.2. Aortic valve. In aortic stenosis of considerable degree 2D shows thichened aortic cusps that open with systolic doming (9). Less distinct forms as in bicuspid aortic valve may be detected only by flow disturbance in systole in the ascending aorta. In severe AS the jet can be followed into the ascending aorta by 2DD, the observable flow phenomena correlate with the degree of obstruction.

In aortic regurgitation the doppler findings of diastolic flow pertubations in the left ventricle are more sensitive than the M-mode findings of mitral or septal flutter in diastole (10).

3.2.3. Mitral regurgitation can be easily diagnosed by the Doppler findings of systolic flow disturbances behind the mitral valve (fig. 4) (11). The degree of regurgitation can be estimated by following the systolic jet into the left atrium (12).

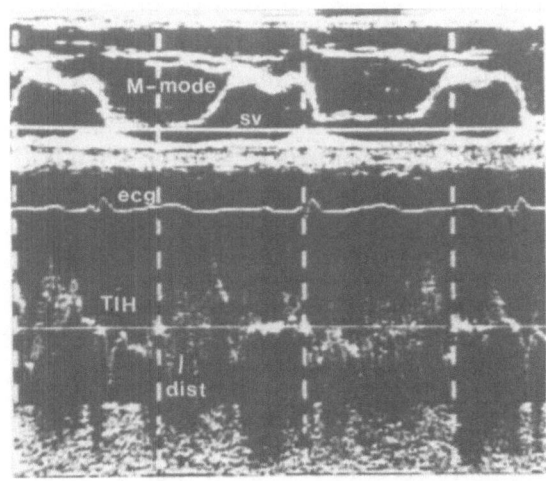

FIGURE 4. Mitral regurgitation in mitral valve prolaps. Midsystolic beginning of flow disturbances (dist.) in TIH behind the mitral valve as indicated in the M-mode by the sample line (sv) within the left atrium.

3.2.4. <u>Tricuspid regurgitation</u> is frequently found in children with right ventricular volume or pressure overload but is also an important hemodynamic factor in Ebstein's anomaly of the tricuspid valve. The diagnosis by 2DD is much more sensitive and specific than by contrast echocardiography (13).

3.3. <u>Heart disease in the neonatal period</u>. A severely ill neonate may be symptomatic because of heart disease. This may be a simple PDA in the preterm baby, a critical AS or some form of complex heart disease. In most cases conventional non-invasive diagnostic methods do not yield enough specificity to establish the correct diagnosis and starting adequate therapy or deciding upon the necessity of further invasive diagnostic procedures.

In 92 symptomatic neonates that were referred to us for cardiologic examination we diagnosed severe congenital heart disease in 44 patients with the use of 2DD. In all cases the basic diagnosis was confirmed by heart catheterization and angiocardiography or by autopsy. Out of 84 different cardiac defects that mostly occured in combination 77 were diagnosed correctly (91% sensitivity). There were 2 false positive diagnoses (97% specificity).

4. DISCUSSION

Pulsed Doppler echocardiography is a valuable supplementation of 2D because it can sense blood flow velocities in a direct way. Thus 2D findings can be further elucidated and cardiac abnormalities can be described in a more hemodynamically orientated way. Limitations of 2D as resolution problems or artefact production can be overcome by 2DD. Our experiences show that the correct and complete diagnosis can be obtained non-invasively in nearly every child with congenital heart disease.

A limitation is the inability to sense high flow velocities in distant structures as stated by the sampling theorem (maximum Doppler shift is half the puls repetition frequency). Another limitation of inadequate spectrum analysis by TIH has been abandoned by introduction of FFT of the Doppler signal.

Future aspects of 2DD concerning measurement of blood flow velocity and volume are promissing.

REFERENCES

1. Satomura, S. 1959. Ultrasonic Doppler method for the inspection of cardiac function. J. acoust. Soc. Am. 29, 1181
2. Baker, D.W. 1970. Pulsed ultrasonic Doppler blood flow sensing. IEEE Trans. Sonics Ultrason. SU—17, 170
3. Jaffe, C.C., Atkinson, P., Taylor, K.J.W. 1979. Physical parameters affecting the visibility of small ventricular septal defects using two-dimensional echocardiography. Invest. Radiol. 14, 149
4. Funabashi, T., Yoshida, H., Nakaya, S., Maeda,T,Taniguchi,N.1981. Echocardiographic visualization of ventricular septal defect in infants and assessment of hemodynamic status using a contrast technique
   Circulat. 64, 1025
5. Bierman, F.Z., Williams, R.G. 1979. Subxyphoidal two-dimensional imaging of the interatrial septum in infants and neonates with congenital heart disease. Circulat. 60, 20
6. Kronik, G., Slany, J., Moesslacher, H. 1979. Contrast M-mode echocardiography in diagnosis of atrial septal defect in acyanotic patients. Circulat. 59, 372
7. Sahn, J.D., Allen, H. 1978. Real-time cross-sectional echocardiographic imaging and measurement of the patent ductus arteriosus in infants and children. Circulat. 58, 343
8. Goldberg, S.J., Areias, J.C., Spitaels, S.E.C., de Villeneuve, V.H. 1979. Echo Doppler detection of pulmonary stenosis by time interval histogram analysis. J.Clin.Ultrasound 7,183
9. Weyman, A.E., Feigenbaum, H., Hurwitz, R.A., Girod, D.A., Dillon, J.C. 1977. Cross-sectional echocardiographic assessment of the severity of aortic stenosis in children. Circulation 55, 773
10. Goldberg, S.J.,Areias, J., Feldman, L., Sahn, D.J., Allen, H. 1979. Lesions that cause aortic flow disturbance. Circulat. 60, 1539
11. Abbasi, A. S., Allen, M.W., deChristofero, D., Ungar, I. 1980. Detection and estimation of the degree of mitral regurgitation by range-gated pulsed Doppler echocardiography. Circulat. 61, 143
12. Miyatake, K., Kinoshita, N., Nagata, S., Beppu, S., Park, J.D. Sakakibara, H., Niura, J. 1980. Intracardiac flow pattern in mitral regurgitation studied with combined use of ultrasonic pulsed Doppler technique and cross sectional echocardiography. Am.J.Cardiol. 45, 155 (1980)
13. Fehske, W., Redel, D. 1980. Erkennung und Beurteilung der Tricuspidalinsuffizienz durch die zweidimensionale Doppler-Echokardiographie. Z.Kardiol. 69,722 (abstr.)

TRANSESOPHAGEAL PULSED DOPPLER MEASUREMENT OF HEMODYNAMICS IN HUMANS

M.K. WELLS AND M.B. HISTAND

INTRODUCTION

Hemodynamic patterns in the major blood vessels of the chest provide valuable information for diagnosing normal and abnormal cardiac function and cardio-pulmonary physiology. For example, quantitative measurements of pulmonary artery or aortic blood velocity can be used to calculate cardiac output, evaluate the mechanical conditions of the heart valves, or detect intervals of disturbed or turbulent flow in these vessels. With the aid of mathematical models which describe pressure/flow relationships in arteries, measurements of arterial blood flow can be used to calculate arterial pulse pressure (1). Measurement techniques employing miniature ultrasound transducers positioned in the esophagus can be used to monitor pulmonary and aortic blood velocity and wall motion and to study their relationship to other physiological parameters. The value of an esophageal approach for measuring hemodynamic parameters in the thorax and for cardiac evaluation has been demonstrated in dogs (2); esophageal endoscopes fitted with ultrasound transducers were used to record aortic wall motion, aortic blood flow and velocity profiles. Instrumentation for obtaining these measurements consists of pulsed ultrasound Doppler velocimeters (PUDVM), pulse echo recorders, and echocardiographic units. This paper describes our experience measuring blood velocity and vessel diameter in the aorta and pulmonary artery of healthy conscious humans and recent advances in determining instantaneous Doppler angle and true velocity using a multiplexed Doppler flowmeter. It is hoped that this information will be useful to physiologists and clinicians and will encourage the ultimate development of truly non-invasive quantitative techniques for measuring hemodynamic parameters.

METHODS

The blood velocity measurements reported here were obtained with a pulsed ultrasound Doppler velocimeter and a miniaturized ultrasound transducer designed to be swallowed and positioned in the esophagus. Design and operation of the PUDVM have been described elsewhere (3,4). The PUDVM operated in a pulse radar-like mode and measured the instantaneous mean velocity of blood cells in a small volume within a blood vessel by sensing the change in frequency (Doppler shift) of ultrasound scattered by the moving cells. Time-varying velocity waveforms at various locations within the vessel cross-section were obtained by electronic range gating. This measurement technique was noninvasive in the sense that blood vessel walls remained intact and no surgery was required. It had the additional advantage of not disrupting the normal blood velocity patterns. For these experiments the PUDVM was operated at either 7.5 MHz or 4 MHz with a pulse length of 8 cycles and a pulse repetition rate of 25 kHz. This permitted a maximum velocity measurement of approximately 100 $cm-s^{-1}$ at a 0° Doppler angle.

An esophageal probe designed for use in man is shown in Figure 1. The probe contained two piezoelectric crystals mounted in a small epoxy tip and attached to a flexible catheter. One of the sensors was mounted with its axis tilted upward 45° from the normal to the catheter axis and was used for the Doppler flow measurements. Its resonant frequency was approximately 7.5 MHz. The other transducer which operated at 4 MHz was mounted perpendicular to the catheter and was used for ultrasound echo ranging. Both transducers were made from 3 mm diameter circular disks of LTZ-2 (Transducer Products, Torrington, CT) and were backed with a 3 mm thick layer of Stycast epoxy (Emerson and Cumings, Inc., Canton, MA).

The epoxy backing was deposited under vacuum and provided mechanical damping for the transducers. The transducer Q was approximately 5. The tip of the probe containing the two ultrasound transducers was approximately 15 mm long and 5 mm in diameter. The catheter was 2.5 mm in diameter and the wall consisted of three layers of spirally wound stainless steel wire of 0.2 mm diameter. The middle layer was wound in a direction opposite to the other two layers. This design provided a high degree of torsional rigidity for directional control

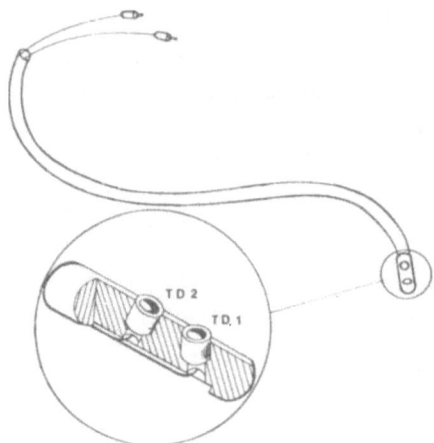

FIGURE 1. Schematic view of an esophageal ultrasound probe consisting
of a 2.5 mm diameter flexible catheter and a 5 mm diameter epoxy tip
containing two piezoelectric transducers. The insert shows the
distal transducer, 1, with its axis tilted upward at 45° and transducer
2 with its axis normal to the long axis of the probe.

during 360° rotation, yet was sufficiently flexible to be reasonably
comfortable for the patient.

Electrical safety of the probe for human use was assured by sub-
jecting each lead to a 200V potential while the probe was immersed in
physiological saline and verifying that the impedance between each lead
and the saline was greater than 100 MΩ. Electrical safety was tested
before and after each recording session.

The power output of the probe was measured using a microbalance.
The average power per unit area when both transducers were operated
simultaneously at a pulse repetition rate of 25 kHz and a pulse length
of 16 cycles was 47.6 mW cm^{-2}, which is below levels reported to damage
tissue(5).

An echo track was used with the 4 MHz sensor to detect aortic and
PA diameter and wall motion. The A-mode signal and tracking gates were
monitored and an analog signal corresponding to time-varying was recorded.

Arterial blood velocity and vessel diameter measurements were attempted in six adult subjects. Swallowing the probe was facilitated by

a sip of water and in some subjects by prior spraying of a topical anesthetic to the back of the throat. Once in the esophagus, the probe could be moved easily in the axial direction or rotated to obtain maximum strength Doppler and echo signals. In one subject, fluoroscopy confirmed good torque control of the probe and showed some longitudinal motion of the transducer with respiration and change in body position. Doppler illumination of an artery was determined by the contour of the velocity waveform and quality of the Doppler audio signal. Pulmonary artery flow was distinguished from aortic flow by injecting boluses of 2 to 6 cm^3 of saline through a cubital vein. Microbubbles in the saline produced momentary increases in the strength of the audio signal and were apparent on the echo tracing as the bolus passed through the ultrasound sample volume. Microbubbles appeared in the PA within 1 to 2 sec after injection and were subsequently cleared by the lung.

RESULTS

A recording of blood velocity in the aorta of a conscious, seated subject is shown in Figure 2(a). The esophageal probe was inserted approximately 27 cm from the incisor and a forward velocity was observed with the ultrasound crystal directed leftward and posteriorly. The characteristic velocity waveform shows a large forward velocity during systole followed by a brief backward velocity during early diastole and little velocity during the remainder of diastole. Intravenous injection of saline failed to alter the Doppler signal indicating that the observed flow was not originating from the pulmonary artery. Furthermore, the flow signal could be followed as the esophageal probe was advanced to a distance of more than 30 cm. These findings confirm that the observed flows were within the aortic arch and descending aorta. Although the precise Doppler angle was unknown, we assumed that the long axis of the probe was parallel to that of the aorta and calculated a peak velocity (based on a Doppler angle of 45°) of 30 cm-S^{-1}. Despite motion artifacts, the aortic blood velocity was also obtained during mild exercise on a bicycle ergometer. During exercise the heart rate doubled and the peak centerline velocity increased to 50 cm-S^{-1} (Figure 2(b)). The pattern during exercise compared to that at rest showed an elevated forward flow and no reverse flow.

126

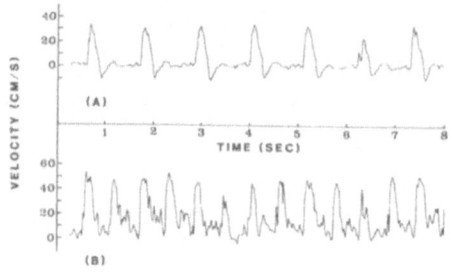

FIGURE 2(a). Centerline velocity measured in the descending aorta. A
   slight (< 10 cm-S^{-1}) reverse velocity occurs during early diastole.
   Maximum forward velocity reached values of about 30 cm-S^{-1}.
   (b) Centerline blood velocity in the descending aorta during bicycle
   exercise. Note the absence of reverse velocity and the elevated heart
   rate.

Using an echo track and the esophageal probe, motion of the far
aortic wall was measured in the descending aorta (Figure 3). The near
wall was too near the transducer to be detected. The far wall had a
mean distance of 27 mm from the transducer and its maximum excursion
with each cardiac cycle averaged 2.0 mm.

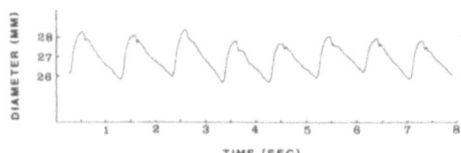

FIGURE 3. Aortic diameter changes measured in conscious man. The vessel
   diameter change was approximately 2 mm and the wall motion waveform
   closely resembled a pressure wave.

A recording of blood velocity from the right pulmonary artery is
shown in Figure 4. The velocity waveform for a single cardiac cycle is
relatively symmetric and is characterized by a cessation of flow during
diastole. Beat-to-beat variations in waveform are noticeable and might
be attributed to relative motion between the esophageal probe and the
pulmonary artery. The orientation of the ultrasound beam realtive to
the axis of the PA was unknown for this case; thus the absolute velocity

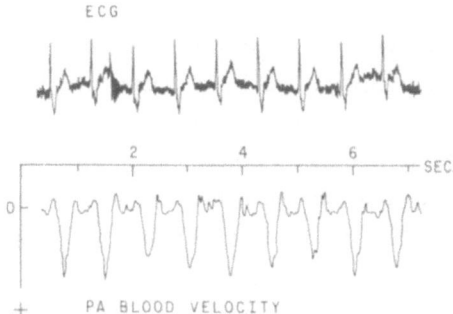

FIGURE 4. Recording of pulmonary artery blood velocity and ECG from a
    conscious human. The velocity waveforms are generally symmetric and
    there is little flow during diastole. In this case, the blood moved
    away from the ultrasound transducer during systole.

could not be calculated. PA blood velocity was verified using the

bubble injection technique.

Figure 5 is a recording of pulmonary artery diameter in the same

subject. The diameter changed by about 4 mm during each cardiac cycle

corresponding to a change in mean diameter of about ± 9%. Sudden fluc-

tuations in the diameter recording seen during diastole are apparently

induced by motion of the heart which causes a relative displacement

between the transducer and PA.

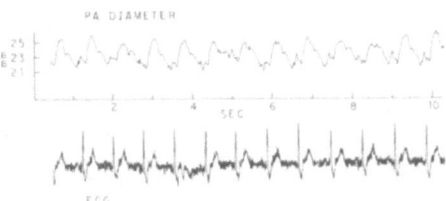

FIGURE 5. Pulmonary artery diameter obtained with an esophageal probe
    and echo track. Mean vessel diameter changed by about ± 9% during
    each cardiac cycle.

DISCUSSION

Using pulsed ultrasound techniques and an esophageal approach, measurement of blood flow in the great vessels within the human chest is limited only by the size of the esophageal transducer and the ultrasound transmission pathways in the chest.

The orientation of the ultrasound beam emitted from the probe in the thorax could be varied by external manipulation. The insertion distance of the marked probe was measured from the incisors. The torque preserving qualities of the three layer cable provided for rotational orientation of the cylindrical probe tip in the esophagus. Although both depth and lateral movement of the probe tip varied with body position and respiration, spatial fixation was sufficient to permit identification of and measurements in the thoracic aorta and pulmonary artery.

To obtain quantitative measurements of blood velocity or blood flow, one must know the angle between the ultrasound beam and the flow axis. Absolute velocity is proportional to the Doppler frequency shift and inversley proportioned to the cosine of the Doppler angle. For transesophageal measurements the orientation of the probe is generally not known. The true Doppler angle can be calculated independently of observed probe-vessel orientations using a triangulation technique and a probe having three transducers arranged in a triangular array and focused at a common point within the vessel (2). Sequential measurements of velocity made with each of the three transducers provide sufficient information to calculate the average Doppler angle and average velocity. If the measurements are made in a sufficiently short interval such that the blood velocity vector and probe-vessel orientation can be considered stationary, the instantaneous Doppler angle and instantaneous true velocity can be obtained. Transducers specifically designed for carrying out this triangulation procedure have been coupled to a three channel multiplexed pulsed Doppler velocity meter to monitor true blood velocity in dogs (6). Real-time measurement of pulsatile blood velocity requires high speed switching of the transducers' driver and receiver circuitry and a microcomputer to process the data. Sequential measurements from the three sensors are obtained during an interval of 32.7 ms (each sensor is operated for 10.9 ms) and the true velocity is computed, displayed and held while new data are acquired. This switching rate allows for faithful reproduction of frequency components in the velocity waveform below about 15 Hz and provides a velocity resolution of 1 cm-S^{-1}. Figure 6 shows a recording of blood velocity measured in the ascending aorta of an anesthetized dog using this multiplexing technique. The direct output shows velocities computed for each transducer switching cycle which is updated every 32.7 ms. A filtered version of this waveform (15 Hz active filter) and an average velocity (100 point running average) are also plotted. Velocity data have been obtained for more than thirty dogs using a three element esophageal probe and multiplexing Doppler and the feasibility of this method for measuring true velocity has been demonstrated. For measurements in humans, a smaller multi-crystal transducer that can be swallowed easily must be designed.

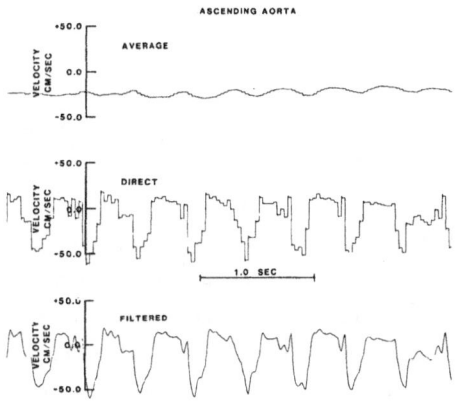

FIGURE 6. Velocity data obtained with the multiplexing Doppler and three element esophageal probe from the ascending aorta of a dog. The waveforms are displayed inverted from their normal orientation. Both average velocity and true instantaneous pulsatile velocity are recorded.

130

With the aid of an esophageal ultrasound probe, it is possible to
monitor hemodynamic parameters in thoracic vessels such as the aorta,
pulmonary arteries, carotid artery, superior vena cava and the pulmonary
veins. Proper identification of these vessels requires an understanding
of the thoracic anatomy including the relative orientation and range
of the vessel from the esophagus, the normal blood velocity waveforms
and the direction of flow. Nevertheless, it is possible to confuse
signals from adjacent vessels especially if the velocity waveforms are
similar and the flow directions the same. The saline injection technique provides a means for verifying when measurements are being made
in the pulmonary arteries. The injections can be repeated without
risk to the patient and produce well defined changes in both the
Doppler and echo signals.

Transesophageal Doppler and echo measurements can be distorted by
movement of the probe within the esophagus and artifacts may appear on
data records as sharp spikes or oscillations. Because of their relatively short duration, however, they do not generally interfere with
the calculation of blood velocity or vessel diameter.

Our studies indicate the feasibility of using an esophageal
approach to obtain hemodynamic data from the aorta and pulmonary
artery in humans. The method is safe, well tolerated by patients and
does not require intra-arterial catheterization or the injection of
radiopaque or radioactive substances. These techniques could be
applied when diagnosing diseases such as coarctation, aneurism and
dissection of the aorta, pulmonary and aortic stenoses, and for
evaluating aortic grafts. In addition, transesophageal ultrasonography
may lead to a noninvasive and direct measurement of cardiac output
that could be used in conscious patients at rest and during exercise.

ACKNOWLEDGMENT

This research was supported by National Institutes of Health
Contract HO1-HR 62920 and Grant RO1-HL 22326.

REFERENCES
1. Wells MK, Histand MB. 1977. Noninvasive measurement of pulmonary
   hemodynamics. Advances in Bioengineering, eds Grood and Smith. ASME,
   New York.

2. Daigle RE, Miller CW, Histand MB, McLeod FD, Hokanson DE. 1975. Non-traumatic aortic blood flow sensing using an ultrasonic esophageal probe. J. Appl. Physiology 38(6).

3. Baker DW. 1970. Pulsed ultrasonic Doppler bloodflow sensing. IEEE Trans. on Sonics and Ultrasonics 3(SU-17).

4. Baker DW, Daigle RE. 1977. Noninvasive ultrasonic flowmetry. Cardiovascular Flow Dynamics and Measurements, eds Hwang and Normann. University Park Press.

5. Ulrich WD. 1973. Ultrasound dosage for experimental use on human beings. U.S. Naval Med. Res. Inst. Report AD 73 1075.

6. Histand MB, Wells MW, Corace RA. 1981. Multiplexed Doppler flow-metry. 1981 Biomechanics Symposium, eds Van Buskirk and Woo. ASME, publication AMD - Vol 43, New York.

TRANSESOPHAGEAL PULSED DOPPLER ECHOCARDIOGRAPHY IN MITRAL AND
AORTIC REGURGITATION

M. SCHLÜTER, B.A. LANGENSTEIN, P. HANRATH

Since its introduction in 1973 (1) range-gated pulsed Doppler echocardiography (PDE) has gained considerable status as a
valuable diagnostic tool in the assessment of various congenital
and acquired malfunctions of the heart. By its ability to
determine direction, nature and timing of blood flow at specific
locations within the cardiac chambers and great vessels the noninvasive evaluation of valvular stenosis and regurgitation as
well as intracardiac and systemic shunts was rendered possible
(2-8).

As in all echocardiography, the standard transthoracic
approach of PDE is frequently compromised by unfavourable configurations of the thorax and its organs which inhibit ultrasonic access to the heart. The physical principles of the
technique impose additional limitations on the applicability of
transthoracic PDE (9).

In this paper we report on our experiences in the investigation of mitral and aortic regurgitation with transesophageal
pulsed Doppler echocardiography (TPDE) which can overcome most
of the aforementioned restrictions.

PATIENTS AND METHOD

A total of 25 patients comprised the study group. They were
divided into two subgroups: 18 had mitral regurgitation (MR)
determined by cineangiography (5 women, 13 men; mean age 45
years), while 12 patients with angiographically proven aortic
regurgitation (AR) constituted the second subgroup (4 women,
8 men; mean age 47 years). Five patients with combined mitral
and aortic regurgitation were members of both groups.

The 7 patients from the AR group without angiographic

evidence of MR served as control subjects for the MR group, while the 13 patients from the MR group without angiographic evidence of AR served as control subjects for the AR group.

Investigations were carried out with a 3.5 MHz transducer attached to the distal end of a standard 9 mm gastroscope (Fig. 1).

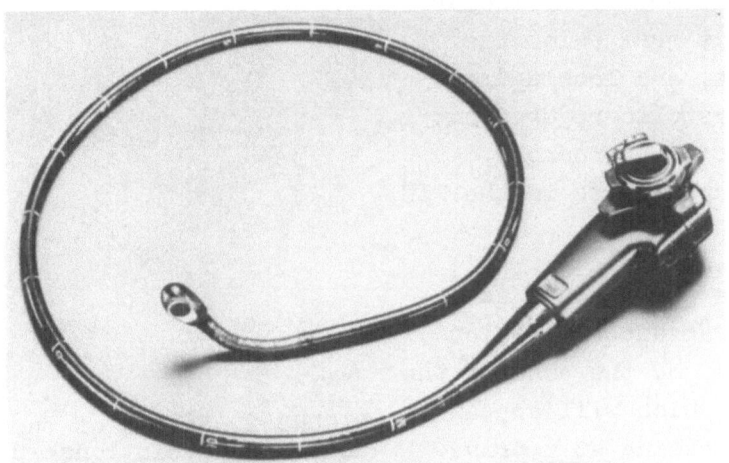

FIGURE 1. The ultrasonic endoscope with the transducer at the distal end and the control unit at the proximal end.

The system was connected to a commercially available echo-Doppler unit (Advanced Technology Laboratories Mod. 500 A). Recordings were obtained as graphic displays (10) with a comprised M-mode diagram showing the location of the Doppler sample volume within the cardiac chambers, a flow pattern in the form of a time interval histogram (TIH), and ECG and PCG tracings for timing purposes.

Prior to the ultrasonic examination, the patient has to undergo a barium x-ray study to rule out a diverticulum of the esophagus, and he must be fasted for about 8 hours. Premedication was 10 mg diazepam i.v. and .5 mg atropine sulfate subcutaneously. The gastroscope can then be introduced blindly with the patient in a supine position.

MR was detected or excluded by placing the Doppler sample volume in the left atrium close to the mitral orifice, and

searching for a systolic regurgitant flow pattern to appear
in the TIH. Incompetence of the
aortic valve was investigated
by placing the Doppler sample
volume in the left ventricular
outflow tract just below the
aortic valve, and looking for
either a diastolic regurgitant
flow pattern or pronounced
diastolic turbulences in the TIH.

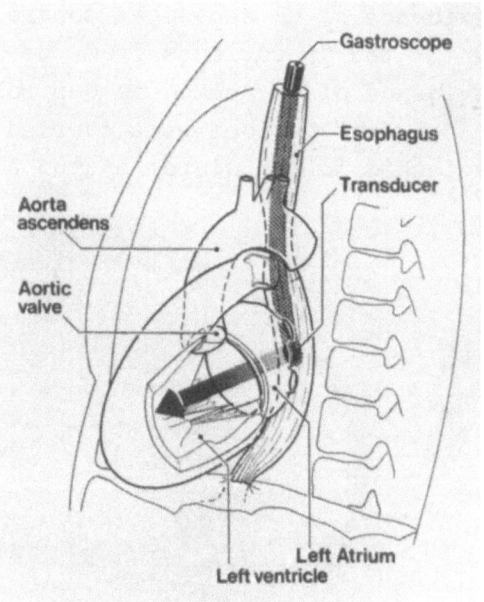

RESULTS

Once the gastroscope is introduced, transducer position
is identified by the echo of the
aortic root which will appear on
the M-mode tracing at a transducer depth of about 40 cm from
the patient's teeth. A further

FIGURE 2. Sketch of the
anatomical relationship
between esophagus and
heart.

downward shift with a slight counter-clockwise rotation will
image the anterior mitral leaflet posterior to the left atrial
posterior wall. From this transducer position, which is sketched
in Fig. 2, MR is readily investigated by scanning the sample
volume across the mitral valve orifice.

Fig. 3 shows a recording from a patient with no evidence of
MR. The top third of the figure displays the comprised M-mode
diagram which is an upside-down version of standard M-mode
patterns. The cardiac structure closest to the transducer is
the left atrial posterior wall, which is followed by the
typical echo trace of the anterior mitral leaflet and by the
dense echo of the anteroseptal left ventricular wall. The
straight horizontal line indicates the position of the sample
volume above the mitral valve in the left atrium.

Below the ECG curve the TIH is registered. The normal
diastolic filling of the left ventricle from the left atrium
(i.e. with blood flow directed away from the esophageal

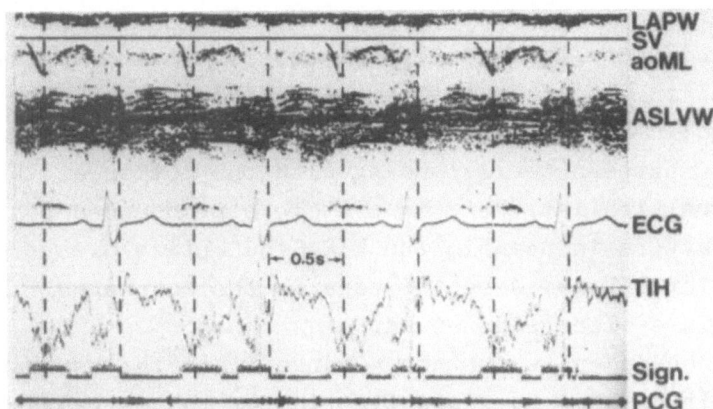

FIGURE 3. TPDE recording from the left atrium of a patient with competent mitral valve. Diastolic flow biphasic negative; no systolic flow. (LAPW: left atrial posterior wall. SV: sample volume. aoML: anterior mitral leaflet. ASLVW: anteroseptal left ventricular wall. TIH: time interval histogram. Sign.: amplitude of Doppler signal).

transducer) is represented as a laminar biphasic flow pattern below the zero-flow baseline. This diastolic flow is in correspondence with the motion pattern of the anterior mitral leaflet in the M-mode diagram. During systole no flow is recorded.

In contrast to this normal mitral flow behaviour, Fig. 4

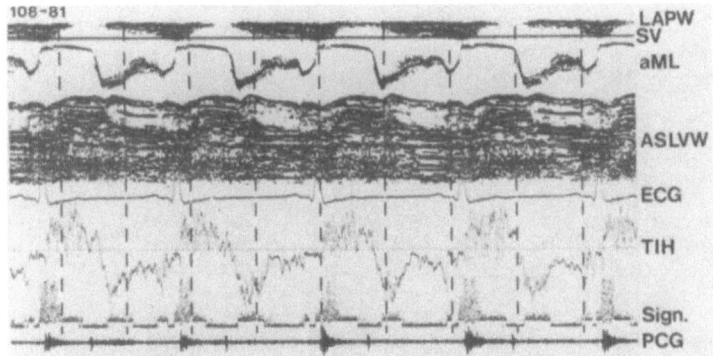

FIGURE 4. Mitral regurgitation. Sample volume in the left atrium. Positive systolic flow pattern indicates regurgitation. (Abbreviations as before).

shows a recording from a patient with MR. The M-mode tracings of Figs. 3 and 4 are principally identical, meaning that the sample volume is placed in the same location in both cases. Again, diastolic filling is represented in Fig. 4 as a biphasic negative flow pattern corresponding with the motion of the anterior mitral leaflet. Yet, in systole a pronounced positive deflection pattern is seen in the TIH, indicative of systolic flow in the left atrium directed towards the esophageal transducer. This is a clear sign of MR.

If the transducer is further advanced into the esophagus from the position used for investigation of the mitral valve and rotated clockwise by a small amount, the left ventricular outflow tract just below the aortic valve can be scanned with the Doppler sample volume from a transducer position slightly above the mitral valve area.

The M-mode diagrams of Figs. 5 and 6 both show the position of the sample volume within the left ventricular outflow tract posterior (with respect to the esophageal transducer) to the anterior mitral leaflet. Fig. 5 is a recording from a patient with no angiographic evidence of AR, whereas Fig. 6 was recorded from a patient with AR of angio grade III. The normal ejection of blood from the left ventricle into the aorta ascendens is represented in both cases by a positive deflection in the TIH.

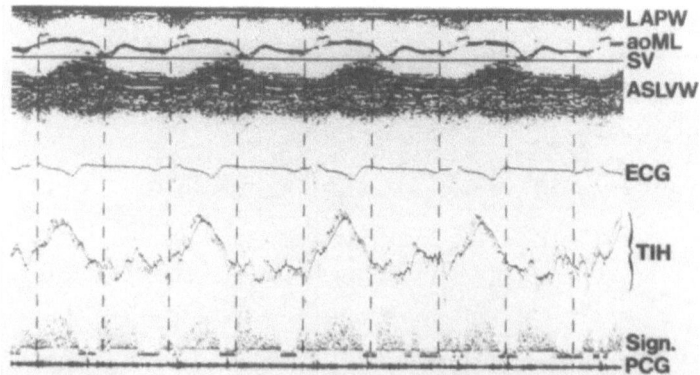

FIGURE 5. TPDE recording from the left ventricular outflow tract of a patient with competent aortic valve. Positive systolic flow; no diastolic flow. (Abbreviations as before).

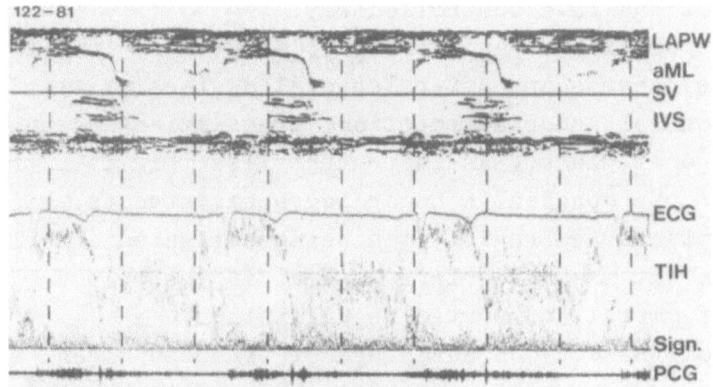

FIGURE 6. Aortic regurgitation. Sample volume
in the left ventricular outflow tract. Marked
diastolic turbulences following regular systolic ejection profile. (Abbreviations as before,
except for IVS: interventricular septum).

In the patient with a competent aortic valve (Fig. 5) no significant diastolic flow is registered.

In contrast, prominent diastolic turbulences starting with
a high negative amplitude well before the opening of the mitral
valve are apparent in Fig. 6. This is indicative of a high-
velocity reflux across the aortic valve, resulting in a turbulent diastolic flow behaviour in the left ventricular outflow
tract. The nature (turbulent) and the timing (pre mitral opening) identifies this flow pattern as pathological and differen-
tiates it from regular left ventricular filling across the
mitral valve.

DISCUSSION

The earliest investigations with transesophageal ultrasonography were undertaken in 1971 with the aim of measuring blood
flow in the thoracic aorta by the continuous-wave Doppler
technique (11). With the advent of range-gated pulsed Doppler
systems, similar measurements were repeated in 1979 (12), and
recently an esophageal transducer was presented for pulsed
Doppler echocardiography (13). The gastroscope-like systems
used by these authors all more or less lacked the means to
manipulate the transducer orientation inside the esophagus into

various directions in a controlled way.

The incorporation of an ultrasonic transducer into the tip of a flexible gastroscope offers several degrees of freedom for transducer control, such as rotation, translation and angulation in two orthogonal planes. An instrument like this is extremely suited for transesophageal echocardiographic studies, since many cardiac structures and regions can be investigated at will by the physician. It is particularly useful in the pulsed Doppler assessment of mitral and aortic regurgitation.

Apart from the obvious advantage of transesophageal echocardiography in obese patients and in those with chronic obstructive pulmonary disease or barrel chests, the close anatomical relationship between the esophagus and the heart yields further advantages for pulsed Doppler examinations of the left atrium and the left ventricular outflow tract.

The short distance between the mitral valve area and an esophageal transducer allows the use of high pulse repetition frequencies and, consequently, enables the measurement of high regurgitant flow velocities in the left atrium. Parallel alignment of the ultrasonic beam axis with the direction of blood flow is easily accomplished by transducer angulation, as is the scanning of the left atrium for localized regurgitant jets without hindrance from ribs or lung tissue. This results in a superior recording quality, and in a sensitivity for detecting MR which is considerably higher than with standard PDE, particularly for cases of mild to moderate MR (14). Also, the investigation of incompetent mitral valve prostheses is greatly facilitated with TPDE.

Ultrasonic examination of the left ventricular outflow tract with TPDE does not allow as high pulse repetition frequencies as in the detection of MR because of the larger distance of this cardiac region from the esophagus, and parallel alignment of ultrasonic beam direction with the blood flow axis is anatomically not possible. Yet, taking into consideration the high regurgitant flow velocities that are frequently present in AR, especially if the aortic valve is stenosed, a certain angle between blood flow and ultrasonic beam is necessary for an

unambiguous (i.e. free of aliasing (15)) Doppler registration
of AR.

It is thus concluded that TPDE is a valuable diagnostic
means in the detection of mitral and aortic regurgitation.

REFERENCES

1. Johnson SL, Baker DW, Lute RA, Dodge HT: Doppler echocardiography. The localization of cardiac murmurs.
   Circulation 1973; 48: 810
2. Quinones MA, Young JB, Waggoner AD, Ostojic MC, Ribeiro LGT,
   Miller RR: Assessment of pulsed Doppler echocardiography in
   detection and quantification of aortic and mitral regurgitation.
   Br Heart J 1980; 44: 612
3. Hatle L: Noninvasive assessment and differentiation of left
   ventricular outflow tract obstruction with Doppler ultrasound.
   Circulation 1981; 64: 381
4. Thuillez C, Theroux P, Bourassa MG, Blanchard D, Peronneau P,
   Guermonprez JL, Diebold B, Waters DD, Maurice P: Pulsed
   Doppler study of mitral stenosis.
   Circulation 1980; 61: 381
5. Goldberg SJ, Areias JC, Spitaels SEC, deVilleneuve VH: Echo
   Doppler detection of pulmonary stenosis by time-interval
   histogram analysis.
   J Clin Ultrasound 1979; 7: 183
6. Waggoner AD, Quinones MA, Young JB, Brandon TA, Shah AA,
   Verani MS, Miller RR: Pulsed Doppler echocardiographic
   detection of right-sided valve regurgitation.
   Am J Cardiol 1981; 47: 279
7. Stevenson JG, Kawabori I, Dooley T, Guntheroth WG: Diagnosis
   of ventricular septal defect by pulsed Doppler echocardiography.
   Circulation 1978; 58: 322
8. Stevenson JG, Kawabori I, Guntheroth WG: Pulsed Doppler
   echocardiographic evaluation of the cyanotic newborn: Identification of the pulmonary artery in transposition of the
   great arteries.
   Am J Cardiol 1980; 46: 849
9. Newhouse VL, LeCong P, Furgason ES, Ho CT: On increasing the
   range of pulsed Doppler systems for blood flow measurements.
   Ultrasound Med Biol 1980; 6: 233
10. Lorch G, Rubenstein S, Baker D, Dooley T, Dodge H: Doppler
    echocardiography. Use of a graphical display system.
    Circulation 1977; 56: 576
11. Side CG, Gosling RG: Non-surgical assessment of cardiac
    function.
    Nature 1971; 232: 335
12. Wells MK, Histand MB, Reeves JT, Sodal IE: Ultrasonic trans-
    esophageal measurement of hemodynamic parameters in humans.
    ISA Transactions 1979; 18: 57

13. Hisanaga K, Hisanaga A, Ichie Y, Nishimura K, Hibi N,
    Fukui Y, Kambe T: Transesophageal pulsed Doppler echo-
    cardiography.
    Lancet 1979; I: 53
14. Schlüter M, Langenstein BA, Hanrath P, Kremer P, Bleifeld W:
    Mitral regurgitation detected by transesophageal pulsed
    Doppler echocardiography (abstr).
    Eur Heart J 1981; 2 (Suppl A): 114
15. Baker DW: Applications of pulsed Doppler techniques.
    Radiol Clin North Am 1980; 18: 79

MEASUREMENT OF REGIONAL ECHO INTENSITY
AS A MEANS OF CARDIAC
TISSUE CHARACTERIZATION

D.G.Gibson, R.B.Logan Sinclair

The idea of using ultrasound to gain information about tissues
beyond simply their position and motion is an attractive one.
Such tissue characterization depends on analyzing the returning
signal, in order to describe in the greatest possible detail the
interaction between ultrasound and targets in the heart (1,2).
It follows, therefore, that there must be a close relation
between tissue characterization and an understanding of the
processes of image formation (3). A number of properties of
tissues have been investigated with this end in view. A large
body of data exists on the velocity of sound in various organs,
and on its variation with the frequency of the incident energy,
and also with the state of preservation of the tissue (4).
Absorption and attenuation have also been studied (5). The
former term refers to energy loss within tissues as heat, and the
latter also includes energy loss by scattering and reflection.
Both these properties are frequency dependent, and the nature of
this dependence may be more informative in identifying
differences between tissues than values at a single frequency.
Although both the velocity of sound and also attenuation or
absorption can readily be studied in vitro, these measurements

require methods based on transmitting ultrasound through the tissue being examined, and thus cannot readily be used in clinical cardiology, where access to the heart is limited by anatomical constraints. For this reason, the most promising approach would appear to be one based on examination of the properties of the reflected energy, whether this is due to backscattering or specular reflection. However, these properties cannot be rigorously considered in isolation, since the amount of energy impinging on a target within the heart clearly depends on absorption by proximal tissues, and the same applies to the returning echo. For a complete description of the process, therefore, these values must be specified for each unit volume of the tissue (6). The problem is a formidable one, although progress towards its solution has been in the study of breast disease, where transmission techniques are possible (7).

If such methods are to be used in clinical cardiology, therefore, there would seem to be room for a simplified approach. We have thus examined the possible value of analyzing of the relative amplitude of the returning echo in various types of heart disease. A number of lines of evidence suggest that this might be of value in detecting collagen within cardiac structures. The possibility that collagen might be a major factor in the genesis of these structural echoes was suggsted by Fields and Dunn on the basis of its elastic properties (7), its Young's modulus being greater than that of other biological tissues except bone by a factor of over 1000. Mimbs et al (8) have measured integrated backscatter after experimental myocadial infarction, and also in experimentally induced daunorubicin cardiotoxicity, and shown its amplitude to be correlated with tissue collagen content. When the tissue was treated with collagenase, backscattering was significantly reduced, although hydroxyprolene levels remained unchanged. In these experiments, similar changes were demonstrable from simple measurement of the amplitude of backscatter at 2.25 MHz, although the scatter was rather wider. Since myocardial collagen is increased in patients with coronary artery disease, left ventricular hypertrophy and a variety of other less common forms of left ventricular disease, and since its presence significantly modifies the diastolic properties of the left ventricle, its detection also has appreciable clinical significance.

A number of problems present themselves if this approach is to be applied to clinical cardiology. The method should be applicable to standard echocardiographic equipment, preferably in real time. This is important, since the rate of data acquisition with two dimensional echocardiography is very rapid, and if it has to be stored in computer memory, or on disk, then only one or two seconds' of display can be analysed. Measurement of absolute values of echo amplitude cannot easily be achieved, so that we have used relative ones, taking the pericardium behind the posterior wall of the left ventricle as an internal standard, which has proved remarkably constant between patients. The parietal pericardium consists of dense masses of collagen tissue (10), so that it is, perhaps, not surpri sing that it reflects ultrasound with considerable intensity. The use of an internal standard, at a constant position within the heart, incidentally goes some way to solving two potential problems, those of the additional effects of path-length and ultrasound frequency on amplitude. The nature of reflection at targets within the heart is clearly significant. In many accounts of the subject, it is assumed to be specular, and if this were indeed the case, then reflected amplitude would depend critically on the relative orientation of interfaces and the ultrasound beam (11). However, when it is remembered that the ventricular cavities can be outlined from the apical approach, it is clear that specular reflection is unlikely to be the dominant mode of image formation, and indeed comparison of 40 targets viewed from apical and parasternal approaches shows little difference in amplitude (13). Clearly, gain settings on the instrument must be standardized. We have found it convenient to avoid use of swept gain except for the first 1-2 cm of near field. It is essential that no form of "image processing" is used, and that the instrument employed has a digital and not a simple optically coupled TV scan converter. The problem of modification of the signal by proximal tissues is more tractible in the heart than with other solid organs, such as liver, due to the uniform properties of blood which occupies the greater part of the cardiac volume. Failure to measure absolute amplitudes is thus compenstaated for by the ability to view the coloured display in real time, so that the eye can approaciate the distribution and texture of the various amplitude levels. It may well be that this, essentially statistical approach is capable of further development.

Figures 1-4 in colour

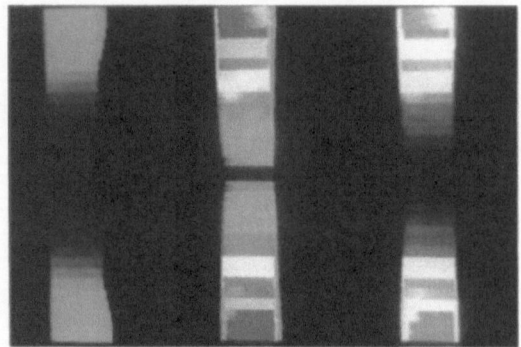

Figure 1: Display of echo amplitude. Left hand panel shows standard grey scale display, middle panel, simple substitution of colour for amplitude, and right, amplitude and colour processing. A standard sequence of colours is used for increasing amplitude.

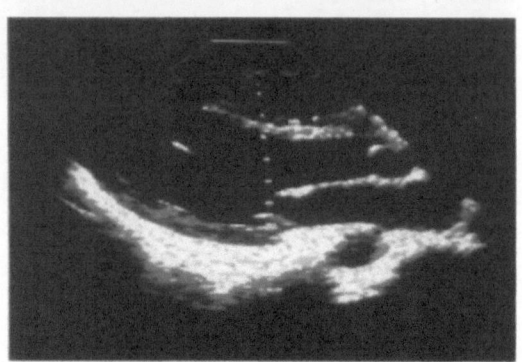

Figure 2: Normal left ventricle in parasternal long axis view. Note that normal myocardium appears green or cyan on display, indicating low echo amplitude.

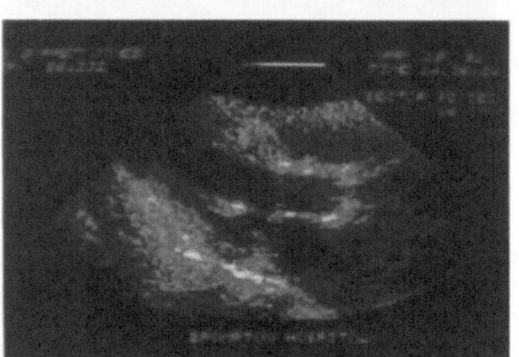

Figure 3: Parasternal long axis view of left ventricle of patient with aortic valve disease. Note high intensity echoes from septum particularly towards the apex, and papillary muscle.

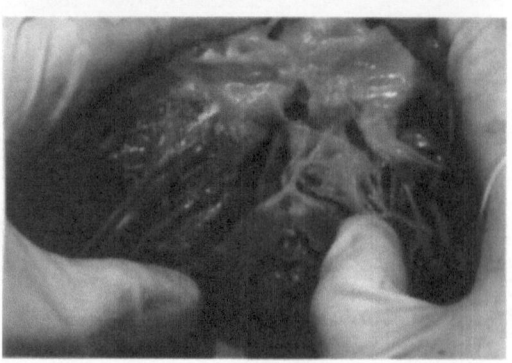

Figure 4: Pathological specimen corresponding to Figure 3. Note fibrosis at apex of papillary muscle.

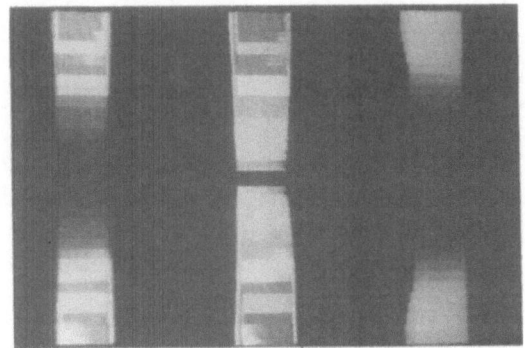

Figure 1: Display of echo amplitude. Left hand panel shows standard grey scale display, middle panel, simple substitution of colour for amplitude, and right, amplitude and colour processing. A standard sequence of colours is used for increasing amplitude.

If regional amplitude on the image is to be investigated, it must be displayed. Although manufacturers provide up to 32 grey scale levels, the dynamic range of currently available displays is not adequate to display more than 7 or 8. In addition, there are psychological difficulties in the perception of grey scale which make it quite unsuitable in this context (12). We have therefore explored the use of colour (13). Simple conversion of amplitude to colour destroys amplitude perspective and the results are totally unacceptable (13). We have therefore retained the overall grey scale, and superimposed colour on it so that both vary with echo intensity. The three methods are demonstrated in Figure 1. This combined approach has a number of advantages. The processing can be done very rapidly, so that it is possible to display the image in real time rather than storing it in computer memory, thus making it very much cheaper as well as more versatile than many previous approaches. Secondly, it is also possible to alter the saturation of the colours, which can thus be gradually removed from the display if they are felt to be obscuring some other feature, such as texture. Colour and amplitude can be processed independently before being combined in the final image. Manufacturers have introduced a number of ways of "enhancing" the image, with a view to improving its subjective qualities. Although no objective evidence has been adduced to support their use, their popularity suggests that they are felt to be of value. Since they usually involve either non-linear amplification or differentiation of the image to make boundaries more apparent, it is clear that their use will distort original amplitude levels. Using the double approach that we have described, it is possible to derive information controlling colour at an early stage of the processing. The grey scale component can then be "enhanced" in whatever way appeals to the fancy of the operator or manufacturer, and then the two signals recombined. In this way, any improvement of image quality is apparent in local brightness, but original echo amplitude levels are preserved in the colour. Finally, it is possible to generate displays showing the distribution of echoes of a single amplitude level, which are of great value in critical analysis of the images.

Preliminary observations on the use of this technique have been described elsewhere (13). Consistent values are obtained from normal hearts, in which the structure reflecting with greatest amplitude is the central fibrous body, at approximately 66% that of posterior pericardium. Normal valve cusps and septal myocardium reflect at approcximately 30-35%, and myocardium in

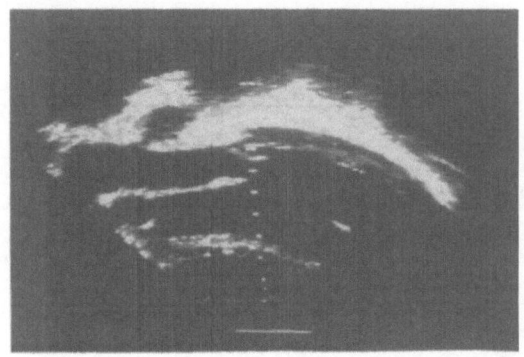

Figure 2: Normal left ventricle in parasternal long axis view. Note that normal myocardium appears green or cyan on display, indicating low echo amplitude.

the posterior wall at 25% (Figure 2). The use of relative amplitudes based on posterior pericardium is supported by the reproducible measurements obtained from components of plastic valve prostheses within the heart, which represent substances of known and constant composition whose properties can be studied in vivo. We also have increasing direct histological evidence to suggest that fibrosis as a major cause of increased echo intensity. This has come from a study of 24 patients in whom echocardiograms were obtained within 1 week of death. These will be described in detail elsewhere. An example is given in Figure 3. The former shows the parasternal long axis view of a patient with aortic valve disease, in whom brightly reflecting targets are demonstrated in the septum, and also in the anterior papillary muscle. Figure 4 shows a corresponding histological specimen , demonstrating fibrosis at the head of the anterior papillary muscle.

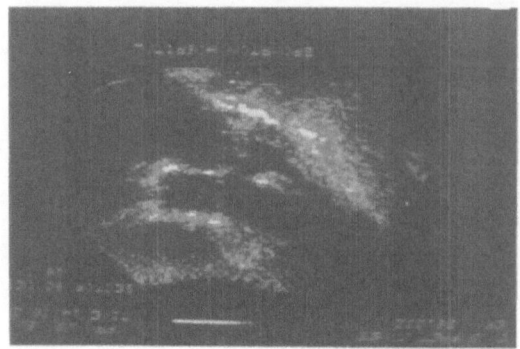

Figure 3: Parasternal long axis view of left ventricle of patient with aortic valve disease. Note high intensity echoes from septum particularly towards the apex, and papillary muscle.

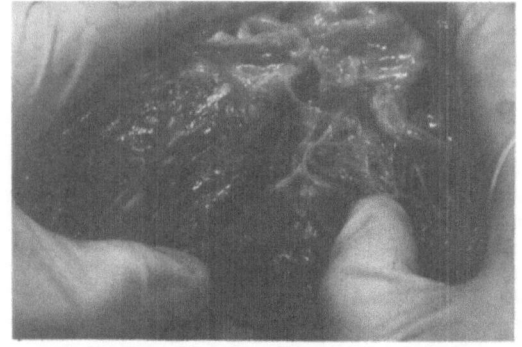

Figure 4: Pathological specimen corresponding to Figure 3. Note fibrosis at apex of papillary muscle.

Similar excellent correlation has been observed in a series of patients with eosinophilic heart disease, confirmed by endomyocardial biopsy (in press). These results thus confirm those of Tanaka et al (14) who also noted a close relation between regional echo amplitude and local fibrosis.

In summary, therefore, it seems that simple analysis of regional echo amplitude is possible using colour and amplitude processing. The technique appears to have the potential of demonstrating collagen tissue, whose detection, particularly within the myocardium, may well have clinical significance. However, this approach to image analysis is a very general one, with its major applications outside cardiology, and probably outside medicine altogether. The use of such a technique, which substitutes some measure of rigour for clinical convenience, thus represents one possible means of developing reliable and practicable techniques of tissue characterization.

REFERENCES

1. Wells PTN. Present status of tissue identification. Echocardiology. Ed Rijsterborgh H. Martinus Hijhoff. The Hague. 1981; pp 455-460.

2. Hill CR. Tissue characterisation. Progress in Medical Ultrasound. Ed Kurjak A Excerpta Medica. Amsterdam. 1980; 1:

3. Chivers RC, Hill CR. Ultrasonic attenuation in human tissue. Ultrasound in Med. and Biol 1975; 2: 25-29.

4. Goss SA, Johnston RL, Dunn F. Comprehensive compilation of empirical ultrasonic properties of mammalian tissues. J Acoust Soc Am 1978; 64: 423-457.

5. Cartensen AL. Absorption of sound in tissues. NBS Spec Pub 525, Washington 1979; 29-36.

6. Duck FA, Hill CR. Mapping true ultrasonic backscatter and attenuation distribution in tissue - a digital reconstruction approach. NBS Spec Pub 525, Washington 1979; 247-251.

7. Johnson SA, Greenleaf JF, Rajagopalan B, Bahn RC, Baxter B, Christensen D. High spatial resolution ultrasonic measurement techniques for characterization of static and moving images. NBS Spec Pub 525, Washington 1979; 235-246.

8. Fields S, Dunn F. Correlation of echographic visibility of tissue with biological composition and physiological state. J Acoust Soc Am 1973; 54: 809-812.

9. Mimbs JW, Yuhas DE, Miller JG, Weiss AN, Sobel BE. Detection of myocardial infarction in vitro based on altered attenuation of ultrasound. Circ Res 1977; 41: 192-198.

10. Ishihara T, Ferrans VJ, Jones M, Boyce SW, Kawanami O,

human parietal pericardium. Am J Cardiol 1980; 46: 744-753.

11. Feigenbaum H. Echocardiography (third edition). Lea and Febiger. Philadephia. 1981

12. Ratliff F. Contour and contrast. Scientific American 1972; 226: 6-90-103.

13. Logan-Sinclair RB, Wong CM, Gibson DG. Clinical application of amplitude processing of echocardiographic images. Br Heart J 1981; 45: 621-627.

14. Tanaka M, Terasawa H. Echocardiography: evaluation of tissue character in myocardium. Jpn Heart J 1979; 43: 367-376.

TISSUE PARAMETER CHARACTERIZATION BY ULTRASOUND: STATE-OF-THE-ART IN CARDIOLOGY

T.D. Franklin, Jr., J.A. Brink, J.L. Cuddeback,
              N.T. Sanghvi, A.E. Weyman

Pulsed-reflected ultrasound has evolved during the past decade into a major non-invasive technique for imaging the dynamic anatomy of the heart and evaluating the velocity, direction and character of intravascular blood flow (1-3). Numerous clinical studies have repeatedly demonstrated the importance of this modality in the diagnostic evaluation of almost every type of cardiac disease from the rarest congenital disorder to the almost ubiquitous syndrome of mitral valve prolapse (1-3). At the more basic research level, several groups have attempted to extend the capabilities of ultrasonic diagnosis to the tissue level in order to develop an in vivo method for determining the ultrastructural basis for functional cardiac disease (4-16). This area of investigation, conventionally termed "tissue parameter characterization" seeks to define the nature of a particular organ or tissue system based on the changes which occur in a sound wave during its physical interaction with that tissue system. In the heart, primary interest has centered around the identification and differentiation of the normal from either the ischemic or infarcted myocardium. While ischemia has been the primary area of interest, there are also a variety of other cardiac structural abnormalities such as the infiltrative, hypertrophic and toxic cardiomyopathies; the various forms of myocarditis; and cardiac tumors and thrombi which offer fertile ground for similar types of studies.

General Methods of Waveform Analysis and Experimental
Models

There are two general approaches to the ultrasonic waveform analysis on which tissue characterization is based.
These include: 1) parametric analysis, in which a specific
characteristic of the sound wave such as its velocity, attenuation as a function of frequency or scattering properties
are measured and related directly to tissue structure, and
2) non-parametric analysis, which relies on pattern recognition and signal processing techniques similar to those used
in voice analysis to define the major spatial and statistical
features of individual waveforms and based on these features
to identify the tissue from which the signals arise (9,17-19).

The majority of studies, to date, have applied the parametric approach and focused on changes which occur in specific
characteristics of the sound wave as a result of its interaction with a tissue sample. Two primary experimental models
have been used in these studies: the transmission model
which examines the changes which occur in the sound wave
during its passage through a sample of myocardium and the
reflection model in which the total energy content or spectral
distribution of energies within the echoes reflected from a
tissue sample are analyzed. Figure 1 compares the experimental models used in transmission and reflection experiments.
In the experimental transmission model (Figures 1A & B) both
a transmitting and receiving transducer are immersed in a
water bath and an ultrasonic pulse is initially transmitted
between the two to define the free field system response.
A sample of unknown tissue is then placed between the two
transducers (B) and its effects on the ultrasonic waveform
measured. In the reflection model (Figure 1C & D) the same
transducer is used as both a transmitter and receiver.
Typically, the pulse is initially reflected off a glass
plate acting as a "perfect reflector" and the system response
of the transceiver measured (C). A piece of myocardium is
then inserted in place of the glass plate and an interro-
gating pulse transmitted into the heart muscle. The energy

154

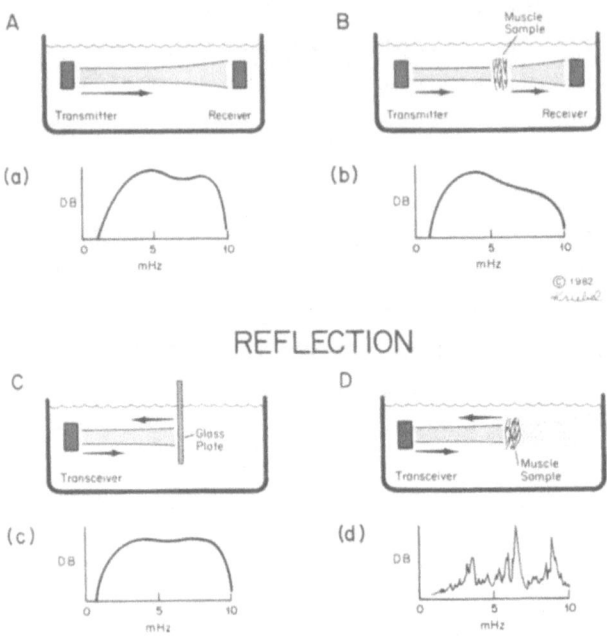

TRANSMISSION

A   B

(a)   (b)

REFLECTION

C   D

(c)   (d)

FIGURE 1   Series of diagrams illustrating the experimental models
used in tissue characterization. In the transmission
model (panels A & B) a transmitting and receiving transducer are initially immersed in a water bath (A).
A pulse is then transmitted from one to the other
to define the system response (a). An unknown sample
of tissue is then placed between the two transducers (B)
and the effects of this tissue sample on the sound
wave compared to the free field and system response (b).
In the reflection model, a single transducer is used
as both the transmitter and receiver (C & D). The
system response in this format is typically defined
using a glass plate or some other "perfect reflector"
(C). An unknown tissue sample is then insonated using
the pulsed echo format and the reflected or back
scattered signal from this sample is plotted as a
function of frequency and compared to that of the
perfect reflector.

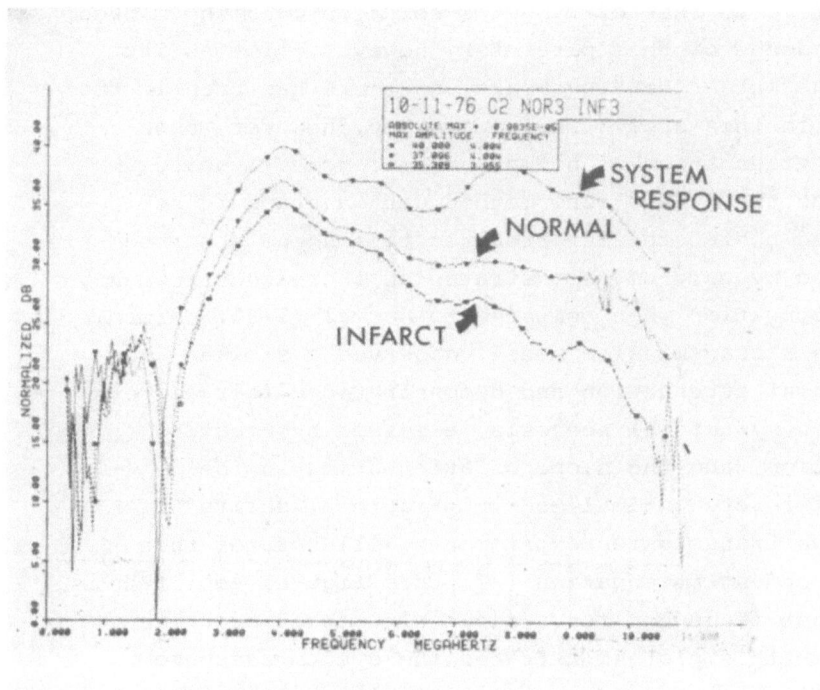

FIGURE 2   Transmission experiment in which the frequency-dependen
            attenuation of normal and infarcted myocardium is
            compared to the free field system response. In the
            uppermost plot, the normalized amplitude of the broad
            banded transducer/receiver pair is plotted against
            frequency. There is a relatively flat response from
            3 to 9 MHz. The middle curve illustrates the frequency
            dependent decrease in amplitude of the signal or
            attenuation which occurs when a sample of normal myo-
            cardium is placed between the transducer and receiver.
            The lower curve indicates the increase in attenuation
            produced when infarcted myocardium is substituted
            for the normal tissue.

to a level close to that of ringer's solution (4). The marked
angular dependence of this parameter, however, limited its
utility in the intact beating heart and there has been little
further work in this area. The same group, however, then
compared the attenuation of normal and infarcted myocardium
in vitro using the pulsed echo method with a standard reflector placed behind the interrogated tissue and observed
that infarcted myocardium demonstrated an increased frequency-
dependent attenuation when compared to normal (5-6). Mimbs,
et al., using a transmission model, observed a similar frequency-dependent attenuation and demonstrated a fair correlation between myocardial necrosis, assessed by creatine
kinase depletion, and the slope of attenuation in the
chronically-infarcted animal model. Figure 2, derived from
one of our own transmission experiments, illustrates this
frequency-dependent attenuation. In this figure, amplitude is
plotted against frequency for a range of 0 to 10 mHz. The
upper curve in this plot illustrates the system response
which, for this transducer/receiver pair is relatively flat
from a frequency of 3-9 mHz. The middle curve illustrates
the attenuation produced when a sample of normal myocardium
is placed in the path of the ultrasonic waveform. Normal
muscle produces attenuation of the signal at all frequencies,
but this is more marked in the higher frequency range. The
lower curve is produced by a sample of infarcted myocardium.
In this case, the overall attenuation is increased, but this
increase in attenuation is more marked in the higher frequency ranges.

A number of early studies of the basic interactions of
ultrasound with tissue suggested that protein, particularly
collagen, was an important determinant of ultrasonic attenuation in soft tissue (23,24). O'Donnell, et al., therefore,
examined the relationship of attenuation to increasing
collagen accumulation in the period from two to six weeks
following acute myocardial infarction (10). They observed
that while collagen was responsible for no more than 15% of
the attenuation observed in normal myocardium, it appeared

content of the reflected echoes can then be measured either absolutely, as a function of frequency (as indicated in the accompanying diagram), or relative to the signal from the perfect reflector. The majority of available data has been generated using the transmission model. Because of the obvious limitations of this method in in vivo studies, however, recent interest has focused primarily on the analysis of pulsed reflected signals.

Parametric Studies

Most experimental cardiac studies to date have utilized the ischemic canine model and examined changes in specific properties of the ultrasonic waveform which result from its interaction with the ischemic myocardium. These changes have then been correlated with sequential changes in myocardial structure during the evolution from acute ischemia to established scar. The major parameters studied include: a) the acoustic impedence which is the product of tissue density and sound velocity, b) attenuation, which is the loss of energy within the sound wave as it passes through tissue and is the result of absorption (conversion of sound energy into some other form of energy, i.e. heat) and scattering, and c) back scatter, which is the amount of energy that is reflected back along the path of the sound wave and can be measured by the transceiver. Scattering, in general, tends to be an omni-directional phenomenon with the result that the back scatter measurement reflects only a small, but presumably representative, portion of the total scattered energy. Both scatter and attenuation vary with frequency and their appropriate analysis requires a broad band transmitted pulse and the analysis of the reflected or transmitted energy as a function of frequency.

The initial application of these methods of analysis to the ischemic myocardium was by Lele, et al. who observed that the acoustic reflectance of infarcted myocardium was consistently lower than that of normal heart muscle, indicating that its characteristic acoustic impedence was lowered to be the major determinant of increased attenuation in regions of established myocardial infarction (10).

Finally, the variation in attenuation from the onset of acute ischemia to the phase of established infarction and scar was examined (25). In this series of studies, two distinct time-related patterns were observed. In the early phases of infarction (15 minutes to 24 hours) a slight decrease in attenuation was noted while in myocardium subjected to ischemic injury for three days or more, attenuation progressively increased. Thus, in the early stages of infarction, edema and cellular dissolution appear to decrease tissue density by dilution of protein constituents and, therefore, reduce attenuation and impedence. During the evolution from necrotic tissue to scar, however, attenuation gradually increases as the tissue collagen content increases and this is progressive overtime up to 11 weeks after infarction.

Since transmission techniques are not readily adaptable to in vivo studies, quantitative techniques for characterizing the echoes arising from within the myocardium, which are presumably scattered by the smaller tissue and muscle components, were needed. Several such methods have been developed or proposed. The first, "interrogated back scatter" measures the difference between the frequency average of the back scattered transfer function over the transducer band width from the interrogated tissue and is expressed in DB down from the back scatter obtained from a nearly perfect reflector.

Using these methods, O'Donnell, et al., demonstrated an increase in interrogated back scatter in the acute phases of myocardial infarction. Further studies in the chronic infarct preparation demonstrated significant increases with time after infarction which were related to the collagen content of the evolving scar tissue as well as to the organizational state of the structural protein.

Since scattering is one of the causes of attenuation, the increase in backscattered energy in chronic infarction is

consistent with the increased attenuation noted in transmission studies. The reported increase in back scatter in
the initial phases of ischemia when attenuation is decreasing is more difficult to reconcile. It may indicate that the
edema which is thought to reduce the magnitude of attenuation
by dilution of protein constituents may do so in a way which
leaves tissue ultrastructure, and hence, scattering, intact.
However, this remains uncertain.

An alternative approach to the analysis of back scatter
relies on the characteristic organizational patterns of normal
and pathologic tissue at the microscopic level. These organizational patterns are assumed to result in a characteristic and relatively consistent spacing of acoustically
different targets within the tissue which, when struck by an
acoustic wave, behave as a series of diffuse scatters due to
their small size relative to the ultrasonic wavelengths. The
small, regularly spaced scatterers can then be predicted
to produce interference patterns which depend quite specifically on the physical parameters (such as the spacings) of
the array. These interference patterns then cause wavelengths within the frequency spectrum of the beam which are
similar to the scatter spacing to be selectively reinforced
while others are subjected to phase cancellation. Ultrasound then may be used to determine the acoustical structure
of tissue based on the selective reinforcement of certain
frequencies when the Bragg scattering condition,

$$n\lambda = 2d \sin \theta,$$

where λ = ultrasonic wavelength
         n = number of wavelengths
         d = distance between scatters
         θ = angle from the horizontal to the
             scattered signal
is satisfied.

Using this concept, the tissue may be characterized by either
finding the frequency (λ) and then varying the angle or by

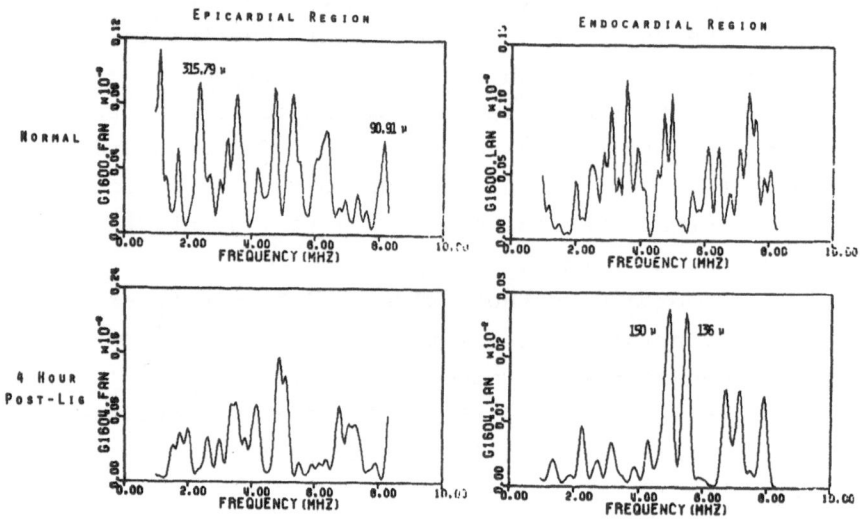

FIGURE 3   Frequency versus amplitude of plots of gated signals
            recorded from the subepicardial and subendocardial
            regions of the myocardium prior to and two hours post
            coronary ligation. Although multiple amplitude peaks
            are noted in each of these frequency domain plots,
            there is clear regularization and a tendency for
            selection of frequencies in the subendocardial window
            at two hours post ligation.

fixing the angle and sweeping the frequency so that differences in path length vary over a number of wavelengths.
Theoretically, either technique should yield a succession of
signal amplitude peaks whose spacing is indicative of the
targets internal structure. Figure 3 is an example which
illustrates the variability in frequency peaks arising from the
subendocardium and subepicardium prior to and two hours after
coronary artery ligation. These plots suggest how peaks occuring
at specific frequencies can be related to internal organ
structure. In this example, the frequency peaks recorded at
two hours post coronary ligation from the subendocardium

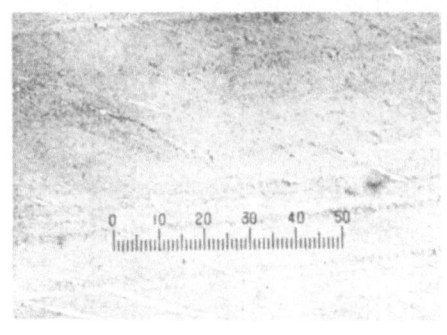

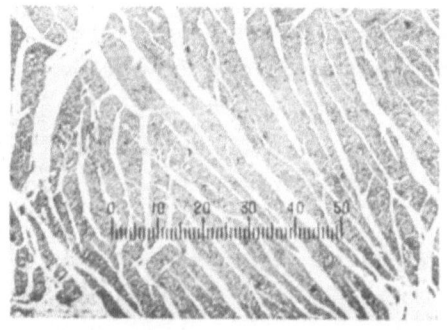

FIGURE 4   Histologic sections taken from the animal studied in
Figure 3. The upper section is derived from an area
of normal myocardium, while the lower panel is taken
from the subendocardium in the ischemic area. There
is a marked difference in the ultrastructural characteristics of the two samples suggesting that edema
within the myocardium may cause some separation of
interfaces there by enhancing the reflectivity and
order of the array.

correspond to wavelengths in the 150-180 µ range. These
distances appear to correspond to repetitive internal spacings between muscle bundles within ischemic tissue which may
separate into a series of regular reflectors due to edema
formation within the area of acute ischemia (Figure 4).

Problems Inherent in Quantitative Analysis

There are a number of problems inherent in quantitative
waveform analysis. These include variation in target

orientation relative to the incident sound wave, phase cancellation and in the _in vivo_ setting the effects of cardiac
and respiratory motion with resultant phasic variations in
the tissue path from the transceiver to the heart and in the
tissue itself. The angle between the target and the sound wave
affects both the amplitude of the reflected signal and its
Fourier transform. The amplitude of the signal diminishes
rapidly at off normal angles decreasing to 1/10 at 6° and
1/100 at 12° (26).

In addition to these absolute changes, variation in the
Fourier transform of the signal also occurs as a result of
phase cancellation due to variations in the path length
that must be traversed by different portions of the wave
from the transmitter and receiver. These can be, in part,
overcome by using a small receiving transducer thereby reducing
the effective beam width or utilizing an acoustoelectric receiver
which measures the net energy in the sound field and thus, is
not affected by distortions in phase. The effects of cardiac
and respiratory motion can, likewise, be controlled by gating
the transmitted pulse and sampling at a specific point in the
cardiac cycle during held respiration. Because of the
complexity of these problems, however, most studies have been
performed in an ideal experimental setting with strict control of sampling angle, optimization of transducer band
width and incorporation of methods to limit the effects of
phase cancellation. In the _in vivo_ setting further control
is necessary to overcome the effects of cardiac motion, and
cyclic changes in tissue perfusion, wall thickness and wall
stress.

Section D Non-Parametric Analysis

Non-parametric statistical analytic methods of waveform
analysis have been used by several groups to characterize
reflected signals from organs other than the heart (17,18,19).
Using these methods, success has been reported in differentiating waveforms arising from different organ systems as
well as in differentiating the normal from the pathologic
state in the same organ. We have recently completed a series
of studies designed to evaluate the ability of these non-

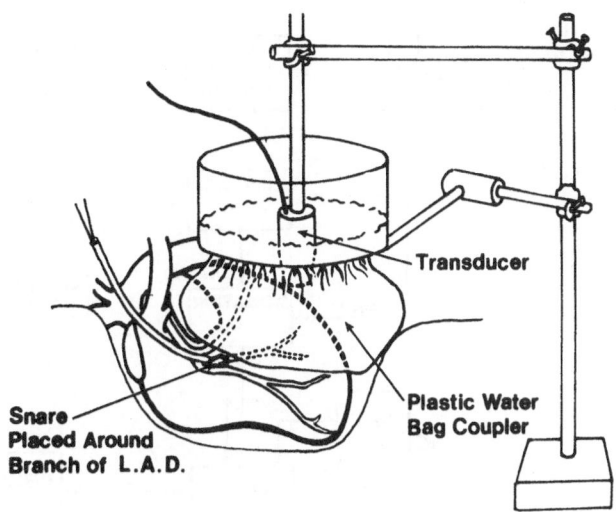

FIGURE 5   Experimental model used for in vivo waveform sampling
            from the acutely ischemic myocardium. In this model,
            the transducer is coupled to the anterior surface
            of the beating heart, using a polyethylene bag filled
            with ringer's solution. The bag is supported by a
            ring stand while the transducer is fixed in space
            so that sampling occurs from a constant area of myo-
            cardium within the ischemic region. The focal zone
            of the transducer is fixed within the heart muscle
            using a fixed distance focus pointer.

parametric statistical methods to characterize waveforms
arising in vivo from normal myocardium and on the basis of
this training experience, to distinguish unknown waveforms
as coming from either normal or acutely ischemic muscle. The
experimental model used in these studies is illustrated in
Figure 5. This model consists of an open-chested canine
preparation in which a pericardial cradle has been created
and the anterior wall of the left ventricle exposed. An
elongated snare is then placed around the left anterior
descending coronary artery or one of its major branches to
permit remote occlusion. A polyethylene bag filled with
ringer's solution and supported by a ring stand is then
placed lightly on the anterior surface of the left ventricle

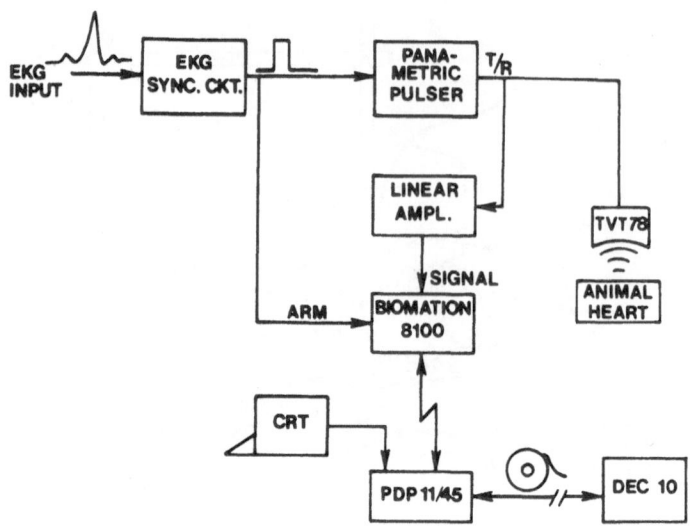

BLOCK DIAGRAM FOR HEART TISSUE CHARACTERIZATION IN VIVO

FIGURE 6   Block diagram of the system used for in vivo tissue
characterization and waveform analysis.   (See text
for details).

to permit coupling of the transducer with the beating heart.
The ultrasonic beam is then aligned such that the beam path
falls within the area of myocardium supplied by the ensnared
vessel and the focal zone of the beam is fixed within the
myocardium using a measured focus pointer.   Ultrasonic pulses
are then transmitted and recorded using the system diagrammed
in Figure 6.   This system consists of a broad banded lead
metaniobate transceiver focused at 84 ± 9 mm at half power
with the half power beam width of 1 mm at the focal point.
The center frequency of the transducer is 8 MHz with a fairly
flat amplitude response from 1 to 8 MHz.   The transceiver is
driven by a Panometrics 50/50 PR pulse receiver which is syn-
dhronized to an EKG trigger to limit recording to a predetermined point in the cardiac cycle.   During the experiments,
whole transmural RF, A-mode waveforms were sampled at 20 NS
intervals into 2048 data points with an 8 BIT amplitude resolution

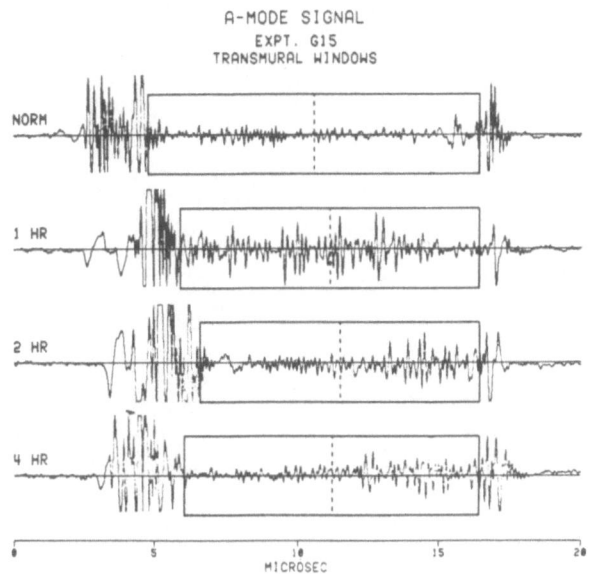

FIGURE 7   A-mode RF signals from the transmural myocardium
            obtained prior to and at one, two and four hours
            post coronary ligation. The subepicardial and
            subendocardial gates are fixed to exclude the specular
            reflections from the epicardium (left) and endo-
            cardium (right). An obvious change in the signal
            amplitudes from within the heart muscle can be
            appreciated between the different sampling periods.

and stored on a biomation 8100 transient recorder. Waveforms were
sampled from the same transmural pathway prior to and at 1,2, and
4 hours post-ligation. In initial experiments, 40 waveforms
were digitized at each of these sampling periods. However, in
later studies a larger data base of 100 waveforms was obtained
during each experimental period. Figure 7 illustrates representative whole transmural RF waveforms obtained from each of
these sampling periods in one experimental study. To eliminate
the specular reflections from the epicardial and endocardial
interfaces, subendocardial windows contain 256 data points
corresponding to a 4 mm tissue depth were manually selected
from each digitized A-mode waveform. The digitized RF data
for each window was then subjected to three transformations to
produce a normalized A-mode signal; a rectified A-mode signal;

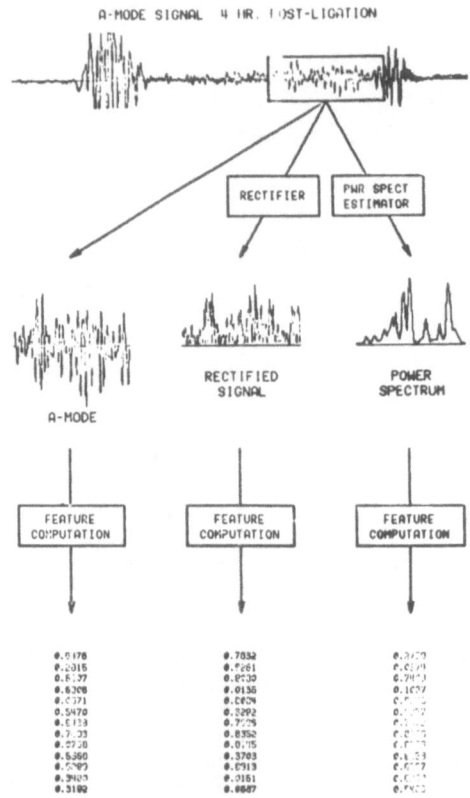

FIGURE 8   An illustration of the three transformations of the subendocardial window of the transmural RF waveform. The transformations include the normalized A-mode, the rectified A-mode and the power spectrum of the RF signal. Each transformation is then subjected to further statistical analysis based on the thirteen features described in Table 1.

and a frequency domain power spectrum. These three transformations were then used to compute three separate sets of 13 features intended to characterize the waveform of each windows ensemble. Figure 8 illustrates the three transformations of these waveforms while the 13 parameters are listed in Table 1. The thirteen features of each transformation were then submitted to a stepwise multivariate discriminate analysis program (SPSS) in order to compute the discriminate function which optimally distinguished the three post-ligation samples from the pre-ligation waveofrm (20,21,

22). Appendix A describes the theoretical basis of this classification routine.

In the multivariate analysis of each group of waveforms, half of the waveforms were randomly chosen as training samples and used for the computation of a discriminate function based on some subset of the 13 features. The remaining waveforms were then used as unknowns. The random selection of the training waveforms was performed twice per transformation of each window's A-mode data ensemble to ensure against spuriosities associated with the randomization. Finally, the computed discriminate function attempted to classify individual unknown waveforms as having originated from normal or ischemic tissue. A total of 7067 unknown waveforms were subjected to stepwise multivariate discriminate analysis. In this series of experiments, the accuracy with which the computed discriminate function could identify individual waveforms as having come from normal pre-ligation myocardium or from ischemic tissue, is listed in Table 2. The best classification accuracy (96.6%) was achieved using the rectified amplitude transformation. The results of the other 2 transformations, however, were not significantly different with the power spectrum transformation showing a 95% discriminate accuracy and the normalized amplitude signal proving accurate in 93%. The combined accuracy of all three transformations was 94.8%. During these studies a clear relationship was noted between the size of the training sample and the accuracy of the discriminate function. In early studies, where only 40 waveforms were used for the training group, accuracies varied from only 75-85%, while with a training group of 100 waveforms, the accuracy improved to greater than 98%.

We then attempted to determine whether the discriminate function improved with increasing time after ligation. These analyses suggested that there was little difference in classification ability between the normal and the one or two hour post-ligation periods, however, there was marked improvement in classification accuracy when the two and four hour post-

168

ligation periods were compared. Thus, 21 of 24, or 87.5% of
the data sets analyzed showed either the same or an increase
in the classification accuracy from the two to four hour post
ligation periods.

Finally, the relative importance of each feature to the
discriminate function was investigated for all subjects. The
results of this analysis are indicated in Table 3. The features
were ranked according to their frequency of participating and
their relative contribution to the discriminate function. It
was noteworthy that in the majority of cases, statistical
features played a more important role in the determination of
the discriminate function than did spatially-related amplitude
functions (D1-D4)* which presumably would be more closely
related to the parametric features such as integrated back
scatter discussed earlier.

These studies indicate that when multiple parameters are
independently utilized to define the most important features
of a group of waveforms, a waveform or signal signature can be
defined which can act as a discriminant function in determining
with surprising accuracy whether individual waveforms arise
from normal or ischemic tissue as early as one hour after
coronary occlusion. They also suggest that statistical
features of the ultrasonic signal, although non-quantitative
are better discriminators of these changes than are pure
amplitude-dependent parameters.

The uniformly optimistic results of these and other
studies suggest that there is sufficient change in an ultrasonic waveform during its interaction with a tissue system
to permit classification of the ultrastructural characteristics
of the tissue. The optimal method for characterizing these
changes, however, remains undefined and the translation of
results obtained in the optimized research setting to the
clinical environment is still a goal rather than a reality.

* See Table I

APPENDIX A

Stepwise Multivariate Discriminant Analysis

The 13 features representing the amplitude, rectified amplitude, and power spectrum waveforms were used to classify each sample waveform into groups (ensembles) representing a priori experimental conditions. The four groups represented the echocardiographic data of pre-ligation and 1, 2, and 4 hours post-ligation. Classification was made according to a linear discriminant function determined by the SPSS computer program for stepwise multivariate discriminant analysis.

Discriminant analysis involves one or more linear combinations of the features, the maximum number of combinations equal to either one less than the number of groups or the number of features, whichever is less. These discriminant functions are of the form:

$$Y_j = v_1 X_1 + v_2 X_2 + \ldots v_n X_n$$

where Y_j is the score of discriminant function j, $\underline{v}$ is the vector of weighting coefficients, $\underline{X}$ is a subset of the 13 features, and n is the number of features included in the stepwise discriminant function, j. Consider X_{ki}, the dependent vector variable for the ith waveform in the kth group; m, the grand centroid or total sample mean; and m_k, the centroid for group k. The matrix of weighted squares and cross-products of deviations of group centroids from the grand centroid will be deemed $\underline{B}$, for "between groups":

$$\underline{B} = \sum_{k=1}^{4} \sum_{i=1}^{N_k} (m_k - m)(m_k - m)^T$$

$$= \sum_{k=1}^{4} N_k (m_k - m)(m_k - m)^T$$

The matrix of squares and cross-products of deviations of waveforms from their group centroids, pooled over all groups, will be deemed $\underline{W}$, for "within groups" Tool

$$\underline{W} = \sum_{k=1}^{4} \sum_{i=1}^{N_k} (X_{ki} - m_k)(X_{ki} - m_k)^T$$

The sum-of-squares of Y for the kth group is denoted by $SS_k(Y)$, and realizing $v^T = v_1 \ v_2, \ v_3, \ \ldots \ v_{13}$, the within-group sum-of-squares of the transformed variable Y is:

$$SS_w(Y) = SS_1(Y) + SS_2(Y) + \ldots SS_k(Y)$$

$$= \underline{v}^T \underline{W} \ \underline{v}$$

Similarly, the between-groups sum-of-squares of the transformed variable Y is:

$$SS_b(Y) = \underline{v}^T \underline{B} \ \underline{v}$$

The ratio of the between-groups to within-groups sums-of-squares of the discriminant function score Y as a function of the vector of coefficients $\underline{v}$ is:

$$\frac{SS_b(Y)}{SS_w(Y)} = \frac{\underline{v}^T \underline{B} \ \underline{v}}{\underline{v}^T \underline{W} \ \underline{v}} = \lambda$$

This ratio, λ, is a criterion for measuring the group differentiation along the dimension specified by the vector, $\underline{v}$. The remaining step for discrimination is to maximize the criterion λ by establishing the optimum coefficient vector, $\underline{v}$. The partial derivative of λ with respect to each component v_i of $\underline{v}$ is taken, setting the result to zero.

$$\frac{\partial \lambda}{\partial \underline{v}} \frac{\underline{v}^T \underline{B} \ \underline{v}}{\underline{v}^T \underline{W} \ \underline{v}} = \frac{2[(\underline{B} \ \underline{v})(\underline{v}^T \underline{W} \ \underline{v}) - (\underline{v}^T \underline{B} \ \underline{v})(\underline{W} \ \underline{v})]}{(\underline{v}^T \underline{W} \ \underline{v})^2} = 0$$

$$= \frac{2[(\underline{B} \ \underline{v}) - (\lambda \ \underline{W} \ \underline{v})]}{\underline{v}^T \underline{W} \ \underline{v}}$$

$$= (\underline{B} - \lambda \underline{W}) \ \underline{v} = 0$$

Assuming that $\underline{W}^{-1}$ exists, multiplying both sides of the above equation by $\underline{W}^{-1}$:

$$(W^{-1} \underline{B} - \lambda \underline{I}) \underline{v} = 0$$

This is of the form:

$$(\underline{A} - \lambda \underline{I}) \underline{v} = 0,$$

the characteristic equation of $\underline{A}$. The solution is readily available, yielding eigenvalues λ_m and associated eigenvectors $\underline{v}_m$ of the matrix A. This solution insures either a maxima or a minima of the discriminant criteria λ, and should be proven to be a maxima with the second order derivative of λ with respect to $\underline{v}$ [21]. The discriminant function is thus completed, with the coefficients specified by vector $\underline{v}$.

TABLE 1

The 13 features used to characterize ultrasound signals reflected from myocardial tissue were computed for the amplitude, rectified, and power transformations of the digitized A-mode signal corresponding to subepi- or subendocardial tissue segments.

1. The first four central moments of the transformed signal (M1, M2, M3, M4);

2. The four spatial distribution measures the signal weights within each quarter of the data window (D1, D2, D3, D4);

3. The skewness and kurtosis of the sample probability density function (SK, KU);

4. The eigenvolume and eigenratio of the joint sample density function of all pairs of successive data values within the data window (EV, ER); and

5. A measure of the range between the likelihood of the most- and least-probable sequence of three data values within the data window (RT).

TABLE 2

Classification Accuracy of Three Transformations

of 13 A-mode Data Sets Taken from Nine Dogs

(Percentages reflect number of intra-subject unknown waveforms

classified correctly)

Transformation	Total Number Correct Waveforms	Percent Correct
Amplitude	2361/2540	93.0
Rectified	2439/2526	96.6
Power Spectrum	2414/2541	95.0
TOTAL	7214/7607	94.8

Table 3 : To study the relative importance of each feature: (A) the frequency with which each feature displays greater than 90 percent relative contribution; (B) the frequency of participation in a discriminant function; and (C) the average relative contribution (percent) are tabulated for each feature per transformation across 68 different classifications for all subjects.

Transformation	Criteria	Features												
		M1	M2	M3	M4	D1	D2	D3	D4	SK	KU	EV	ER	RT
AMPLITUDE	A	8	2	6	1	4	2	—	4	2	4	37	14	—
	B	36	30	36	30	23	31	20	29	35	52	53	41	35
	C	28.1	16.8	28.5	16.2	20.4	14.5	12.3	20.3	14.6	27.9	61.5	44.6	12.5
RECTIFIED	A	16	4	5	1	8	—	5	6	12	2	19	7	1
	B	43	43	34	40	30	34	36	30	46	38	42	34	39
	C	41.4	24.5	25.9	19.1	24.2	15.0	22.2	26.8	35.0	23.8	43.0	32.8	8.4
POWER SPECTRUM	A	21	5	15	2	19	1	3	6	7	6	4	—	1
	B	61	41	39	39	41	31	30	30	36	30	41	49	33
	C	51.4	30.4	45.6	25.0	44.3	20.8	16.5	26.0	27.4	24.6	25.6	17.8	6.8

References

1. Weyman AE. 1982. Cross-Sectional Echocardiography, Philadelphia, Lea & Febiger.

2. Feigenbaum H. 1981. Echocardiography, 3rd edition, Philadelphia, Lea & Febiger.

3. Hatle L, Angelsen B. 1981. Doppler Ultrasound in Cardiology - Physical Principles and Clinical Applications. The Foundation of Scientific and Industrial Research at the Norwegian Institute of Technology, May.

4. Lele PP and Namery J. 1972. Detection of myocardial infarction by ultrasound. IN: Proceedings of ACEMB, Americana Hotel, Bal Harbour, FL p. 135.

5. Lele PP, Mansfield AB, Murphy AI, Namery J and Senapati N. 1976. Tissue characterization by ultrasonic frequency-dependent attenuation and scattering. IN: Ultrasonic Tissue Characterization, M. Linzer ed., NBS Spec. Publ. No. 435, U.S. Government Printing Office, Washington, D.C., p. 153.

6. Lele PP and Senapati N. 1977. Chapter 3 - The frequency spectra of energy backscattered and attenuated by normal and abnormal tissue. IN: Recent Advances in Ultrasound in Biomedicine, Vol. 1, DN White, ed., Research Studies Press, Forest Grove, OR, p. 55-85.

7. Mimbs JW, Yuhas DE, Miller JG, Weiss AN and Sobel BE. 1977. Detection of myocardial infarction in vitro based on altered attenuation of ultrasound. Circ Res 41(2):192.

8. Miller JG, O'Donnell M, Mimbs JW and Sobel BE. 1977. Ultrasonic attenuation in normal and ischemic myocardium. Presented at the 2nd International Symposium on Ultrasonic Tissue Characterization, June 13-15, National Bureau of Standards, Gaithersburg, MD.

9. Franklin TD, Sanghvi NT, Fry FJ, Egenes KM and Weyman AE. 1977. Ultrasonic tissue characterization studies of ischemic and infarcted myocardium. Presented at the 2nd International Symposium on Ultrasonic Tissue Characterization, June 13-15, National Bureau of Standards, Gaithersburg, MD.

10. O'Donnell M, Mimbs JW and Miller JG. 1979. The relationship between collagen and ultrasonic attenuation in myocardial tissue. J Acoust Soc Am 65(2):512.

11. O'Donnell M, Mimbs JW, Sobel BE and Miller JG. 1977. Ultrasonic attenuation of myocardial tissue - dependence on time after excision and on temperature. J Acoust Soc Am 62(4): 1054, October.

12. O'Donnell M, Bauwens D, Mimbs JW and Miller JC. 1979. In vivo detection of acute myocardial ischemia in the dog by quantitative ultrasonic backscatter. IN: Proceedings of 4th Intl. Symposium on Ultrasonic Imaging and Tissue Characterization. NBS, Gaithersburg, MD, June 18-20, p 9.

13. Mimbs JW, O'Donnell M, Bauwens D, Miller JG and Sobel BE. 1979. Characterization of the evolution of myocardial infarction by ultrasonic backscatter. Circulation 60(4): II-17, October.

14. Bauwens D, O'Donnell M, Miller JG and Mimbs JW. 1979. Detection of acute myocardial ischemic in vivo with quantitative backscatter. Circulation 60(4):II-17, October.

15. Joynt LF. 1979. A stochastic approach to ultrasonic tissue characterization. Ph.D. Thesis, Dept. of Electrical Engineering, Stanford University, Stanford, CA. Prepared under NIH Grant 5P50-GM17940, June.

16. O'Donnell M, Mimbs JW and Miller JG. 1981. Relationship between collagen and ultrasonic backscatter in myocardial tissue. J Acoust Soc Am 69(2):580, February.

17. Preston K, Czerwinski MJ, Skolnik JL and Leb DE. 1979. Recent developments in obtaining histopathological information from ultrasound tissue signatures. IN: Ultrasonic Tissue Characterization II. M. Linzer ed., NBS Spec. Publ. No. 525, U.S. Government Printing Office, Washington, D.C., p 303.

18. Czerwinski MG. 1976. Quantitative ultrasonic signal analysis. M.S. Thesis, Dept. of Electrical Engineering, Carnegie-Mellon University, Pittsburg, September.

19. Lerski RA, Smith MJ, Morley P, Barnett E, Mills PR, Watkinson G and MacSween RNM. 1981. Discriminant analysis of ultrasonic texture data in diffuse alcoholic liver disease. Ultrasonic Imaging 3:164, April.

20. Nie NH, Hall CH, Jenkins JG, Steinbrenner K and Bent DH. 1975. Statistical Package for the Social Sciences, New York, McGraw-Hill.

21. Cooley WW and Lohnes PR. 1971. Multivariate Data Analysis, New York, John Wiley and Sons, Inc.

22. Tatsuoka MM. 1971. Multivariate Analysis: Techniques for Educational and Psychological Research, New York, John Wiley and Sons, Inc.

23. Field S and Dunn F. 1973. Correlation of echographic visualizability of tissue with biologic composition and physiologic state. J Acoust Soc Am 54: 809.

24. O'Brien WD. 1977. Role of collagen in determining ultrasonic propagation properties in tissue. Acoust. Hologr 7: 37.

25. O'Donnell M, Mimbs JW, Sobel BE and Miller JG. 1979. Ultrasonic attenuation in normal and ischemic myocardium. IN: Ultrasonic Tissue Characterization II, M. Linzer, ed., National Bureau of Standard, Spec. Publ. No. 525, U.S. Government Printing Office, Washington, D.C.

26. Howry DN. 1957. Techniques used in ultrasonic visualization of soft tissue. IN: Ultrasound in Biology and Medicine, E. Kelly, ed., (American Instit. of Biologic Science, Washington, D.C.).

Anatomical Profile and Evaluation of the
Left Ventricular Function in Hypertrophic Cardiomyopathy
by 2-dimensional Echocardiography

G. BIAMINO, U. SCHWIETZER and M. SCHARTL
Kardiopneumologische Abteilung Klinikum Steglitz, FU Berlin

The hypertrophic cardiomyopathy (HCM) may be a heredo-familial disorder and is probably connected with a genetic defect on the basis of
either a mendalian dominant or an autosomal-dominant trait with almost
complete penetrance (1,2). A typical pathological characteristic of this
disease is a hypertrophy of myocardial fibres. The distribution of hypertrophy regarding the left ventricle always includes the interventricular
septum (3,4,5,6). In the case of an obstruction of the left ventricular
outflow tract a displacement of the anterior papillary muscle' is present.
Until the clinical introduction of the M-mode echocardiography an objective diagnosis could only be made by hemodynamic measurements in connection with angiocardiography. The non-invasive echocardiographic technique
has been used as a safe and convenient tool and has played a major role
in current progress in knowledge of hypertrophic cardiomyopathy (HCM).
In addition to non specific signs, related to the hypertrophic state,
typical M-mode patterns were introduced to define HOCM (fig. 1):

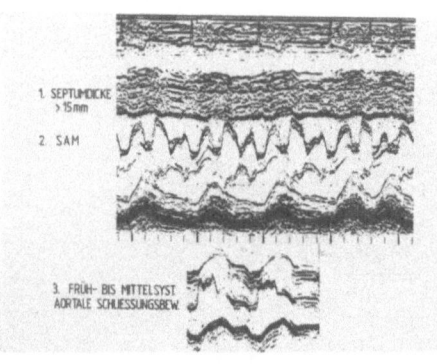

FIGURE 1:
Typical signs for HOCM in
M-mode recordings.

1. thickness of the interventricular septum ranging over 15 mm; 2. systolic anterior movement (SAM) of parts of the mitral valve apparatus;
3. midsystolic closure movement of the aortic valve; 4. a thickness ratio
septum to left ventricular posterior wall larger than 1.3.

Subsequent reports have demonstrated, that the sensitivity of M-mode is high for these signs, however the degree of specificity is not reliable enough. For instance a marked hypertrophy of the ventricular wall occurs also in arterial hypertension and aortic valve stenosis. Furthermore, the right sided endocardial delimitation of the interventricular septum often appears blurred so that the evaluation of thickness depends on the subjective setting of the time-gain-compensation. In consequence this value is not necessarily reliable in predicting the presence or magnitude of left ventricular outflow tract obstruction. It has moreover been shown, that an obstruction of the left ventricular outflow tract can occur in the absence of a symmetric septal hypertrophy as well as a systolic anterior movement of parts of the mitral valve sustaining apparatus (7,8,9,10,11,12,13,14). On the other hand this M-mode finding has been observed in the case of HCM without measurable left ventricular gradient (7,15). Finally recent data suggest that the incidence of the midsystolic closure in HOCM is with 40% not high (16). The 2-dimensional sector scan echocardiography allows dynamic images of the heart in multiple cross sectional planes, integrating various elements of single dimensional echocardiography in a spatial orientation. The aim of this study was to analyse whether the use of 2-D echo gives a better qualitative and quantitative diagnosis of HCM. Particularly the anatomical localisation of the intraventricular obstruction was to be compared to the hemodynamic measured pressure gradient. Furthermore, this study was to contribute to the understanding of the mechanism of SAM and its relation to the degree of obstruction.

Methods

32 patients with the suspected diagnosis of HCM on the basis of clinical, electrocardiographic, phonocardiographic and M-mode signs were examined using 2-DE. The patients were studied in the supine and/or lateral position, using a real time phased array sector scanner (RT 400 Roche, 80°). In connection with an Irex II system simultaneous recordings of one or two M-mode echos were possible. Images were recorded on 3/4 inch reel-to-reel video tape (Umatic system). The analysis of the stored images was performed during play back in real time and/or by frame to frame. With the help of a 35 mm camera single frame photographs of the video monitor were taken.

Study procedure

The 2-DE analysis included the following standard planes: 1. parasternal position: the long axis, the short axis at the level of the left
ventricular outflow tract as well as of the mitral valve and the papillary muscle; 2. apical position: 4-chamber view and left ventricular
long axis; 3. subcostal position: 4-chamber view.

Results

The early to midsystolic starting abnormal anterior motion of parts
of the mitral valve apparatus is a frequent to nearly constant finding
in patients with HOCM in the presence of a pressure gradient at rest. It
has been used to evaluate and estimate the severity of left ventricular
outflow tract obstruction (17). Other reports could not confirm these
results. Nevertheless, an explanation of the M-mode shape of SAM particularly in regard to its late systolic return in direction to its initial
position is not well understood. In our study we observed in 75% of the
cases a SAM. A clear analysis of this movement is only possible in the
parasternal long axis view. The variability of the pattern in 2-DE is
so large, that only a general description of this phenomenon is possible.

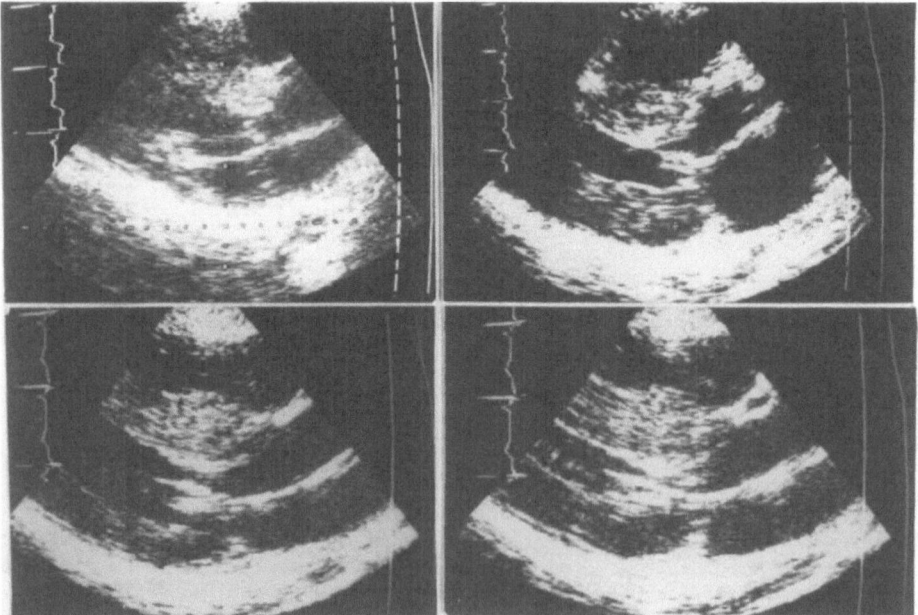

FIGURE 2: Different patterns of SAM in patients with HOCM, long axis
view. The last two pictures show different phases of one ejection period.
(time interval 160 msec)

Neither duration nor degree of SAM correlate with the severity of obstruction. As earlier studies have postulated the SAM is the resultant of the
anterior displacement of the chordae tendineae, edges of the papillary
muscle on the one side and/or of the anterior mitral leaflet on the other
side. Different theories have been discussed: 1. the Venturi effect
(18,19); 2. a vigorous contraction of the posterior basal left ventricular wall, forcing the anterior and posterior mitral leaflet into the
left ventricular outflow tract (20,21,22). A third hypothesis (23,24,25)
corresponds to our experience in this study and demands a hypertrophy
of the interventricular septum, connected with a malalignment of the
anterior papillary muscle (fig. 3).

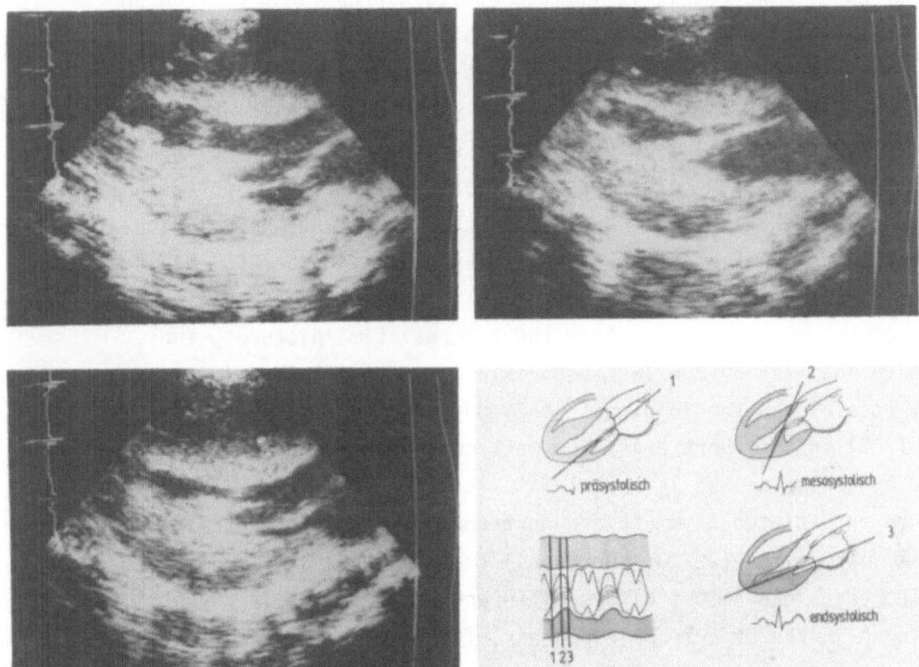

FIGURE 3:
Early, mid and late systolic displacement of the papillary muscle
(for details see text).

Directly after the beginning of the ejection period the papillary muscle changes its axis to an anterior superior position displacing the region of attachment of the chordae tendineae to the free edge of the mitral valve. The late systolic posterior directed movement of SAM may be connected with the late systolic emptying of the apical part of the left ventricle. This event leads to a change of the axis of the papillary muscle from the anterior superior to the initial posterior superior direction. Consequently the top of the papillary muscle tilts to the back so that the SAM structures are displaced in the posterior direction, away from the transducer.

One dimensional echocardiography has focused attention on some aspects of HOCM. However, it is limited by its narrow field of view and lack of spatial orientation. In contrast, biplane angiography allows a visualisation of ventricular walls but does not permit an adequate assessment of the dynamic abnormalities of ventricular walls and valves (20,18,27,28,29,26,30,31). Because of its tomographic character the 2-D technique offers the unique possibility to analyse in a spatial way the contraction behaviour of the walls to each other and the relationship between the walls and the valves. This delineation of HOCM has been increased by the technical improvement, which permits the selective recordings of one or two M-modes from the 2-D real time pictures. The qualitative analysis of the left ventricle with the 2-D technique was not only possible in the long axis (85%) but also in a satisfactory percentage (70%) in the short axis. The most comprehensive results were obtained by analysing the left ventricle in the apical views. In our experience an isolated asymmetric hypertrophy of the interventricular septum is less common (12% of our cases) than has been stressed in previous studies, since almost always different parts of the left ventricle are included in the hypertrophic process. This fact comes to be especially evident in the apical 4-CV, as demonstrated in fig. 4 and 5.

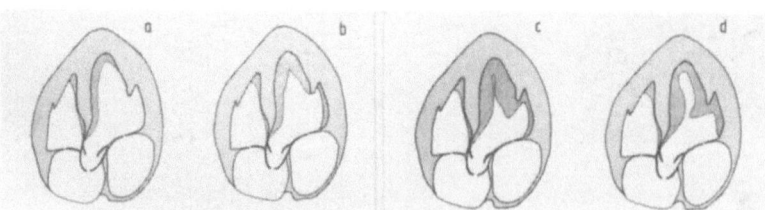

FIGURE 4: Schematic variations of HCM

This schema emphasizes that, besides the almost obligatory hypertrophy of the interventricular septum, the apical areas of the left ventricle are also often involved.

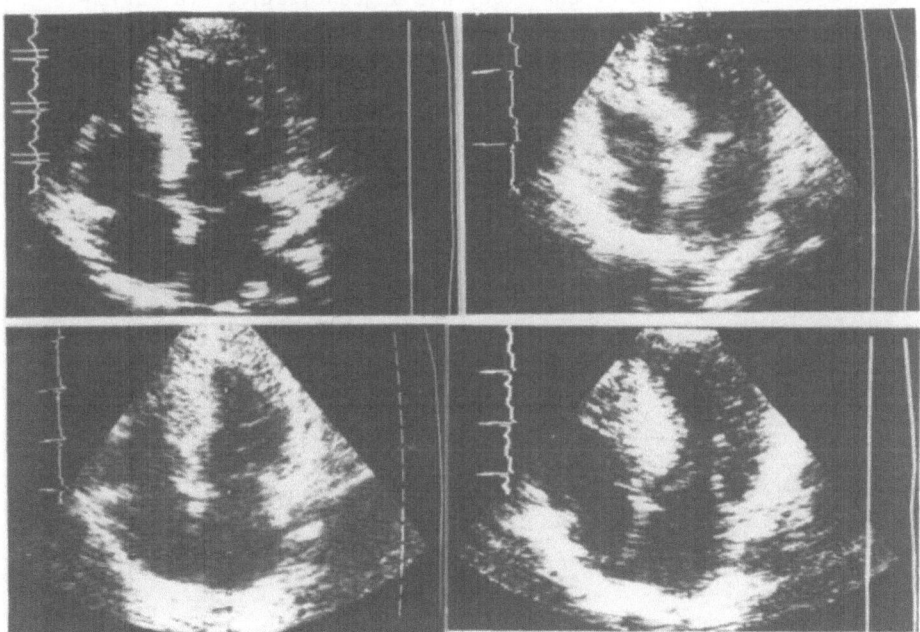

FIGURE 5:   4-CV in HCM

The qualitative analysis of the 4-CV demonstrated, that not the displacement of the mitral valve apparatus into the LVOT but obviously much more the existence of a both hypertrophic and anatomically malorientated papillary muscle is the basic requirement for the development of a intraventricular pressure gradient. The hypertrophic papillary muscle narrows dynamically the reduced intraventricular cavity in an hour-glass fashion and in that way determines the pressure gradient. However, it is not possible to estimate the extend of the hemodynamically measured pressure gradient from such pictures. The reason for this lack of correlation lies in the anatomical substratum of the relatively often observed global hypertrophy of the left ventricle. In such cases an hour-glass narrowing of the left ventricular outflow tract is not observed in systole, but a nearly complete occlusion of the distal and apical parts of the left ventricle. This contraction pattern provokes pressure gradients measurable during heart catheterisation.

Our studies confirm the extreme variability of the anatomical pictures of this disease. In our opinion the presence of an obstruction only depends on the coincidental distribution of hypertrophy so that a strict differentiation between HOCM and non obstructive forms of cardiomyopathy can not be reliably made. One aim of our study was a quantitative evaluation of the contraction pattern of the left ventricle in HCM. The computerized evaluation of the left ventricle function shows, that in comparison to normals the investigated patients with HCM have both smaller endsystolic and enddiastolic diameters in the long axis view, whereas the fractional shortening is usually higher than normal ones (fig. 6).

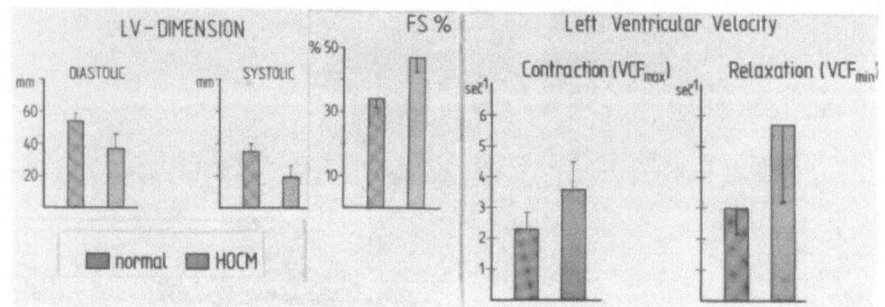

FIGURE 6: FS%, min. and max. V_{CF} of the LV in HCM in comparison to normals.

On the basis of the 4-CV the calculated volumes of the HCM patients were rather low ranging around 70 ml enddiastolic and 25 ml endsystolic, with a resulting ejection fraction of 65%. The mean V_{CF} values as well as the maximal contraction and relaxation velocity calculated from M-mode recordings were increased in patients with HCM (fig. 6). The segmental analysis of the left ventricle is made more difficult and in several cases impossible because of the banana like configuration of the left ventricle. As a consequence it is not possible to establish the maximal long axis of the left ventricle in systole and diastole, which would be a basic requirement for a superposition of the systolic and diastolic silhouette of the left ventricle.

Conclusions

The introduction of the 2-DE has stimulated the investigation of HCM and is still playing a major role in the current progress of knowledge of this disease. The possibility to scan large segments of the heart in its dynamic function enables the observer to integrate the

different views to an almost complete spatial picture of the left ventricle. This very sophisticated possibility of a qualitative analysis
unfortunately does not lead to a corresponding quantitative evaluation
of the intraventricular pressure gradient, and also does not permit a
segmental assessment of the left ventricular function which could give
a general evaluation of the degree of this disease.

REFERENCES

1. Emanuel R, Withers R , O'Brien K: Dominant and recessive modes of
    inheritance in idiopathic cardiomyopathy. Lancet 2:1065, 1971.

2. Henry WL, Clark CE, Epstein SE: Asymmetric septal hypertrophy
    (ASH): The unifying link in the IHSS disease spectrum. Observation
    regarding its pathogenesis , pathophysiology and course. Circu-
    lation 47:827, 1973

3. Olsen EGJ: Cardiomyopathies. In Edwards JE and Brest AW, Eds.,
    Clinical-pathologic Correlations 1, Cardiovascular Clinics,
    Philadelphia, 1972, F.A. Davis Company, 4:240.

4. Teare D: Asymmetrical hypertrophy of the heart in young adults,
    Br Heart J 20:1, 1958.

5. Olsen EGJ: Morbid anatomy and histology in hypertrophic obstruc-
    tive cardiomyopathy. In Hypertrophic Obstructive Cardiomyopathy,
    Wolstenholme GEW and O'Connor M, Eds., London, 1971, Ciba Foun-
    dation Study Group No. 37, J. & A. Churchill, p. 183.

6. Davies MJ, Pomerance A, Teare RD: Pathological features of hyper-
    trophic obstructive cardiomyopathy (HOCM), J Clin Pathol 27:529,
    1975.

7. Chahine RA, Raizner AE, Ishimori T, Montero AC: Echocardiographic,
    haemodynamic, and angiographic correlations in hypertrophic cardio-
    myopathy. Br Heart J 39:945-953, 1977.

8. Criley JM, Lennon PA, Abbasi AS, Blaufuss AH: Hypertrophic cardio-
    myopathy. In Clinical Cardiovascular Physiology, Levine HJ, Ed.,
    New York, Grune & Stratton, 1976, p. 771.

9. Raizner AE, Chahine RA, Ishimori T, Awdeh MR: The clinical corre-
    lates of left ventricular cavity obliteration. Am J Cardiol 40:
    303-309, 1977.

10. Rossen RM, Goodman DJ, Ingham RE, Popp RL: Echocardiographic
    criteria in the diagnosis of idiopathic hypertrophic subaortic
    stenosis. Circulation 50:747-751, 1974.

11. Feizi O, Emanuel R: Echocardiographic spectrum of hypertrophic
    cardiomyopathy. Br Heart J 37:1286-1302, 1975.

12. Roy P, Tajik AJ, Giuliani ER, Gau GT: An unusual case of idio-
    pathic hypertrophic subaortic stenosis. Mayo Clin Proc 51:159-162,
    1976.

13. Come PC, Bulkley BH, Goodman ZD, Hutchins GM, Pitt B, Fortuin NJ: Hypercontractile cardial states simulating hypertrophic cardiomyopathy. Circulation 55:901-908, 1977.

14. Mintz GS, Kotler MN, Segal BL, Parry WR: Systolic anterior motion of the mitral valve in the absence of asymmetric septal hypertrophy. Circulation 57:256-263, 1978.

15. King JF, DeMaria AN, Miller RR, Hilliard GK, Zelis R, Mason DT: Markedly abnormal mitral valve motion without simultaneous intraventricular pressure gradient due to uneven mitral septal contact in idiopathic hypertrophic subaortic stenosis. Am J Cardiol 34: 360-366, 1974.

16. Chahine RA, Raizner AE, Nelson J, Winters WL, Miller RR, Luchi RJ: Mid systolic closure of aortic valve in hypertrophic cardiomyopathy. Am J Cardiol 43:17-23, 1979.

17. Maron BJ, Epstein SE: Hypertrophic cardiomyopathy. Recent observations regarding the specificity of three hallmarks of the disease: asymmetric septal hypertrophy, septal disorganization and systolic anterior motion of the anterior mitral leaflet. Am J Cardiol 45: 141-154, 1980.

18. Henry WL, Clark CE, Griffith JM, Epstein SE: Mechanism of left ventricular outflow obstruction in patients with obstructive asymmetric septal hypertrophy (idiopathic hypertrophic subaortic stenosis). Am J Cardiol 35:337, 1975.

19. Wigle ED, Adelman AG, Silver MD: Pathophysiological considerations in muscular subaortic stenosis. In Hypertrophy Obstructive Cardiomyopathy, Wolstenholme GEW, O'Connor M, Eds., London, J & A Churchill, 1971, p 63.

20. Criley JM, Lennon PA, Basi AS, Blaufuss AH: Hypertrophic cardiomyopathy. In Clinical Cardiovascular Physiology, Levine HJ, Ed., New York, Grune & Stratton, 1976, p 771.

21. Criley JN, Lewis KB, White RI Jr, Ross RS: Pressure gradients without obstruction. A new concept of "hypertrophic subaortic stenosis". Circulation 32:881, 1965.

22. White RI Jr, Criley JM, Lewis KB, Ross RS: Experimental production of intracavitary pressure differences. Possible significance in the interpretation of human hemodynamic studies. Am J Cardiol 19: 806, 1967.

23. King JF, Reis RL, Bolton MR, DeMaria AN, Zelis R, Mason DT: Superior-to-inferior septal hypertrophy in IHSS: the fundamental determinant of obstruction. (abstr) Circulation 48 (suppl IV): IV-6,1973.

24. Reis RL, Bolton MR, King JF, Pugh DM, Dunn MI, Mason DT: Anteriorsuperior displacement of anterior papillary muscle (APM) producing obstruction and mitral regurgitation in IHSS: operative relief by posterior-medial realignment of APM following ventricular septal myectomy. Circulation 48 (suppl IV): IV-74, 1973.

25. King JF, DeMaria AN, Reis RL, Bolton MR, Dunn MI, Mason DT: Echocardiographic assessment of idiopathic hypertrophic subaortic stenosis. Chest 64:723, 1973.

26. Flamm MD, Harrison DC, Hancock EW: Muscular subaortic stenosis: prevention of outflow obstruction with propranolol. Circulation 38: 846, 1968.

27. Roelandt J: The cardiomyopathies. In Practical Echocardiology, White D, Ed., Forest Grove, Oregon, Research Studies Press, 1977, pp 187-200.

28. Popp RL: Echocardiographic assessment of cardiac disease. Circulation 54:538, 1976.

29. Tajik AJ, Giuliani ER: Echocardiographic observations in idiopathic hypertrophic subaortic stenosis. Mayo Clin Proc 49:89, 1974.

30. Adelman AG, McLoughlin MJ, Marquis Y, Auger P, Wigle ED: Left ventricular cineangiographic observations in muscular subaortic stenosis. Am J Cardiol 24:689, 1969.

31. Redwood DR, Scherer JL, Epstein SE: Biventricular cineangiography in the evaluation of patients with asymmetric septal hypertrophy. Circulation 49:1116, 1974.

NEW ECHOCARDIOGRAPHIC POSSIBILITIES IN THE ETIOLOGICAL
DIAGNOSIS AND THERAPY OF PERICARDIAL DISEASES
IVO CIKES

A number of articles have proven echocardiography as the
most reliable, safest and simplest method currently available
in evaluating patients with pericardial effusion (1-6). It has
obvious advantages over other techniques because of its noninvasive nature, high sensitivity, possibility of bedside examination and repeatability.

Although a conclusive diagnosis may be obtained in a few
minutes, to avoid false positive and false negative diagnosis,
some technical and anatomical pitfalls must be recognised (3-6).
However, with the considerable experience and skill of the
examiner, the incidence of false positive and false negative
studies is extremely low.

Good axial resolution makes M-mode echocardiography superior in qualitative diagnosis (pericardial thickening, small
effusion, constrictive hemodynamics). Two-dimensional echocardiography providing multiple cross-section planes of the
entire pericardial sac and surrounding structures is superior in assessing the amount, distribution and loculation of
pericardial fluid and particularly in avoiding diagnostic
pitfalls. As neither M-mode nor two-dimensional echocardiography provide reliable criteria for the diagnosis of cardiac
tamponade and constrictive pericarditis, they still remain
clinical and hemodynamic diagnoses (4-6).

Until recently, in pericardial diseases echocardiography
was limited to the detection of pericardial effusion and rough
semiquantitation of the pericardial fluid. Lately, further
advances have been made in the echocardiographic evaluation
of patients with pericardial diseases. It has been shown
that this technique can provide data about the pathology of

pericardial lesion. These data may help in making clinical decisons in patients with pericardial diseases. Furthermore, under echocardiographic guidance some diagnostic and therapeutic procedures such as pericardiocentesis, percutaneous pericardial biopsy and pericardial fenestration can be performed.

Intrapericardial Masses

In patients with pericardial effusion frequent findings at autopsy are pericardial adhesions, pericardial fibrinous deposits and tumorous infiltrations. Until recently these structures could not be detected in vivo. Using two-dimensional echocardiography it was shown that echo-producing structures within the pericardial sac could be visualised (7-15). In four series, 18 out of 39 described patients had surgical or autopsy findings which corresponded well with those described by echocardiography (7,9,11-15).

Over the last four and a half years we have found intra-pericardial masses in 19 patients with pericardial effusion of various etiology (7,8,10,12,13,15) (Fig. 1). They were presented as bridging bands extending from the epicardium to the pericardium, freely vibrating bands attached only to the pericardium or epicardium and shaggy or lumpy structures on the epicardial and/or pericardial surface (Fig. 2). Tumorous masses in patients with primary or metastatic pericardial tumours were presented as cauliflower-like or bizarre masses protruding from the pericardium into the pericardial sac. (Fig. 3). In patients with bridging intrapericardial bands suggested loculation of pericardial fluid can be confirmed by the lack of postural fluid redistribution or by contrast study with rapid instillation of 2-5 ml of sterile saline or pericardial fluid itself (6,13). It is much more difficult to image intrapericardial masses with the M-mode technique (Fig. 4).

The echocardiographic finding of intrapericardial masses improves our understanding of the pathology of underlying lesions and they may be relevant in solving clinical problems

190

in patients with pericardial effusion.

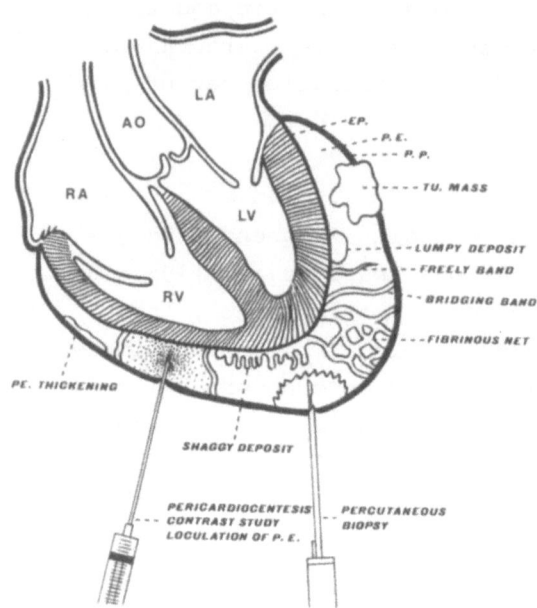

Fig. 1. Schematic presentation of echo-producing masses within pericardial space detected by two-dimensional echocardiography. Ep = epicardium, Pp = parietal pericardium.

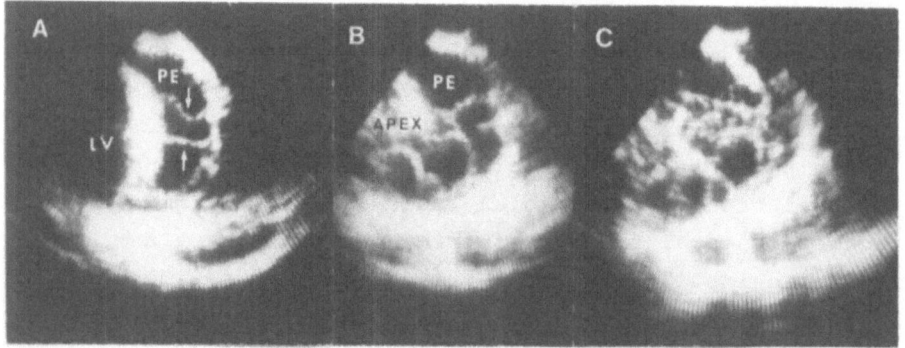

Fig. 2. A. Cross-section of the left ventricle (LV) at the level of chordae tendineae showing bridging bands (arrows) extending from epicardium to parietal pericardium. B. Section at apical level with adhesive bands dividing pericardial sac into few compartments. C. Section below cardiac apex showing impressive adhesive net in pericardial sac.

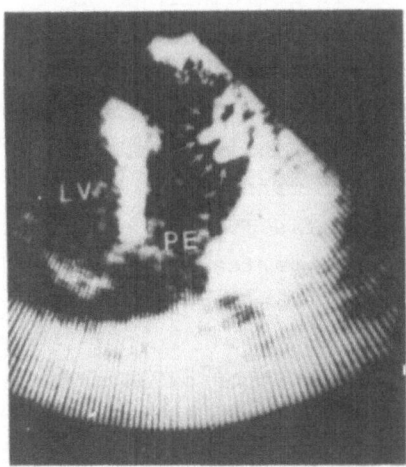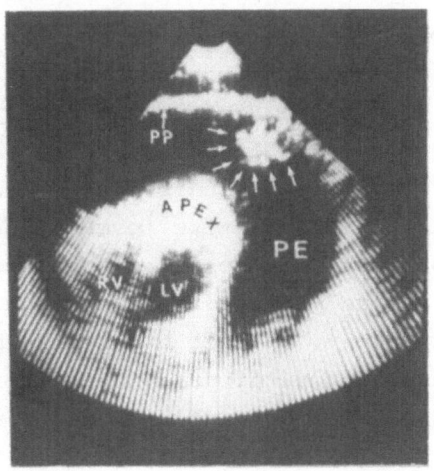

Fig. 3. Tumorous bizarre and cauliflower-like masses on the parietal pericardium protruding in the pericardial fluid (arrows) in a patient with pericardial mezothelioma. Histological diagnosis was obtained by percutaneous pericardial biopsy guided by two-dimensional echocardiography and proven at surgery. LV = left ventricle, PE = pericardial effusion, RV = right ventricle, PP = parietal pericardium.

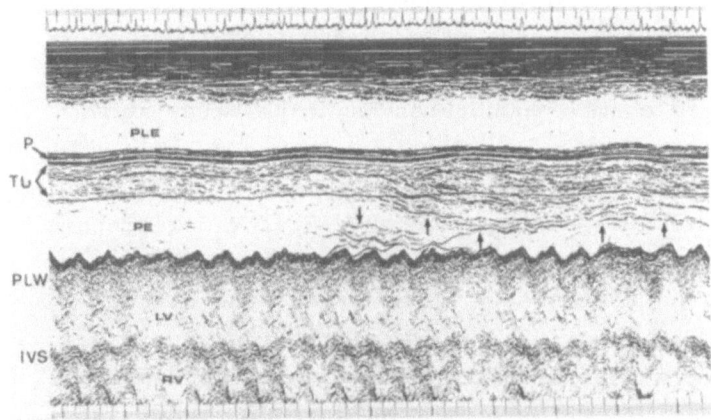

Fig. 4. M-mode echocardiogram from patient with pericardial mezothelioma. Coexistent pericardial (PE) and pleural (PLE) effusion was recorded from posterior thoracic wall. The parietal pericardium (P) with large tumorous mass (Tu) is demonstrated between the two effusions. Long echoes in the pericardial fluid (arrows) are residues of microbubbles from contrast echopericardiography. PLW = posterior left ventricular wall, LV=left ventricle, IVS = interventricular septum, RV = right ventricle.

On the basis of echocardiographic-pathologic correlations obtained so far, large cauliflower-like or bizarre pericardial masses are strongly suspect to be tumours, band-like structures suggest pericardial adhesions, while lumpy and shaggy epicardial or pericardial echoes speak in favour of fibrinous deposits. In some patients this echocardiographic finding may indicate effusive-constrictive forms of pericarditis (9,11). A definite etiological diagnosis can be obtained by pericardiocentesis or percutaneous pericardial biopsy guided by two-dimensional echocardiography. Target biopsy of imaged masses can be performed under echocardiographic control. Recognition of loculated effusion is important when planning pericardiocentesisl

Pericardiocentesis

Although pericardiocentesis has been used since 1840 (16) it is still a procedure with a high risk of morbidity and mortality.

The complications reported include cardiac chamber puncture, with or without tamponade, laceration of coronary vessels, ventricular fibrilation and other ventricular or atrial arrhythmias, cardiac arrest, pneumothorax, vasovagal reactions, infection, bleeding, perforation of the stomach and non-productive pericardiocentesis (17,18). It is believed that the number of non-registered cardiac chamber punctures is higher than those registered.

It is difficult to compare the few studies dealing with the risks involved in pericardiocentesis because of the differences in diagnostic criteria of pericardial effusion, the environment in which pericardiocenteses were performed, the site of the pericardiocentesis, steps taken to minimize the hazards (ECG, plastic catheters replacing the needle, echo-guidance), the hemodynamic status of patients, the duration of the study, and follow-up of patients (17-20). The seriousness of the problem is illustrated by Kotte and McGuire (19); they reported on 21 cardiologists and surgeons experienced in pericardiocentesis who had seen 18 deaths during this procedure.

Several attempts to diminish the potential risk of pericar-

diocentesis are reported. Fluoroscopic guiding of the needle
for pericardiocentesis is not a reliable method, because it
cannot differentiate pericardial effusion from cardiac mass.
In 1956 Bishop and co-workers (21) used the pericardiocentesis
needle as an exploring electrode to detect the injury currents
during the contact of the electrode tip with the heart. This
technique became unwarrantedly popular for it is not absolutely
safe; it may give a spurious feeling of safety, however, and
usually registers already existing injury. In 1966 a soft plastic catheter was introduced to replace the needle or guidewire
after entering into the pericardial space. Plastic catheters
may be introduced over or through the needle or guidewire (21-
26).

The introduction of echocardiography in routine diagnosis
of pericardial effusion is probably the most important advance
in minimizing the hazards of pericardiocentesis. Besides the
reliable diagnosis of pericardial effusion, it also provides
other data important for the safety or pericardiocentesis, such
as semiquantitation, distribution and loculation of pericardial
fluid. It is therefore essential for the selection of patients
and of the optimal puncture site for pericardiocentesis. A spe-
cal transducer with the hole in the center to direct the needle
during pericardiocentesis under A- and M-mode echocardiographic
control was used by Goldberg and Pollock in 1972 (27). The needle tip was seen in the A- and M-mode display as an echo arising
at the needle tip - fluid interface. In one out of their six
patients in whom the procedure was performed, they experienced
ventricular puncture. As is seen from the literature, this method was of no further interest in cardiology. The main disadvantage of pericardiocentesis guided under the control of A- and
M-mode is the lack of spatial orientation.

In order to ensure safe therapeutic or diagnostic pericardiocentesis we have, over the last four years, been guiding the
introduction of the needle for pericardiocentesis using two-
dimensional echocardiography and have applied this method in
17 cases of pericardial effusion (7,8,10,12,13,15). All the
patients had semiquantitatively moderate to large pericardial
effusion. For safe pericardiocentesis it is essential to posi-

tion the needle in the scanning plane. If a portion of the needle is out of the scanning plane, part of the needle body could be misinterpreted as the needle tip, as illustrated in Figure 5.

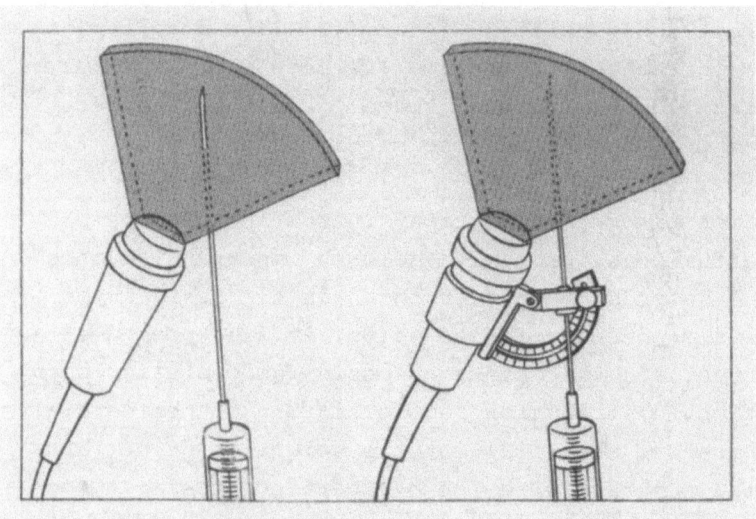

Fig. 5. The drawing shows a puncture or biopsy adaptor mounted to the phase array sector scan transducer ensuring the position of the needle to be always in the scanning plane. Without the adaptor a part of the needle can be out of the scanning plane (left drawing) resulting in the misinterpretation of the needle tip position. The needle could be guided at an adjustable angle to the transducer.

The position of the needle tip can be confirmed by a contrast study - rapid instillation of 2-5 ml of sterile normal saline or pericardial fluid through the needle. If a contrast jet appears at the presumed needle tip, it may be considered as the true tip. (Fig. 6). Besides the classical subxyphoid approach (28) in patients with concomitant pleural effusion we performed pericardiocentesis through the posterior or lateral thoracic wall. We found this approach to be most convenient provided large pleural effusion assures a large echo-free corridor toward the parietal pericardium. In addition the largest

amount of pericardial fluid usually collects behind the left
ventricular posterior wall and the cardiac apex moves away
from the needle in systole lowering the risk of cardiac damage.

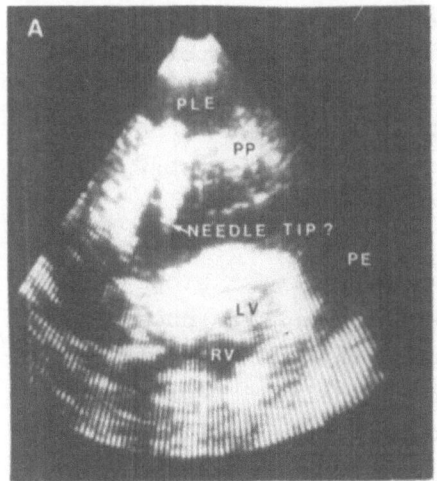
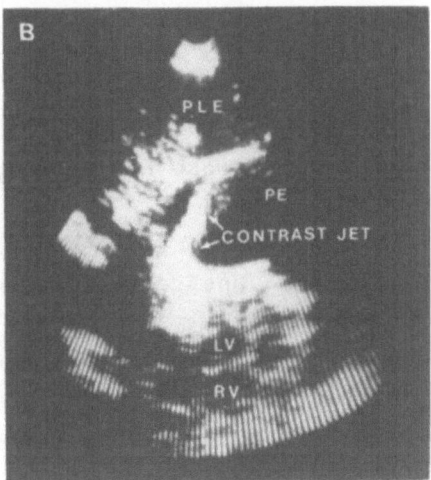
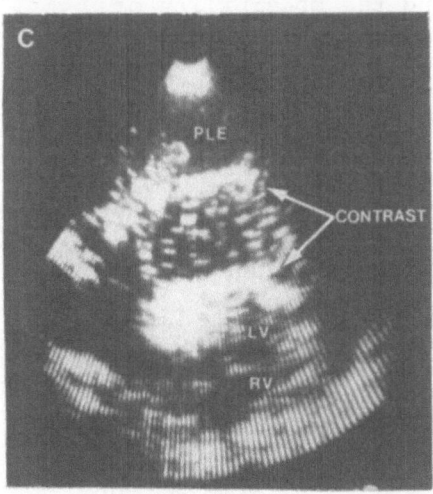

Fig. 6. The presumed needle tip (panel A) may be confirmed
by contrast echopericardiography. The patient had concomitant
pleural effusion and puncture was performed by posterior thoracic approach through the pleural effusion. If contrast jet
appears at presumed needle tip, it may be considered as true
tip (panel B). Panel C shows microbubbles spread in the pericardial sac. LV = left ventricle, RV = right ventricle, PP =
parietal pericardium, PLE = pleural effusion, PE = pericardial effusion.

After entering the pericardial sac, the needle should be replaced by a plastic catheter. The position of the needle or
catheter could be monitored continuously during the procedure
and repositioned if found necessary. In 1 out of 17 patients
from our study group a complication - ventricular puncture
with intrapericardial bleeding - occurred, requiring immediate thoracotomy. In this patient the apical approach was
used because an enlarged nodular liver thwarted the subxyphoid
approach.

In order to ensure that the needle is always in the scanning
plane we recently constructed a special puncture or biopsy
adaptor mounted to the phased array sector scan transducer
(see Figure 5). The needle is introduced through the guide
channel in the adaptor and advances to the desired target under direct monitoring on the oscilloscope. The puncture adaptor ensures the needle guidance and needle position is always
in the scanning plane, thus eliminating the possibility of
misinterpretation of the needle tip. The needle can be positioned in the scanning plane at an adjustable angle by means
of a flexible guide channel holder. Because the puncture
needle is angled relative to the ultrasound beam, the entire
length of the needle in the scanning plane is imaged (Fig. 7).
If a transducer with a central lumen is used only the needle
tip is visualised, because the echo arises at the needle tip -
fluid interface.

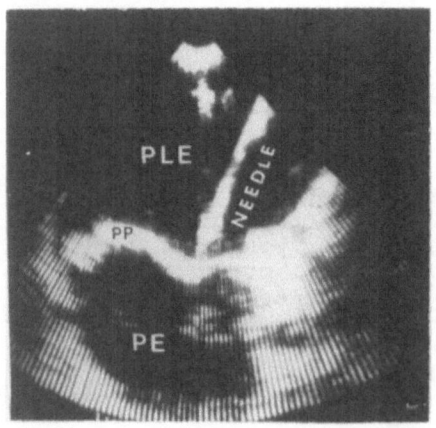

Fig. 7. The needle for pericardiocentesis is seen in its entire length from posterior thoracic wall in patient with large
pleural and pericardial effusion.
The needle is passing through
large echo-free space of pleural
effusion to the parietal pericardium (PP). PE = pericardial
effusion, PLE = pleural effusion.

In addition to constituting a danger of misinterpreting the
needle tip, manual adjustment of the needle in the scanning
plane without an adaptor is a time consuming procedure. Attention should be given to preparing the patient, to adequately
sterilising the instruments and electrical safety precautions
should be taken. It is our opinion that the technique described could eliminate the risk of cardiac damage during pericardiocentesis.

Percutaneous Pericardial Biopsy and Fenestration

An etiological diagnosis can be obtained in less than one
third of cases by analysing pericardial fluid removed during
diagnostic pericardiocentesis (29). Thus in many cases of pericardial effusion thoracotomy with pericardial biopsy remains
the definitive diagnostic solution. In recurrent pericardial
effusion with tamponade during thoracotomy a pericardial window can be created and pericardial fluid drained into the pleural space.

In an attempt to avoid thoractomy and general anaesthesia
for histologic diagnosis of pericardial lesion in patients
with pericardial effusion we introduced a new technique of percutaneous pericardial biopsy and pericardial fenestration under
two-dimensional echocardiographic guidance (13,30). The same
technique as described for pericardiocentesis was used. Pericardial biopsy was performed in six patients, while pericardial window was created in two patients. In patients with concomitant left pleural effusion, the posterior or lateral thoracic approach was preferred as in pericardiocentesis. (Fig. 8).
A disposable Trucut Travenel biopsy needle with a 15.2 cm
cannula length and 20 mm specimen notch was used. In patients
with coexistent left pleural effusion after the pericardial
speciment was taken the remaining window was enlarged and pericardial fluid drained, under higher pressure, into the pleural space. Pericardial window created during pericardial biopsy for pericardial decompression could save repeated pericardiocentesis in recurrent pericardial effusion with tamponade (Fig.9).
In all patients an adequate tissue specimen was obtained for

histological analysis and a proper histological diagnosis was made. So far no complications have been observed. However, a large series of patients is necessary to determine the safety of the described procedure. It is believed that in the future the new adaptor described above will refine and hasten the biopsy technique and make it even safer.

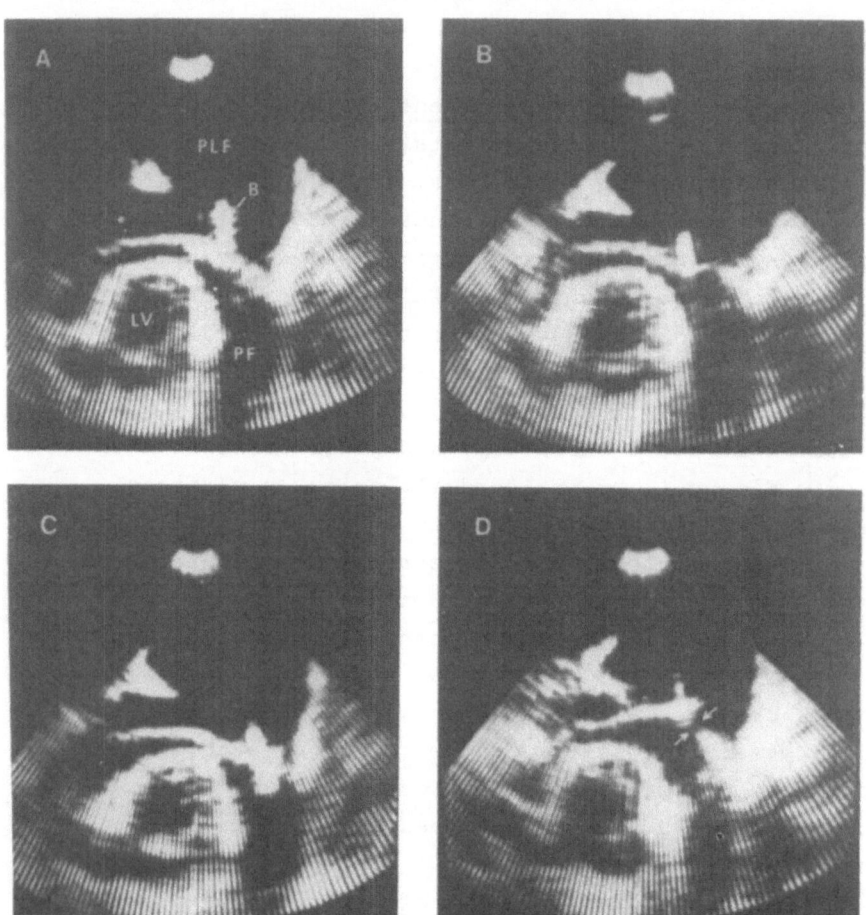

Fig. 8. Sequential frames during percutaneous pericardial biopsy from the posterior thoracic wall in the patient with pleural(PLE) and pericardial effusion (PE). A. Bioptom (B) has reached parietal pericardium. B. Invagination of parietal pericardium. C. Bioptom passing through parietal pericardium. D. Tent-like formation of the parietal pericardium during biopsy. Arrows show the pericardial window previously performed.

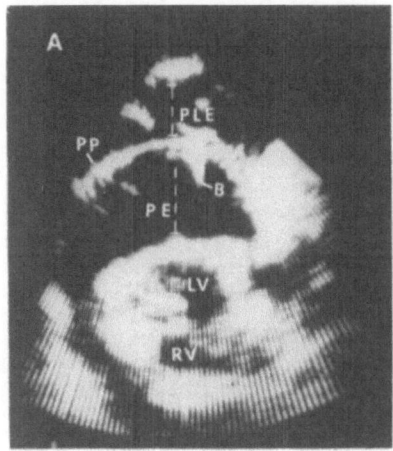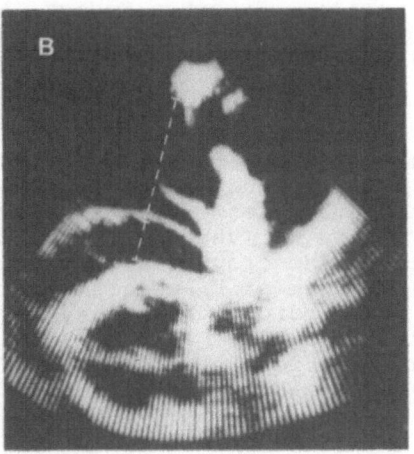

Fig. 9. As a consequence of pericardial biopsy and fenestration, large pericardial fluid under high pressure drained into
the pleural space. Thus a large pericardial effusion (A) diminished and small pleural effusion (B) increased. PE = pericardial effusion, PLE = pleural effusion, PP = parietal pericardium, B = bioptom, LV = left ventricle, RV = right ventricle.

REFERENCES

1. Edler I. 1955. Diagnostic use of ultrasound in heart dis-
    ease. Acta Medica. Scand. 152 (Suppl. 308), 32.
2. Feigenbaum H, Waldhausen JA, Hyde LP. 1965. Ultrasound
    diagnosis of pericardial effusion. JAMA 191,711.
3. Tajik AJ. 1977. Echocardiography in pericardial effusion.
    Am.J.Med. 63, 29.
4. Feigenbaum H. 1981. Echocardiography, 3rd ed., Lea &
    Febiger, Philadelphia.
5. Horowitz MS, Schultz CS, Stinson EB, Harrison DC, Popp RL.
    1974. Sensitivity and specificity of echocardiographic
    diagnosis of pericardial effusion. Circulation 50, 239.
6. Martin RP, Rakowski H, French J, Popp R. 1978. Localisa-
    tion of pericardial effusion with wide angle phased array
    echocardiography. Am.J. Cardiol. 42,904.
7. Cikes I. 1980. Two-dimensional echocardiography in the
    diagnosis of pericardial effusion and adhesive pericarditis.

In: Recent Advances in Ultrasound Diagnosis 2, pp.306-316
(ed. A. Kurjak), Excerpta Medica, Amsterdam-Oxford-Princeton.
8. Cikes I, Cikes N, Pustisek S. 1979. Dvodimenzionalni ehokar-
diografski prikaz fibrinoznog perikarditisa i perikardijal-
nih adhezija u bolesnice sa sistemskim lupus eritematodesom,
Zbornik radova kardioloskih sekcija ZLD i ZLH , Zlatar.
9. Chang S, Chang JK. 1980. Cross-sectional echocardiography
and progressive constrictive pericarditis. In: Recent Advances in Ultrasound Diagnosis 2, pp. 317-322 (ed.A.Kurjak)
Excerpta Medica, Amsterdam-Oxford-Princeton.
10. Cikes I, Cikes N, Ivancic R. 1980. Two-dimensional echocardiography in the diagnosis of pericardial and pleuropericar-
dial adhesions. In: Proceedings of the International Cong-
ress on Echocardiography, Rome.
11. Martin RP, Bowdan R, Filly K, Popp RL. 1980. Intrapericardial abnormalities in patients with pericardial effusion:
findings by two-dimensional echocardiography. Circulation
61,568.
12. Cikes I, Cikes N, Drinkovic N, Jelic I, Pustisek S.1981.
Two-dimensional echocardiography in the detection of intrapericardial masses in pericardial effusion (abstract),4th
Symposium on Echocardiography, p.6,Rotterdam.
13. Cikes I, Ernst A. 1981. New possibilities in echocardiographic diagnosis of pericardial diseases. In: Recent Advances
in Ultrasound Diagnosis 3, pp. 377-386. (ed. A. Kurjak,
A. Kratochwil), Excerpta Medica, Amsterdam-Oxford-Princeton.
14. Chandraratna PAN, Aronow S. 1981. Detection of pericardial
metastases by cross-sectional echocardiography. Circulation
63, 19.
15. Cikes I. 1982. Echocardiography in pericardial disease.
In: Progress in Medical Ultrasound 3 (ed. A. Kurjak), Excerpta Medica, Amsterdam-Oxford-Princeton.
16. Schuh F. 1941. Erfahrungen über die Paracentese der Brust
und des Herzbeutels. Med.Jahrb.d.k.k. Oster-Staates Wien
(Neuste Folge 24) 33,388.
17. Wong B, Murphy JA, Chang CJ, Hassenein K, Dunn M. 1979.
The risk of pericardiocentesis, Am.J.Cardiol. 44,1110.
18. Krikorian JG, Hancock EW. 1978. Pericardiocentesis. Am.J.
Med. 65, 808.
19. Kotte JH, McGuire J. 1951. Pericardial paracentesis. Mod.
Conc.Cardiovasc.Dis. 20, 102.
20. Kilpatrick ZN, Chapman CG. 1965. On pericardiocentesis.
Am.J.Cardiol. 16, 722.
21. Bishop LH, Estes EH, McIntosh HD. 1956. The electrocardiogram as a safeguard in pericardiocentesis. JAMA 62, 264.
22. Nordenstrom B. 1966. Percutaneous catheterisation of the
pericardium. Acta Radiol. 4, 662.
23. Glancy DL, Richter MA. 1975. Catheter drainage of the pericardial space. Cathet.Cardiovasc.Diagn.2,311.
24. Masumi RA, Rios JC, Ross AM, Ewy GA.1968. Technique for
insertion of an indwelling intrapericardial catheter. Br.
Heart J. 30, 333.
25. Owens WC, Schaefer RA, Rahimtoola SH. 1975. Pericardiocentesis: Insertion of a pericardial catheter. Cathet.
Cardiovasc. Diagn. 1, 317.

26. Wei JY, Taylor GJ, Aschuff SC. 1978. Recurrent cardiac tam-
    ponade and large pericardial effusions: Management with an
    indwelling pericardial catheter. Am.J.Cardiol. 42, 281.
27. Goldberg BB, Pollock HM. 1973. Ultrasonically guided peri-
    cardiocentesis. Am.J.Cardiol. 31, 490.
28. Marfan AB. 1911. Ponction du péricarde par l'épigastre.
    Ann.méd.chir.inf. 15, 529.
29. Hancock EW, Krikorian JG. 1977. Benefits and risks of peri-
    cardiocentesis, 1970-1976. Proceedings of the Association
    of University Cardiologists, Phoenix, Arizona.
30. Ernst A, Cikes I, Persic T, Cepelja Z. 1981. Percutaneous
    pericardial biopsy and fenestration guided by echocardio-
    graphy, Abstracts, 4th European Congress in Ultrasonics
    in Medicine, Dubrovnik, p.67, Excerpta Medica, Amsterdam.

THE EFFECT OF ANTIHYPERTENSIVE DRUGS UPON LEFT VENTRICULAR
FUNCTION AT REST AND DURING EXERCISE.

S.Corallo - Cardiac Department - Univ.Hosp. "L.Sacco" - Mila
no - Italy.

The ability to evaluate the morphology and function of
the Left Ventricle (LV) has been one of the principal factors
in the increasing application of the Echocardiography.

Although LV dimensions measured by standard M-mode Echocardiography and used to estimate ventricular volumes, are
subjected to potential errors in calculations, simple dimensions of the Left Ventricle can provide an estimate of the
overall LV size and performance in a large percentage of patients, provided that no segmental disease affects the ventricle (1). This applies particularly well to Arterial Hyper
tension (AH) in which before Echocardiography it was difficult
to detect early cardiac complications, as increase in left
atrial dimension and LV wall thickness and mass (2).

Echocardiography in Arterial Hypertension.

The echocardiogram appears to be superior to the routine
chest X-Ray and the standard 12 lead ECG for detecting early
cardiac abnormalities in AH patients. LV systolic function
as assessed by fibre shortening (FS), ejection fraction (EF),
mean velocity of fibre shortening (M VCF) and LV walls velocity of excursion (LVW velocity) can show significant alterations in AH Pts. (2-3-4-5-6-7-8-9). Incoordinate wall move
ment and nonuniformity of LV structure and function were also
described (10). Moreover diastolic ventricular abnormalities,
as reduction of rapid filling and slow LV relaxation have
been referred (11-12-13).

Echocardiographic assessment of drugs effects in Arterial
Hypertension.

The effects of drugs on LV size and function in AH patients

evaluated echocardiographically, have brought interesting in
formation. Atenolol, a cardioselective Beta-adrenergic blocking agent with no intrinsic sympathomimetic activity, given
orally to a group af AH patients with normal LV size and fun
ction, did not produce changes in fractional shortening, ejec
tion fraction, normalized VCF, and end diastolic volume index,
showing no effects on LV size or function (14). Acebutolol and
propranolol did not induce depression of resting left ventri
cular function in patients with normal or near normal LV
function at rest (15-16). In another group of patients the
Echocardiographic follow up showed a reduction of LV hypertro
phy produced by antihypertensive theraphy (17). A regimen
consisting of chlortalidone, hydralazine and propranolol reduced mean blood pressure, heart rate, and mean VCF, in AH
patients with coronary artery disease or aortic dissection,
showing that reflex cardiac stimulation induced by hydralazine
is neutralized by propranolol, and that this decrease of LV
contractility can be safe in seriously ill patients (18).

Dynamic Exercise Echocardiography.

Recently Dynamic Exercise Echocardiography (DEE) has been
introduced for assessing LV size and performance (19-20-21-
22-23). Time-motion made possible to obtain estimates of LV
diameters intermittently or continously before, during or after an effort, without risk or discomfort to the subject,
noninvasively and repeteably. Therefore it became particular
ly feasible for screening LV performance in AH patients, as
well as in patients follow up in order to assess early LV fun
ction impairment and to evaluate the effects of therapy (19-
23-24-).

Two homogeneous groups of normal subjects and uncomplicated and untreated AH patients were studied by means of DEE
at rest and during bicycle ergometer graded sitting exercise
to exhaustion (24). LV echocardiograms were recorded at rest
and at two minutes intervals during effort and recovery. All
patients tolerated well the test without disturbances or
symptoms. The Echo parameters which responded better to exer
cise were mean VCF, interventricular septum and LV posterior

wall velocity; LV Diastolic Diameter (LVDD). At lower level of effort an increment in contractility was observed, due mainly to LV shortening rate and to heart rate. At peak exercise LVDD, Shortening Fraction and Ejection Fraction increased significan tly in response to a Frank-Starling effect. In the AH patients, a part from the differences in blood pressure, LV wall thickness and LV mass, LV behaviour did not differ from normal group during exercise and recovery, thereof excluding an early impairment of LV function, in that phase of the disease. It con firmed also the role of LV hypertrophy as compensatory mechanism of the increased peripheral resistance due to AH.

DEE was also used in a group of normal subject to test LV performance before and after B-adrenergic blockade, with propranolol administered orally for two weeks (25). Proprano lol decreased heart rate and blood pressure at rest in the subjects and slightly increased end-diastolic size, but did not alter left ventricular performance during effort. In fact, no significant difference between any of the measures examined between the first and second control exercise studies,after Beta-blocade, was shown.Propranolol was then concluded to have little, if any intrinsic depressant effects on the myocardium. Its major action on the heart was postulated to be competitive, B-adrenergic blockade, which is more manifest during periods of intense sympathetic stimulation.

Our preliminary DEE studies with Beta blockers in normal as well as in uncomplicated AH patients seem to confirm the exposed data, and therefore the safety of Beta blocking therapy, associated with efficacy in the treatment of AH. The same applies to the diuretics,also used for long term.

CONCLUSION.

From what exposed we conclude that M-mode Echocardiogra phy is a sensitive and reproducible technique for evaluating LV size and behaviour under a variety of conditions in subjects with symmetrically contracting left ventricle such as normal and hypertensive patients. Dynamic Exercise Echocardiography appears to be a reliable non invasive method for assessing

LV performance. It can be suggested for screening AH patients
in order to assess early LV function deterioration and to e-
valuate the effects of theraphy.

REFERENCES

1. Feigenbaum H. in - Braunwald E. (1980): Heart Disease -
   Saunders - Philadelphia - p.26-147
2. Savage D.D., Drayer J.I., Henry W.L., Laragh J.H. et al.
   (1979): Echocardiographic Assessment of Cardiac Anatomy
   and Function in Hypertensive Subjects - Circulation 59,4,623
3. Dreschr E., Austenat J., Gunther RH., Purfurst W.O., Hujer
   W. (1980): Echocardiography in hypertension. Dimension and
   mass of the left ventricle. Comparison with controls and
   sportsmen. - G.Ital.Cardiol. 10:843-50
4. Pisarczyk M.J., Ross A.M. (1976): Cardiac measurements in
   Hypertension: Echocardiogram, Electrocardiogram and X-Ray
   comparations. Am.J.Cardiol. (ABS) 37:162
5. Reichek N., Devereux R.B. (1981): Left ventricular hypertrophy relationship of Anatomic, Echocardiographic and
   Electrocardiographic findings. Circ. 63:1391
6. Schmid P., Simon G., Dickhut H.H., Keul J. (1979): Echocardiographic results in female athletes, nonathetic women
   and patients with arterial hypertension-Herz - 4- (5):438:43
7. Safar M.E., Lehner JP, Vincent MI, Plainfosse MT, Simon AC
   (1979) - Echocardiographic dimensions in borderline and
   sustained hypertension - Am.J.Cardiol. 22; 44 (5):930-5
8. Cohen A,Hagan AD, Watkins J., Mits J. et Al.(1981) -
   Clinical correlates in hypertensive Patients with Left Ven
   tricular hypertrophy diagnosed with Echocardiography. Am.
   J.Cardiol. - 47 (2):335-41
9. Guazzi M., Fiorentini C., Olivari M.T., Polese A. (1979):
   Cardiac load and function in hypertension - Ultrasonic and
   Hemodynamic study. Am.J.Cardiol. 22:44 (5): 1007.
10.Bibra H., (1981): Evaluation of incoordinate wall movement
   in Hypertensive Subjects. Eur.H.Journal 2 suppl A - abs 51
11.Hanrath P., Mathey D.G., Siegert R., Bleifeld W. (1980):
   Left Ventricular relaxation and filling pattern in different

forms of Left Ventricular Hypertrophy. An Echocardiographic
study. Am.J.Cardiol. 45:15

12. Venco A., Barzizza F., Grandi A., Pozzoli M. et al (1981):
Echocardiographic assessment of hypertensive-diabetic
heart disease. Eur.H.Journal - 2 - suppl. A ABS 52

13. Drelinski G.R., Frolich ED, Dunn F.G., Messerli F.A. et al
(1981): Echocardiographic diastolic ventricular abnormality in hypertensive heart disease: atrial emptying index.
Am.J.Cardiol. 47 (5): 1087-90.

14. Ibrahim HM, Madkour MA, Mossallah R. (1980): Effect of
Atenolol on Left Ventricular function in hypertensive
Patients - Circulation 62 (5); 1036-45

15. Bett J.H., Dryburgh L., Hetherington D.E. (1980):Echocar-
diographic comparison of haemodynamic effects of Metoprolol
and Propranolol - Br.Heart J. 43 (5):541-5.

16. Chandraratna P.A., Aronow WS, Laddu A. (1980): Effects of
Acebutolol and Propranolol on Left Ventricular performance
assessed by Echocardiography - Clin.Pharmacol.Ther. 27 (4):
460-3

17 Hill L.S., Monaghan M., Richardson P.J.: Regression of left
Ventricular hypertrophy during treatment with antihyperten
sive agents. Br. T.Clin.Pharmacol.

18. Moyer J.P.,Pittman AW, Belasco RN, Woods J.W. (1979): Echo
cardiographic assessment of the effect of an antihypertensi
ve regimen on Left Ventricular performance. Am.J.Cardiol.
43 (3):594-9

19. Sugishita Y., Koseki S. (1979) Dynamic Exercise Echocardiography - Circulation 60,743.

20. Weiss J.L. Weisfeldi M.L., Mason S.J. (1979): Evidence of Frank
Starling   effect in man during severe semisupine
exercise - Circulation 59,655.

21. Crawford M.M., White D._., Amon K.W. (1979): Echocardiographic evaluation of Left Ventricular size and performance during handgrip, supine and upright bycicle exercise. Circulation 59,1188.

22. Hanrath P., Matsumoto M.: Transesophageal Echocardiography:
a new method for the evaluation of Left Ventricular perfor-

mancd during dynamic exercise (1981)
in A.Kuriak, A.Kratochwil - Recent advances in Ultrasound
diagnosis 3 - Exerpta Medica - Amsterdam p. 393.

23. Corallo S., Broso G.P., Sega R., et al.: Value and limits
of exercise Echocardiography in normal and pathological
conditions (1981).
IN A.Kuriak, A.Kratochwil - Recent advances in Ultrasound
diagnosis 3 Excerpta Medica - Amsterdam - p. 428.

24. Corallo S., Sega R.,Pirastu A. et al (1981): Exercise Echocardiography in the study of Left Ventricular behaviour in
normal and hypertensive subjects - Eur.Heart J. Vol.2
suppl. A - 221

25. Crawford M.H., Lindenfeld J., O'Rourke R.A. (1980): Effects
of oral Propranolol on Left Ventricular size and performance during exercise and acute pressure loading. - Circulation 61, (3), 549.

FUTURE ASPECTS IN THE TECHNOLOGY OF ECHOGRAPHY

N. BOM

1. INTRODUCTION

It is virtually impossible to describe even a limited
number of technological developments that might be used in
echocardiography in the time-course of a short lecture.
The spectrum of such a subject will range from miniaturi-
zation of instrumentation and micro-technologies within
the transducer itself to application of digital subtraction methods as presently introduced in X-ray. This
lecture will be restricted to four areas where
technological advances do set definite trends in
echocardiography.

Presently much effort is given to improve poor echo
information for instance by time averaging techniques.
However, it seems important to consider first all
possibilities to improve the echo signal itself. This
might be done by more careful transducer design.

Attention should also be given to allow easy
instrument handling. Correct gainsetting is carried out
manually by the operator through a time-gain lever
setting. Instead of this manual method it is presently
possible to automatically match the wide variation in echo
amplitude to the documentation requirements. This and
other technological developments are drastically changing
M-mode handling and documentation.

Introduction of computers and large memories will
have their effect on image enhancement and parameter
extraction of two-dimensional (2D) real-time data. This,
and the limitation of application in 3D will be discussed.

2. THE TRANSDUCER

The transducer is the "eye" (or rather the ear) of the instrument and therefore deserves full attention. Of course it is our wish to sample the heart with a very well defined (narrow) sound beam. No "noise" (echoes) should interfere from any direction other than the main axis of the beam.

Diskshaped transducers are used in mechanical sector-scanners. The disk geometry creates a soundbeam with the advantage that it does not show much sensitivity outside the main lobe. The beam, however, is not all that narrow. With a diskshaped transducer the focussing capabilities are restricted. Focussing may be obtained only in a single zône by application of a lens or by using a curved transducer face.

An electronic sectorscanner operates with many (say 32) small parallel elements in a rectangular format in the transducer head. This creates a large flexibility and therefore focussing at various depths becomes possible. Of course also focussing at any selected fixed depth may be possible. In figure 1 an electronic sectorscan image focussed at 8 cm depth (see A and C) and unfocussed (see B) are compared.

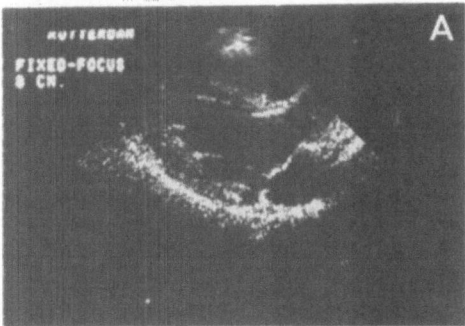
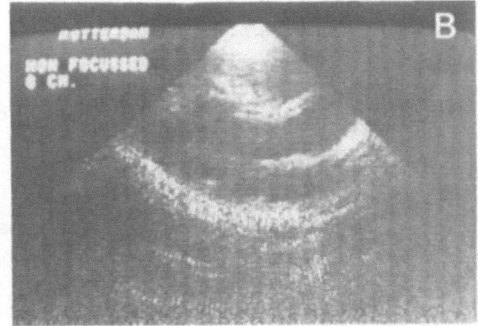
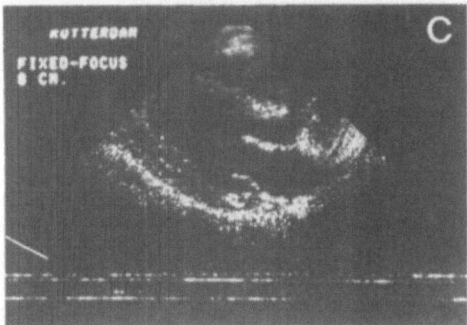
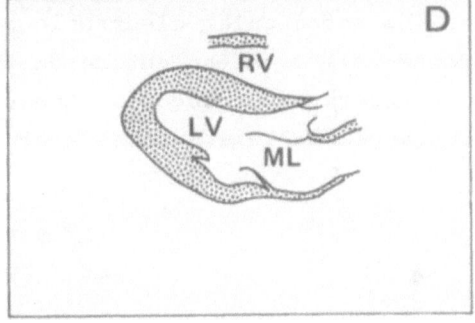

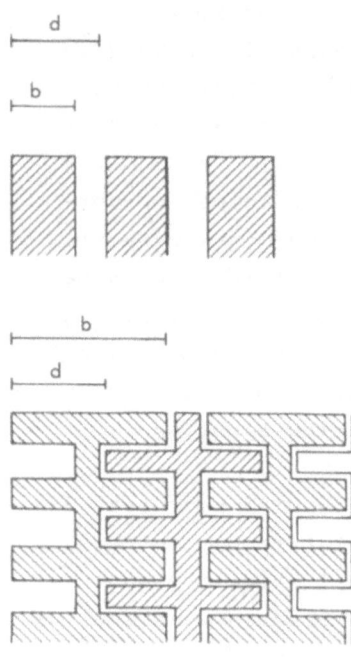

ANTI-ALIASING

In figure 2 three small elements of a sectorscan transducer are shown (top). The periodicity of many elements does introduce off-axis "noise" sometimes described as grating lobe or aliasing. This aliasing may be suppressed with introduction of certain element shapes (figure 2: bottom). New technologies to achieve this are being developed.

Up to now little attention has been paid to "narrow-ness" of the beam in the plane perpendicular to the image plane. The rectangular electronic sectorscan transducer may focus well over the entire depth in the image plane. It does however, not focus in the plane perpendicular to the image plane. This must be kept in mind!

An annular transducer is a transducer consisting of
a series of rings which together form a disk. Such a
transducer might be used in a mechanical sector scanner.
This solution would in principle combine flexible
focussing with a narrow beam in all planes.

Complete flexibility as to beam direction and
focussing would in principle be obtainable by mozaic
transducers. This complicated approach would only be
called for if - in future - continuous monitoring of
cardiac motion were called for. The than required
automatic target following procedures seem too far away
to even be considered today.

3. AUTOMATIC GAINSETTING

Echo amplitude depends on a variety of factors. The
wide range of echo amplitudes requires an elaborate and
flexible time gain amplification in order to match the
wide dynamic range of echoes to the smaller dynamic
capabilities of the final registration paper or display
tube. Automation may help a great deal in overcoming the
need for expert knowledge in how to set the appropriate
time gain curve. It allows the examiner to focus on probe
handling only. Various methods have been described to
obtain automatic gain setting. An obvious one has been
to use information from a previous echo arrival over the
entire depth to set the gain for the next echo sweep. The
gain is to be automatically increased in areas where echo
amplitude is small. When this simple approach is carried
out by an automatic gain control mechanism, only moderate
results are obtained. A better approach has been to use
the average echo amplitude information over a number of
"depth windows". By this technique it became possible to
obtain M-mode tracings indistinguishable from optimal
hand-set recordings. An example is shown in figure 3.

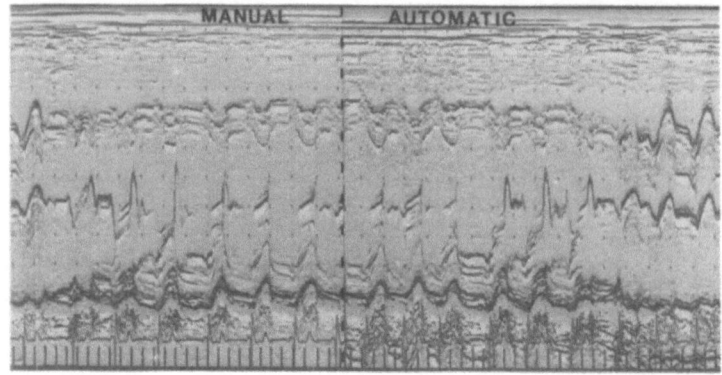

It is expected that in future similar techniques will improve two-dimensional images as well. Present results in this field have only shown limited effect.

4. M-MODE HANDLING

Automatic reading of written information is now slowly introduced in many non medical areas. When we keep in mind that present use of such reading is limited to "black on white" information such as postal codes the tremendous problems with automatic recognition of echo data with its large grey scale can be envisaged.

Many attempts are known in extracting automatically data from M-mode registrations. The most futuristic approach has been to let the computer follow the echo pattern for later automatic interpretation. Sofar this has failed to be of any practical usefulness because of difficulties to teach a machine to follow the "wiggles".

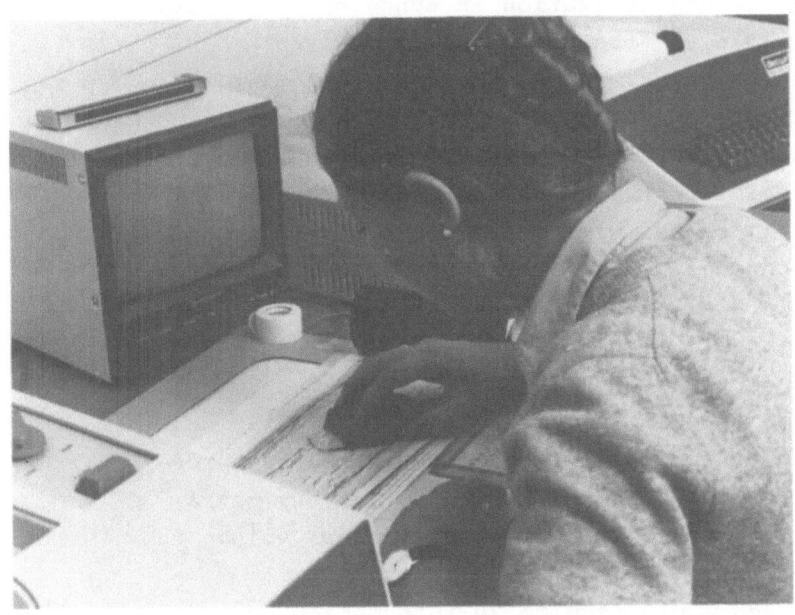

A more practical approach is shown in figure 4.
With a digitizer the echosignal of most cardiac structures
can be well traced by an experienced echographer. Data are
subsequently available for the measurement report. All
this is carried out off-line.

One step forward is the integration of M-mode into a
video memory and micro computer system. Calculation can
than be carried out during the patient study and report as
well as hard copy of the registration become available
during the study itself. Still the operator skill is
required for proper structure identification on the
screen.

This approach allows cheap documentation and rapid
results. The measurements may be directly transmitted
to the hospital's computerized patient files. This may
represent an important technological trend.

5. COMPUTERIZED ECHOGRAPHY

The purpose of computerization in echography is often two-fold: to "clean up" the image and to derive quantitative information. Two-dimensional real-time echocardiograhic images are often disturbed by a granular structure caused by random signals. Time-gating and averaging over similar frames at corresponding points within the e.c.g. signal will improve the signal to noise ratio. This technique, with or without various filter methods has been applied by some research groups. To a certain extent the image quality can be improved. All applications, however, are limited to research only.

The discussed image improvement concerns the two-dimensional aspect. One step further would be the three-dimensional information of the heart. So far any extrapolation from 2D data to 3D parameters such as volume has suffered criticism.

Proper approach would require 2D information over many well defined planes through the cardiac chambers. Several investigators have explored this three-dimensional reconstruction from two-dimensional echocardiographic images. The method calls for precise knowledge of transducer position. This has proved not to be a simple task and it requires many new techniques and algorithms. We must be careful to well balance such efforts with the clinical usefulness of results.

6. CONCLUSION

The general trend of image processing as experienced in many fields such as digital subtraction in X-ray will no doubt effect diagnostic ultrasound. The wide variation in transducer aiming directions necessary for cardiac study will strongly limit any routine approach. First applications might be in the area of contrast echocardiography.

With progress of technology many efforts will be made to simplify the entire echo study from recording to

analyses. Data from M-mode will become more quickly
availabe in a format which fits the hospital patient
documentation system.

It should be realized that at the very beginning of
the echo-chain (the transducer) already unnecessary noise
is introduced and much available information is thrown
away.

It might be more profitable to avoid pollution of the
signal instead of putting much effort in its reconstruction afterwards. Future technological developments will
tell us what can be done.

ACKNOWLEDGEMENT

Subjects described in this lecture have been documen-
ted in more detail elsewhere. The automatic gain system by
C.T. Lancée and J.A. Blom: "M-mode scanning with automatic
gain control" in: Echocardiology, Martinus Nijhoff
Publishers, ed. H. Rijsterborgh, 1981. The M-mode analyses
part by N. Bom and C.T. Lancee in "New Techniques", in:
Progress in Medical Ultrasound Volume 2/1981, Excerpta
Medica, ed. A. Kurjak.

The advantage of transesophageal M-mode echocardiography in comparison
with external echocardiography to detect segmental wall motion
abnormalities in coronary artery disease

Masunori Matsuzaki, M.D. and Reizo Kusukawa, M.D.

Echocardiography is one of the most useful noninvasive procedures for
evaluation left ventricular regional wall motion 1-8. In patients with
severe obstruction of left anterior descending coronary artery (LAD) abnormal interventricular septal (IVS) motion may be seen by "conventional
echocardiography" 3,5,6,8-10. However, this does not indicate that LAD
lesions always lead to abnormality of the IVS motion. Jacobs et al 5,
Gordon and Kerber 11, and Kolibach et al 12, have documented that about
half of their patients with severe lesions of the LAD had normal echocardiographic IVS motion.

Corya et al 4,8, also measured left ventricular anterior wall (LVAW)
motion echocardiographically, and found that abnormal LVAW motion is
closely correlated to the presence of an LAD lesion (66%). However, an
LVAW echogram is sometimes difficult to obtain in patients with coronary
artery disease. Especially in the presence of severe obesity or chronic
obstructive lung disease, LVAW echocardiogram cannot easily be obtained
through a conventional technique.

To obtain an LVAW echocardiogram more easily and dependably, we developed the esophageal echocardiography. In this study (1); we evaluated
the relationship between LVAW motion measured by esophageal echocardiography and that measured by conventional echocardiography and examined
the reliability of the esophageal technique in measuring LVAW motion by
comparing it to left ventriculographic findings (2); we examined the reliability to analyze the motions of IVS obtained by conventional echocardiography and LVAW obtained by esophageal echocardiography in predicting the presence or absence, as well as the location of LAD lesion.

METHODS

Patients. Forty-seven patients who underwent esophageal echocardiography
in Yamaguchi University Hospital were studied. Thirty-three of these

patients were found to have coronary artery disease. The other 14 patients were included in the control group.

Twenty-one of 33 patients with coronary artery disease (Table 1) were studied to compare the LVAW motion measured by esophageal echocardiography with that measured by left ventriculography. Further, in thirty patients with significant LAD disease (75% stenosis) diagnosed by selective coronary arteriography, we examined the reliability to measure the motion of IVS and LVAW in predicting the presence as well as the location of LAD lesion. This group consisted of 7 women and 23 men, ages 32-75 years, and were classified into three groups: Group 1; 12 patients with LAD lesion proximal to the major septal branch and with a history of anteroseptal myocardial infarction (ASMI) (Prox.with ASMI), mean age 58.7 years. Group 2; 8 patients with proximal LAD lesion and without prior ASMI (Prox.without ASMI), mean age 60.7 years. Group 3; 10 patients with LAD lesion distal to the major septal branch, mean age 60.7 years (Table 2). All patients in group 3 had histories of ASMI (Dis.with ASMI). In 14 control subjects, coronary artery disease and other cardiac conditions that could cause abnormal LVAW motion were precluded.

Cardiac catheterization and selective coronary arteriography were performed in all patients with coronary artery disease and in six of 14 control subjects.

Echocardiography

All patients were examined immediately before the cardiac catheterization studies with a commercial echocardiograph (Aloka Model SSD-80 or SSD 110S) using a 2.25 MHZ, 10mm nonfocused transducer. Conventional echocardiography was performed to obtain IVS and LVAW echograms in the supine or in the left lateral decubitus position using previously described technique.

Esophageal echocardiography was performed using 3.0-MHZ, 6mm nonfocused transducer attached to the tip of a gastrocamera (Model V,Olympus Camera Co.Ltd.13,14,15. To compare the esophageal echocardiographic LVAW motion with left ventriculographic finding systolic LVAW excursion was measured in the 20 patients with coronary artery disease, and classified into five groups: hyperkinetic - excursion 14mm; normakinetic 8-13mm; hypokinetic 3-7mm; akinetic 2mm; and dyskinetic - outward motion in systole. The normal upper and lower ranges (13 and 8) of the excursion of the LVAW were assumed to be the values of the mean ±2SD in the control

218

TABLE 1. *Comparison of Left Ventricular Anterior Wall Motions Obtained by Left Ventriculography with Those by Esophageal and Conventional Echocardiography*

Pt	Age (years)	Sex	Diagnosis	Eso. echo Motion	Eso. echo Excursion (mm)	Ant. echo Motion	Ant. echo Excursion (mm)	LVG LVAW	CAG % internal area reduction
1	61	F	Anteroseptal MI	A	2	NO	NO	A	LAD 99, RCA 75
2	61	F	Anteroseptal MI	A	2	NO	NO	A	LAD 100
3	59	M	Anteroseptal MI	A	2	A	0	A	LAD 99, CX 75
4	52	F	Anteroseptal MI	A	4	D	0	D	LAD 75
5	63	M	Anteroseptal MI	NO	NO	H	4	H	LAD 75
6	48	M	Anteroseptal MI	A	2	NO	NO	H	LAD 100
7	52	M	Anteroseptal MI	A	2	NO	NO	A	LAD 100
8	55	M	Anteroseptal MI	A	2	A	0	H	LAD 90, CX 90
9	44	M	Anteroseptal MI	A	2	NO	NO	A	LAD 75
10	69	M	Anteroseptal MI	H	5	NO	NO	A	LAD 99
11	60	M	Anteroseptal lateral MI	H	7	H	5	H	LAD 90, CX 75
12	63	M	Inferior MI	H	6	D	0	N	LAD 99, CX 75
13	75	F	Inferior MI	N	8	NO	NO	H	LAD 99, CX 90, RCA 75
14	69	M	Inferior MI	N	11	NO	NO	H	LAD 75, CX 75, RCA 99
15	32	M	Inferior MI	N	10	H	7	H	LAD 75, CX 75, RCA 99
16	62	F	Posterior MI	N	14	NO	NO	N	RCA 100
17	56	M	Inferior MI, angina pectoris	D	1	NO	NO	N	RCA 75
18	68	M	Angina pectoris	H	6	H	4	D	LAD 100, CX 100, RCA 99
19	50	M	Angina pectoris	N	8	NO	NO	H	LMC 100
20	62	M	Angina pectoris	H	5	A	2	N	LAD 75
21	68	M	Unstable angina	N	8	NO	NO	H	LAD 99, CX 75, RCA 75
								N	RCA 75

Abbreviations: Eso. echo = esophageal echocardiography; Ant. echo = conventional echocardiography; LVG = left ventriculography; CAG = coronary arteriography; MI = myocardial infarction; A = akinetic; H = hypokinetic; N = normokinetic; D = dyskinetic; NO = not obtained; LVAW = left ventricular anterior wall; LAD = left anterior descending coronary artery; LMC = left main coronary artery; CX = circumflex coronary artery.

TABLE 2. *Comparison of Left Ventricular Anterior Wall Motion on Esophageal Echocardiography and Left Ventriculography*

LVAW eso. echo.	LVAW angiogram Hyper- and normokinetic	Hypokinetic	Akinetic	Dyskinetic	Total
Hyper- and normokinetic	4*	2	—	—	6
Hypokinetic	1	5*	—	—	6
Akinetic	—	1	6*	—	7
Dyskinetic	—	—	—	1*	1
Total	5	8	6	1	20

*Agreement of wall motion obtained by the two methods.
Abbreviations: LVAW = left ventricular anterior wall; eso. echo. = esophageal echocardiogram.

group.

In thirty patients with LAD disease
the LVAW excursion, mean systolic
shortening velocity and the time interval between Q wave on ECG and the
beginning of the inward (Q-C interval)
were measured, and also the excursion
and Q-C interval of the IVS were measured with conventional echocardiography (Figure 1). These parameters
from LVAW and IVS echograms were compared between the group of patients
with proximal LAD disease and that
with distal LAD disease to evaluate
the ability of the echograms obtained
by these two procedures in predicting
the location of LAD lesion.

Left Ventriculography and Coronary
Arteriography

Left ventriculography was performed
by contrast injection using a Thomson
6- or 9- inch image intensifier and
Arritechna (R35-90) 35mm cinecamera in
30° right anterior oblique position,

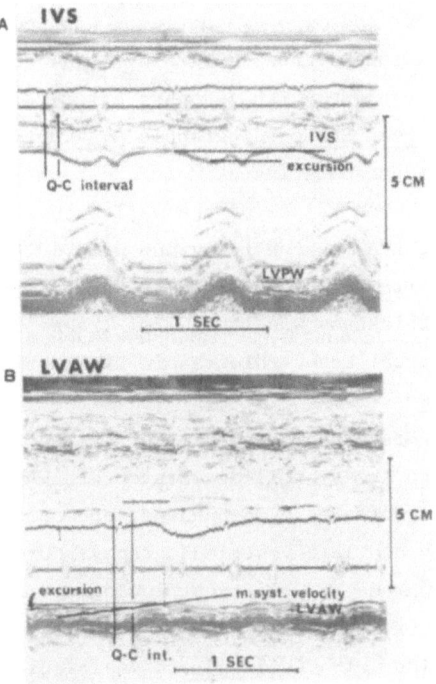

Fig. 1 A : Measurements from the echogram of the interventricular septum (IVS) obtained by conventional
anterior echocardiography.

B : Measurements from the echogram of the left
ventricular anterior wall (LVAW) obtained by
esophageal echocardiography.

LVPW : left ventricular posterior wall.

filming at 48 frames/sec. The outlines of the ventricle at end-diastole
and at end-systole were traced from projected image of the cinefilm and
superimposed on the same paper. The spine and ribs were used at the fixed
points for the tracing. Selective coronary arteriography was performed by
the Sones technique, and injections were filmed in multiple views. We
classified the patients with LAD lesion into two groups according to the
location of the lesion (proximal and distal groups.

Conventional and esophageal echocardiograms, ventriculograms and coronary arteriograms were reviewed and analyzed independently by four spe-
cialists without clinical information. Statistical analyses were made by
using an unpaired T-test.

RESULTS

With the esophageal echocardiographic technique, the LVAW echogram was
recorded satisfactorily in 43 of the 47 patients (11 of the 14 normal

subjects and 32 of 33 patients with coronary artery disease). With the
conventional echocardiography, LVAW echograms were recorded in only eight
of 21 patients with coronary artery disease (Table 1).

Esophageal Echocardiographic LVAW Motion the Control Group

A representative example is shown in Figure 2.

The mean values of the wall excursion and the mean systolic velocity
of the LVAW in control group were $10.8^{\pm}1.7$mm (range 8-13mm) and $34.3^{\pm}5.2$
mm/sec(range 28-41 mm/sec) respectively. The mean value of the diastolic
wall thickness was $11.2^{\pm}0.7$mm (range 9-12.5mm) 15.

Esophageal Echocardiographic LVAW Motion in Patients with Coronary Artery
Disease

Figure 3 shows examples of LVAW motion in each group classified according to the systolic excursion of LVAW. Table 1 is a comparison of LVAW
motion detected by esophageal echocardiography, conventional echocardiography and left ventriculography. Correlation between esophageal echocardiograms and left ventriculograms is shown in Table 2. In 16 of 20
patients, the evaluation of LVAW motion by esophageal echocardiography
coincided with that in left ventriculography. With conventional echocardiography, the classification of LVAW motion agreed with that of left
ventriculography in only three of eight patients. In all patients except
one (case 4 in Table 1), excursion of LVAW was much less with conventional echocardiography than that obtained by esophageal echocardiography.

Figure 4 is a comparison of LVAW motion measured by conventional echocardiography with
that by esophageal
echocardiography in
a 63-year old man
with three-vessel
disease (case 12 in
Table 1). Left ven-
triculography proves
hypokinetic motion
of the LVAW, and
the finding is in
good agreement with
that of esophageal
echocardiography.

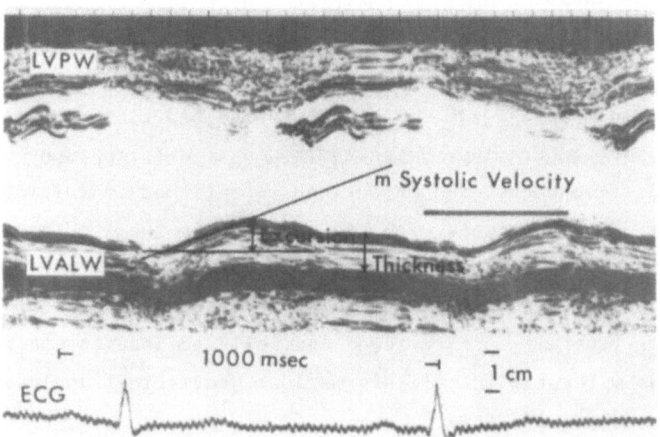

Fig. 2. Esophageal echocardiographic LVAW motion
in a normal subject.

However, with conventional echocardiography, the LVAW echocardiogram shows sligh-tly outward motion during systole. Thus, in this case the abnormal motion of the LVAW is overestimated by the conventional approach.

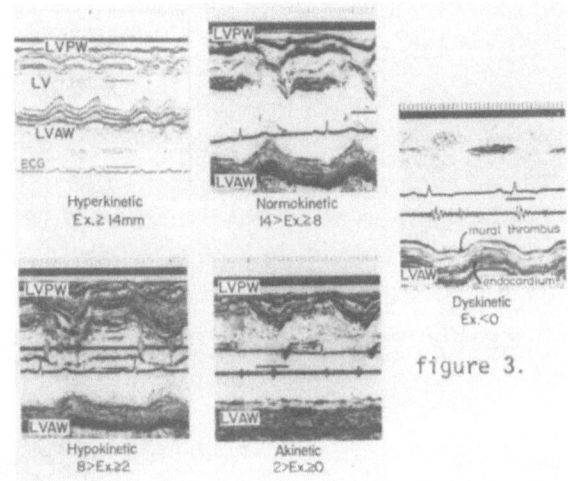

figure 3.

Prediction of the Location of Left Anterior Descending Coronary Artery Disease by Anterior and Esophageal Echocardiography 16.

Anterior and esophageal echocardiographic measurements in normal subjects and patients with LAD disease are shown in Table 3.

Comparison of IVS excursion and LVAW excursion

In all the patients with LAD disease, 18 of 30 (60%) had normal IVS excursion of more than 3mm (8 out of 20 patients with proximal LAD disea-se and all the patients with distal LAD disease). However, these patients except two (93%), had abnormal excursion of the LVAW less than 8mm lower limits of the normal range described above (Figure 5). LVAW excursion in all patients with LAD disease, with or without anteroseptal myocardial infarction, was significantly less than that of normal subjects (proximal with ASMI : P 0.01, proximal without ASMI : P 0.05, distal with ASMI : P 0.01). There was no significant difference between the LVAW excursion of proximal group and that of distal group. However, in comparison with patients with ASMI, significant difference of the LVAW excursion was seen between two groups (Proximal : $2.5^{\pm}1.6$mm, Distal : $4.2^{\pm}2.6$mm, P 0.05) (Table3). Of the proximal group with ASMI, all patients except one, had abnormal LVAW excursion of 3mm or less.

The sum of systolic excursions of the IVS and the LVAW (total excur-sion) was compared between the proximal and distal group (Table 3 and Figure 6). The total excursions in patients with LAD disease (Proximal : $8.7^{\pm}6.3$mm, Distal : $11.0^{\pm}3.8$mm) were significantly lower than that of normal subjects ($16.0^{\pm}2.5$mm) (P 0.01, P 0.01, respectively). In patients with ASMI, right panel in Fig.6, the sum of excursions of the two walls was significantly different between two groups (Proximal : $4.6^{\pm}3.0$mm, Distal: $11.0^{\pm}3.8$mm, P 0.01). In 10 of 12 patients with proximal LAD

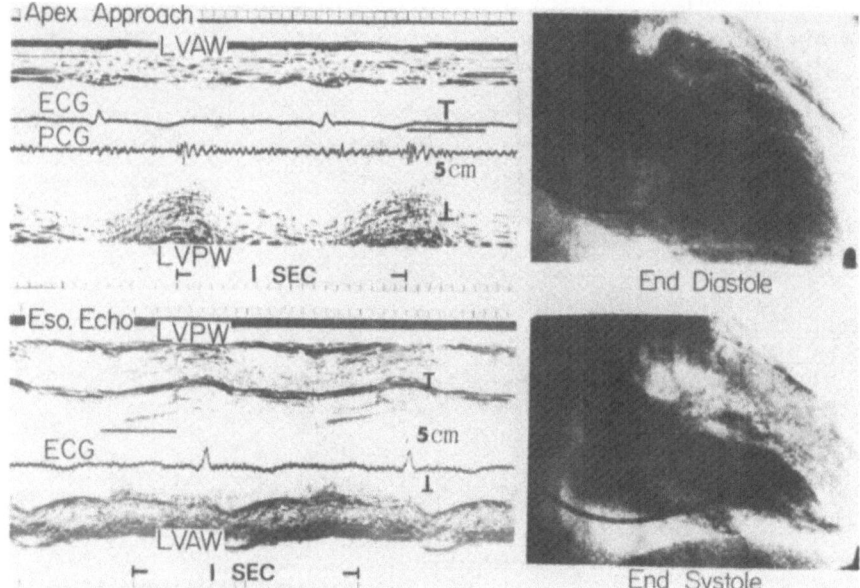

FIGURE 4. *Comparison of the left ventricular anterior wall (LVAW) motion obtained by conventional echocardiography (apex approach) and that by esophageal echocardiography in a patient with inferior myocardial infraction (case 12 in table 1).*

disease and ASMI, the total excursion was 5.5mm or less.

Comparison of Q-C interval of IVS and that of LVAW

Figure 7 showed the comparison of Q-C intervals of IVS and those of LVAW in the proximal (left panel) and the distal groups (right panel).

In patients with proximal group, a comparison of Q-C intervals of the IVS and those of the LVAW showed no significant difference. However, in patients with distal group, the Q-C intervals of the LVAW were longer

Table 3. Conventional and esophageal echocardiographic measurements in normal subjects and patients with coronary artery disease

		Normal	Prox	Prox with ASMI	Prox without ASMI	Dis with ASMI
IVS Ex	(mm)	6.4 ± 0.8	4.3 ± 3.3^a	$2.4\pm2.1^{a,a}$	7.0 ± 3.0	6.5 ± 2.4
LVAW Ex	(mm)	10.8 ± 1.7	4.7 ± 3.3^a	$2.5\pm1.6^{a,d}$	7.9 ± 2.2^b	4.2 ± 2.6^a
IVS Q-C Int	(msec)	82 ± 18	118 ± 47^b	$136\pm43^{a,c}$	90 ± 40	84 ± 32
LVAW Q-C Int	(msec)	84 ± 23	121 ± 44^b	144 ± 31^a	86 ± 38	142 ± 23^a
LVAW m syst vel	(mm/sec)	34.3 ± 5.2	17.4 ± 13.7^a	$11.1\pm9.5^{a,d}$	26.9 ± 14.0	15.4 ± 6.8^a
Total Ex	(mm)	16.0 ± 2.5	8.7 ± 6.3^a	$4.6\pm3.0^{a,c}$	14.9 ± 4.8	11.0 ± 3.8^a
N		11	20	12	8	10

(mean±SD)

IVS=interventricular septum; LVAW=left ventricular anterolateral wall; Ex=systolic excursion; Int=interval; m syst vel=mean systolic velocity; Total Ex=IVS Ex+LVAW Ex in systole; Normal=normal subjects; Prox= patients with proximal lesion of the left anterior descending artery; Dis=patients with distal lesion of the left anterior descending artery; ASMI=anteroseptal myocardial infarction.

a: $p<0.01$ (normal vs each group), b: $p<0.05$ (normal vs each group), c: $p<0.01$ (Dis with ASMI vs Prox with ASMI), d: $p<0.05$ (Dis with ASMI vs Prox with ASMI)

223

than those of the IVS significantly.

Mean Systolic Shortening Velocity of the LVAW in Patients with LAD Disease

Same as the excursion of the LVAW, mean systolic velocity of the LVAW in proximal group with ASMI ($11.1^{\pm}9.5$mm/sec) was significantly smaller than that in distal group ($15.4^{\pm}6.8$mm/sec) (P 0.02).

Cases

Figure 8 shows a representative case with distal LAD disease. The IVS echogram demonstrates normal excursion (8mm) and the normal Q-C interval (50mm/sec). However, the esophageal echogram reveals akinesis of LVAW motion (2mm in excursion), decreased mean systolic velocity (10mm/sec), and prolonged Q-C interval of 160mm/sec. These findings correspond well to the left ventriculographic findings.

Figure 9 shows conventional echogram (Ant.Echo), esophageal echogram (Eso.Echo), left coronary arteriogram and left ventriculograms in a 63-year old man with ASMI. Left coronary arteriogram shows severe

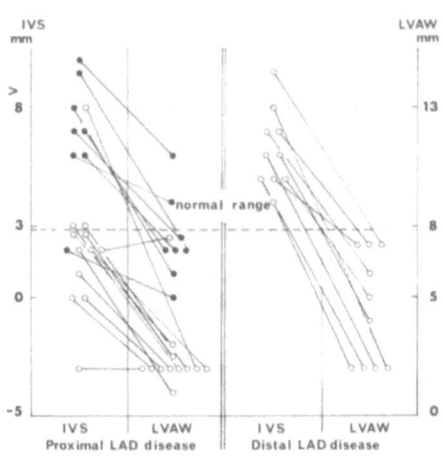

o anterior infarction , • non-anterior infarction

Fig. 5 Comparison of interventricular septal (IVS) and left ventricular anterior wall (LVAW) systolc excursion in patients with proximal left anterior descending coronary artery (LAD) disease and those in distal LAD disease.

stenosis of the LAD proximal to the major septal branch. Both of the IVS and the LVAW have less excursion and prolonged Q-C intervals. Left ventriculograms reveal the akinesis of LVAW and hypokinesis of IVS.

DISCUSSION

Echocardiography is one of the most valuable noninvasive techniques for evaluating regional wall dynamics 1-18. The location of abnormal echo motion generally corresponds to the area distal to the severe stenosis of the coronary artery 5. However, it is sometimes difficult to assess the entire segment of the left ventricle with conventional echocardiography. Corya et al 4, recorded LVAW echoes in 50 of 54 patients with coronary artery disease using conventional echocardiography with the transducer on the chest wall. In their study, the correlation of the LVAW echo-

224

cardiogram with the left ventriculogram was examined, with agreement
found in only 66% of the cases. One
explanation for this poor correlation
was that the areas examined were not
always the same.

In our study, LVAW echo motion that
was interpreted as normal by Corya'a
definition was further classified as
hyperkinetic, normokinetic or hypokinetic, while abnormal LVAW motion as
defined by Corya was classified as
akinetic or dyskinetic. In 16 of these
20 (80%), the classification of LVAW
motion by esophageal echocardiography
coincided well with that by left ventriculography. LVAW echoes recorded by
conventional echocardiography were

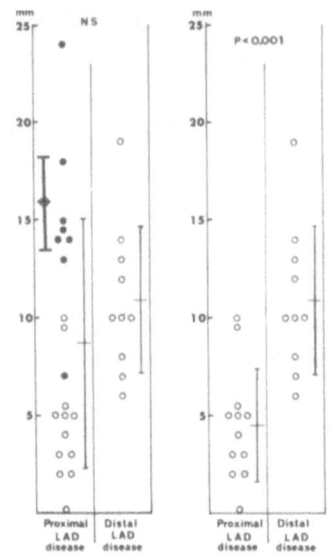

Fig. 6 Comparison of total excursions (IVS excursion plus LVAW excursion) in proximal group and that in distal group.

satisfactory in only eight of 21 patients (38%). All eight of these patients had abnormal LVAW motion on the conventional echocardiogram, but
the LVAW motion classification by conventional echocardiography was compatible with that obtained by left ventriculography in only three patients
(37%). Moreover, LVAW in seven of the eight patients whose LVAW echoes
were recorded by conventional echocardiography showed less systolic excursion compared with that shown
in those recorded by esophageal
echocardiography. Previous investigators 17,   have pointed
out that the anterior shift of
the whole heart occurring during
systole may cause underestimation
of the systolic excursion of the
LVAW. Leighton et al.   used left
ventriculography and documented
that systolic excursion of the
LVAW did not differ greatly from
that of the left ventricular pos-

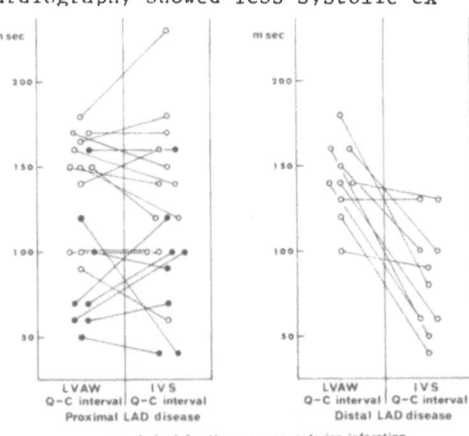

Fig. 7 Comparison of LVAW Q-C interval and IVS Q-C interval in patients with LAD disease.

terior wall. Our data are consistent with this observation. The esophageal transducer probably could move along with the whole heart motion in each cardiac cycle, which would minimize the artifact of underestimation of LVAW motion.

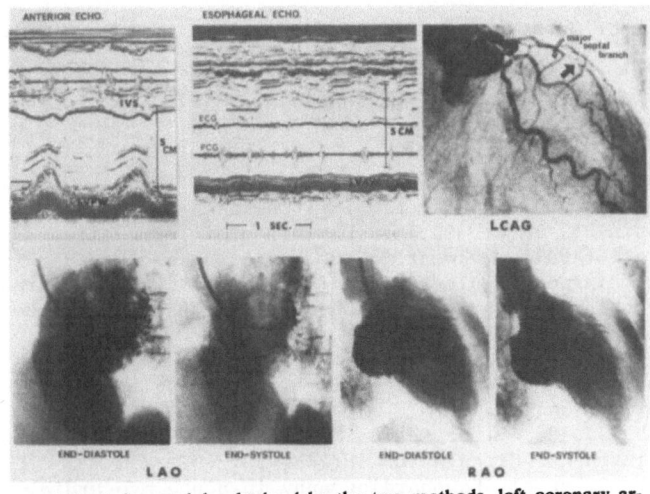

Fig. 8. Echograms of the left ventricle obtained by the two methods, left coronary arteriogram and left ventriculograms from a patient (69 years old male with ASMI) with distal left anterior descending coronary artery lesion.

Thus, our results emphasize that the projection of an ultrasonic beam from the intraesophageal transducer would be a better approach for accurate evaluation of LVAW motion compared with the conventional approach.

In this study, to measure the LVAW motion with esophageal echocardiography was more meaningful in predicting the presence of LAD disease than to measure the IVS motion. Especially, the sum of the LVAW and the IVS excursion was a good parameter to know the location of the LAD lesion in patients with prior ASMI. In experimental studies outward motion of the ischemic wall increased during isovolumetric contraction (aneurysmal bulging 17,18. In addition to those findings, our results indicated that in the ischemic wall the time interval increased significantly

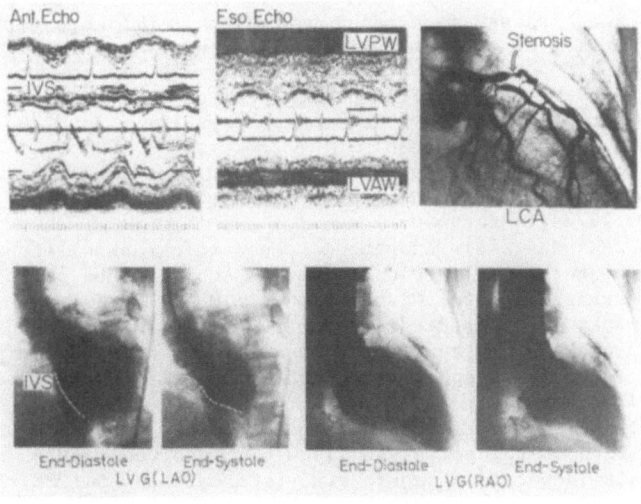

Fig. 9. Echograms of the left ventricle by the two methods, left coronary arteriogram and left ventriculograms from a patient (63 years old male with ASMI) with proximal LAD lesion.

226

between the Q wave on the ECG and the onset of inward wall motion (Q-C interval). Therefore, this time interval was thought to be one of useful parameters to find an ischemia of ventricular wall.

REFERENCES

1. Inoue K, et al. Ultrasonic measurement of left ventricular motion in acute myocardial infarction. Circulation 43:778, 1971.
2. Ratshin RA, et al. Serial evaluation of left ventricular volumes and posterior wall movement in the acute phase of myocardial infarction using diagnostic ultrasound. (abstr) Am J Cardiol 29:286, 1972.
3. Feigenbaum H: Echocardiography. Philadelphia, Lea & Febiger, 1972, pp 199-209.
4. Corya BC, et al. Anterior left ventricular wall echoes in coronary artery disease. Linear scanning with a single element transducer. Am J Cardiol 34:652, 1974.
5. Jacobs JJ, et al. Detection of left ventricular asynergy by echocardiography. Circulation 48:263, 1973.
6. Corya BC, et al. Echocardiography in acute myocardial infarction. Am J Cardiol 36:1, 1975.
7. Baxley WA, et al. Abnormal regional myocardial performance in coronary artery disease. Prog. Cardiovasc Dis 13:405, 1971.
8. Corya BC: Echocardiography in ischemic heart disease. Am J Med 63:10, 1977.
9. Joffe CD, et al. Echocardiographic diagnosis of left anterior descending coronary artery disease (abstr) Am J Cardiol 35:146, 1975.
10. DeMaria A, et al. Left anterior descending involvement in coronary disease, detection by abnormal ventricular septal motion on echocardiogram. Clin Res 22:272A, 1974.
11. Gordon MJ, et al. Interventricular septal motion in patients with proximal and distal left anterior descending coronary artery lesions. Circulation 55:338, 1977.
12. Kolibash AJ, et al. The relationship between abnormal echocardiographic septal motion and myocardial perfusion in patients with significant obstruction of the left anterior descending artery. Circulation 56:780, 1977.
13. Matsuzaki M, et al. Clinical application of esophageal echocardiography to the mitral valve prolapse syndrome. Jpn J Med Ultrasonics 31:89, 1977 (in Japanese)
14. Matsuzaki M, et al. Assessment of left ventricular anterior wall motion. A new application of esophageal echocardiography. J Cardiography 8:113,1978 (in Japanese)
15. Matsuzaki M, et al. Esophageal echocardiographic left ventricular anterolateral wall motion in normal subjects and patients with coronary artery disease. Circulation 63:1085, 1981.
16. Matsuzaki M, et al. Prediction of the location of left anterior descending coronary artery disease by anterior echocardiography and esophageal echocardiography. J of Cardiography 11:401,1981 (in Japanese with English abstract).
17. Kerber RE, et al. Effects of acute coronary occlusion on the motion and perfusion of the normal and ischemic interventricular septum:an experimental echocardiographic study. Circulation 54:928, 1976.
18. Kerber RE, et al. Correlation between echocardiographically demonstrated segmental dyskinesis and regional myocardial perfusion. Circulation 52:1097, 1975.

THE EVALUATION OF LEFT VENTRICULAR FUNCTION BY TRANSESOPHAGEAL M-MODE EXERCISE ECHOCARDIOGRAPHY

M. MATSUMOTO, P. HANRATH, P. KREMER, W. BLEIFELD, T. MAEDA,
K. YASUI, M. INOUE, and H. ABE

Dynamic exercise M-mode and two-dimensional echocardiography provides important informations over the response and cardiac reserve of the left ventricle against exercise(1-8). However, the application of standard transthoracic echocardiography to the exercise often contains difficulties in maintaining good images due to exaggerated respiration and chest wall motion. To overcome these problems the present authors have manufactured a new trans-esophageal echo transducer system using a gastroscope and applied it to the dynamic exercise test of the left ventricular function.

STUDY DESIGN

The usefulness of the present method in the evaluation of in-exercise left ventricular performance was studied in normals and patients with cardiac diseases of a wide spectrum as the first part of the study. Considering the result of the first part of the study that the patients with aortic regurgitation are good candidates for this study the numbers of patients with aortic regurgitation as well as normal subjects were expanded and studied as the second part of the study.

MATERIALS

The first part study population consisted of 14 patients with coronary artery disease without left ventricular dyskinesis, 4 with aortic regurgitation, 4 with congestive cardiomyopathy, 3 normals, 3 with congenital heart diseases and 3 with mitral

*Dr. Matsumoto was a research scholar of the Alexander von Humboldt Foundation in years 1979 and 1980 at the University of Hamburg.

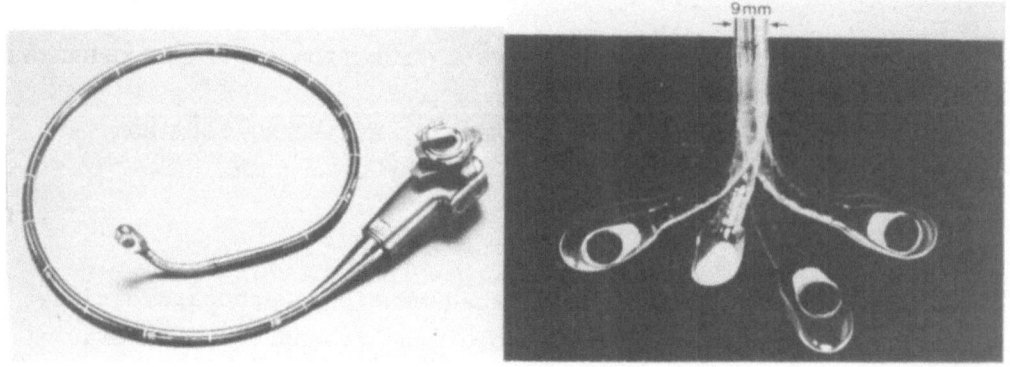

FIGURE 1. Our transesophageal M-mode echo transducer system.

regurgitation. For the second part of the study 11 patients
with aortic regurgitation and 7 normals were added. Forty-nine
total study population consisted of 32 males and 17 females
ranging from 19 to 72 years in age with an average of 47±12.

METHODS

Transesophageal echocardiography

A commercially available medium focused esophageal
transducer (3.5MHz, 10mm diameter) was incorporated into the
tip of a gastroscope(figure 1). The manipulation of the probe,
such as angulation, rotation and up and down movement, was
under the examiner's control. Transesophageal M-mode echocardiograms were recorded with a Picker Echoview System 80C
and Aloka SSD 110 on a continuous strip chart recorder at a
paper speed of 50 and/or 100mm/sec. Prior to the insertion of
the probe intravenous administration of atropine sulfate(0.5mg)
and local anesthesia of the throat with Xylocaine Spray were
performed. A transesophageal M-mode echocardiogram of the left
ventricle was obtained after proceeding the probe about 40cm
from the mouth where aortic valve was visualized and by further
downward movement plus counterclockwise rotation of the probe
as reported by the present(9-11) and other authors(12)(figure 2).
The echocardiographic identification as well as confirmation of

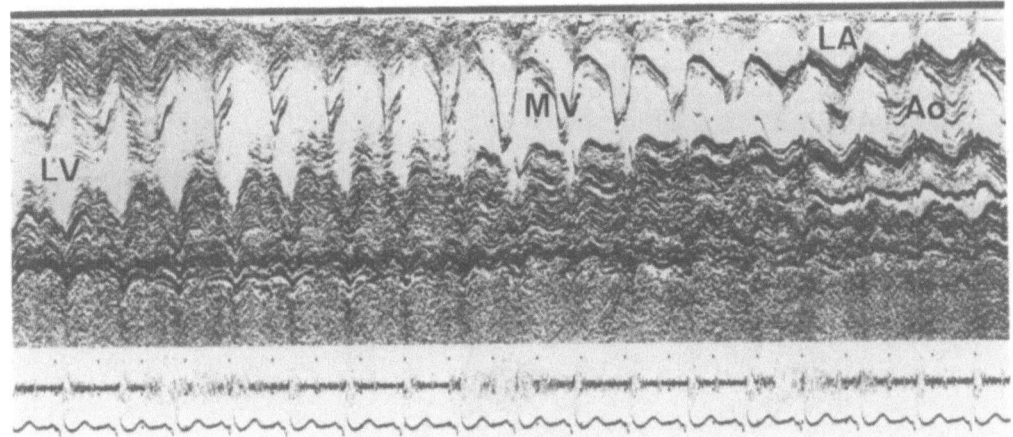

FIGURE 2. Transesophageal echocardiographic M-mode scan from the left
ventricle to the aorta. LV=left ventricle, MV=mitral valve, Ao=aorta

the spatial relationship of the probe to the left ventricle
were carried out during left ventriculography in selected
patients(figure 3). It should be noted that transesophageal
echocardiograms exhibit a mirror image of standard transthoracic
echocardiograms. Echocardiographic indices of the left ventricle
calculated were enddiastolic diameter(Dd), endsystolic diameter
(Ds), fractional shortening(FS), maximal velocity of circumferential fiber shortening(Vcf max), and lengthening(Vlr max).
These indices were calculated by a digital computer from three
successive cardiac cycles before exercise, each minute during
and after exercise.

Bicycle exercise test

Supine bicycle exercise was initiated at a work load of
150kpm/min. The load was increased by 150kpm/min every three
minutes until symptoms such as fatigue, limiting dyspnea and
angina were developed.

RESULTS

1. Success rate of imaging the left ventricle during exercise

Recording of the left ventricle during maximal exercise
was successful in 46 of consecutive 49 patients(94%). The stability, rotation and angulation of the probe were under examiner's

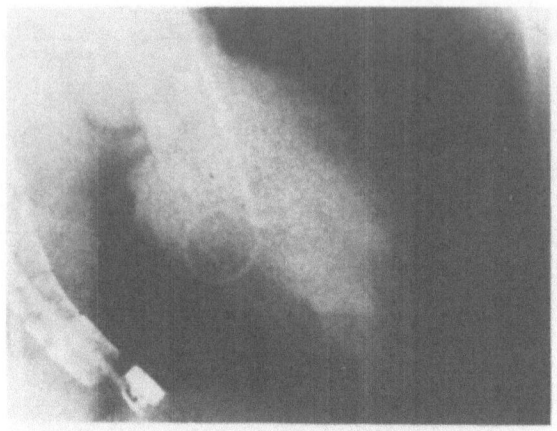
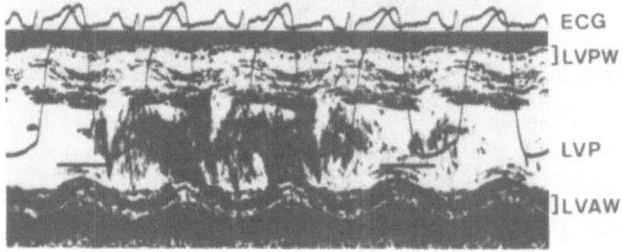

ECG
]LVPW
LVP
]LVAW

FIGURE 3. Simultaneous left ventriculogram and transesophageal echocardiogram.

control. The echo images were not disturbed by respiration nor movement of the chest wall even under severe exercise and the left ventricle was visualized satisfactory throughout exercise as shown in figure 4.

2. A preliminary study of exercise transesophageal echocardiography in patients with cardiac diseases of a wide spectrum.

A pilot study has been carried out to know the types of diseases to which the application of the present method is useful. In figure 5 changes in heart rate(HR), enddiastolic dimension(Dd), endsystolic dimension(Ds), fractional shortening(FS), velocity of maximal circumferential fiber shortening(Vcf max) and lengthening (Vlr max) before exercise(C), during maximal exercise(E,E') and one minute after exercise(A) in 8 patients with coronary artery disease(CAD), 4 patients with aortic regurgitation(AR), 3 normals (N), 3 patients with congestive cardiomyopathy(CCM) and 3 patients with congenital heart diseases are exhibited. E' represents the

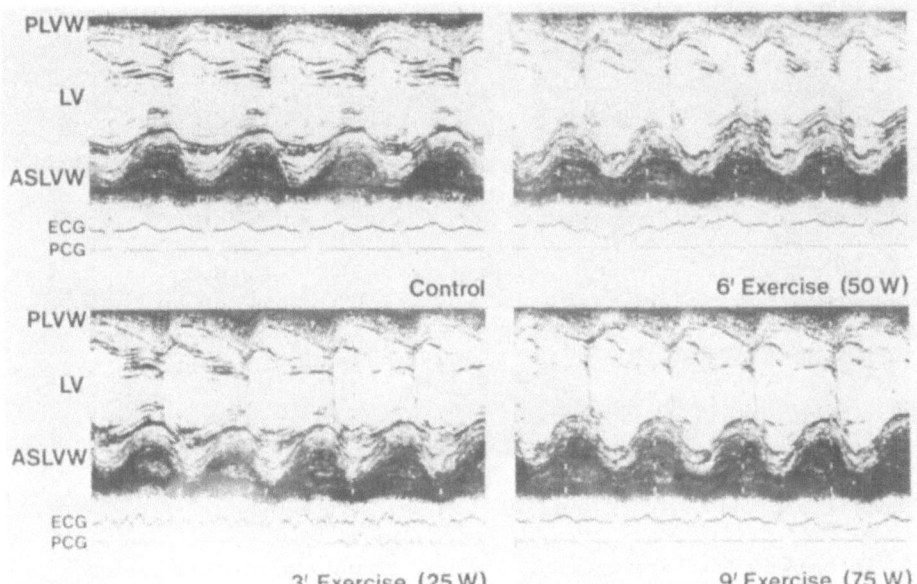

FIGURE 4. Transesophageal echogram of the left ventricle at different
stages of exercise in a normal subject. PLVW=posterior left
ventricular wall, ASLVW=anteroseptal left ventricular wall

mean value for only those patients who could continue the
examination until one minute after exercise. The average duration
was 5.0±2.1 minutes and the maximal work load in average was 389±
144kpm/min. Although the statistical significance was not tested
due to the small number of patients in each group, the following
marked changes were observed as shown in figure 5:1) Ds(36±7→
46±7mm), FS(43±5 → 33±7%), Vlrmax(4.9±1.1 → 3.8±1.3circ/sec) in
aortic regurgitation, 2) Vcf max(3.0±o.6 → 3.9±0.6circ/sec) in
normals, 3) FS(37±0 → 30±1%) in congenital heart diseases, 4)
Vlrmax(3.0±0.5 → 4.6±1.4circ/sec) in congestive cardiomyopathy.

3. Contrast study of left ventricular response to exercise
in normal subjects and aortic regurgitation.

The response of the left ventricle to exercise in different
directions in normals and aortic regurgitation has driven us to
a further investigation in these two groups in a expanded number
of subjects, 10 normals and 15 patients with aortic regurgitation.

3.1. Normal control subjects. Influences of dynamic exercise
in 10 normal subjects(5 males and 5 females, 38±14 years in age)

232

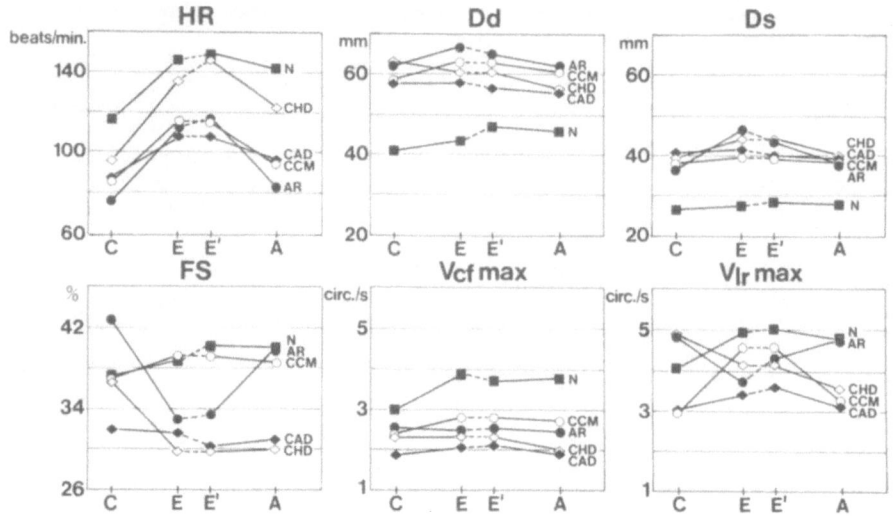

FIGURE 5. Changes in echocardiographic indices during exercise in patient
groups of various cardiac diseases.

are summarized in figure 6. Pressure rate biproduct increased
from 13±2 to 20±3mmHg·min^{-1}·10^3(p<0.001). In accordance with
the increase in heart rate and blood pressure, left ventricular
dimension decreased continuously from 51±5 to 48±6mm(p<0.05)
under maximal exercise. The fractional shortening increased
continuously from 37±4 to 43±5%(p<0.001) at the end of exercise.

3.2. Aortic regurgitation. Fifteen patients with aortic
regurgitation(9 males and 6 females, 36±12 years in age ranging
19-61) were studied as symptomatic(8) and asymptomatic(7) patient subsets. Echocardiograms in a representative case with
symptomatic aortic regurgitation at rest and maximal exercise
are shown in figure 7. Left ventricular enddiastolic diameter
was markedly enlarged already at rest to 76mm and was further
increased to 82mm at maximal exercise. Fractional shortening
decreased from 41% at rest to 37% at the end of exercise.
Pressure-rate product were increased significantly in both
subsets at the end of exercise(p<0.001), but there were no
significant difference between the two subsets. Enddiastolic
dimension during maximal exercise showed significant changes
only in the asymptomatic subset(55±4 ⟶ 51±6mm, p<0.05) and not

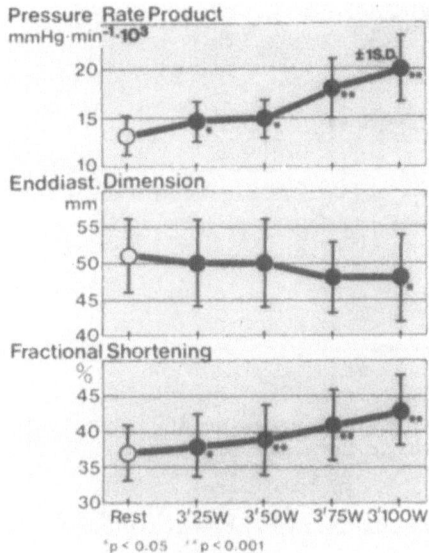

FIGURE 6. Effects of dynamic exercise in ten normal subjects.

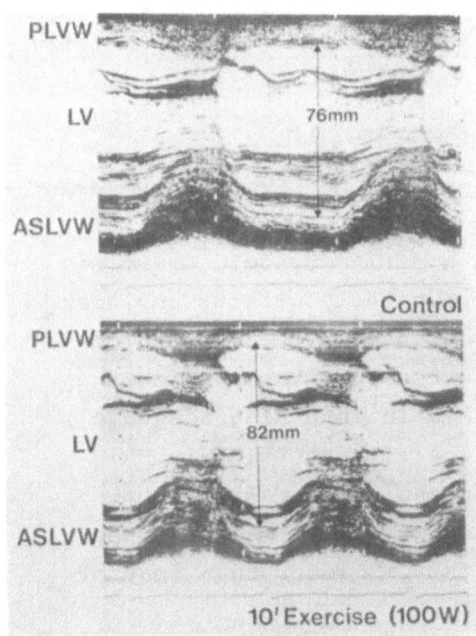

FIGURE 7. Transesophageal echogram of the left ventricle at rest and maximal exercise in symptomatic aortic regurgitation.

234

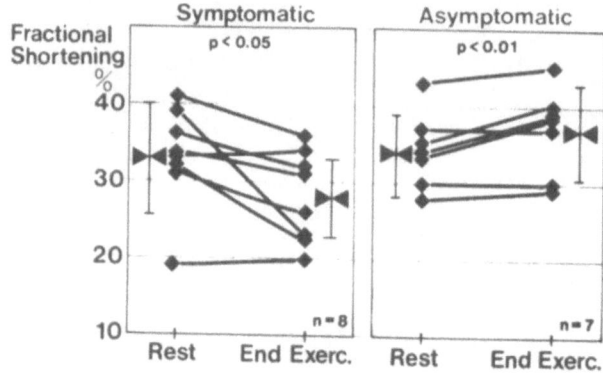

FIGURE 8. Fractional shortening at rest and maximal exercise in symptomatic
and asymptomatic patients with aortic regurgitation.

in the symptomatic subset($69\pm20 \rightarrow 67\pm20$, N.S.). Fractional
shortening was within a normal range at rest in both subsets
except one symptomatic case(figure 8). During maximal exercise,
however, symptomatic subset exhibited significant decrease in
fractional shortening($33\pm7 \rightarrow 28\pm5\%$, $p<0.05$) and the asymptomatic
subset showed significant increase to the contrary($34\pm5 \rightarrow 37\pm6\%$,
$p<0.01$).

Discussion
   Echocardiography has recently been applied for the assessment
of left ventricular function during dynamic exercise(1-8).
Left ventricular size and performance during dynamic exercise
can be evaluated noninvasively and repeatedly without any risk
and alteration of the physiologic response of the myocardium
to the exercise. However, exercise echocardiography using the
parasternal approach contains problems in obtaining adequate
images for analysis as reported in the literature(2-8). This
is mainly caused by hyperventilation and chest wall motion.
The average success rate of recording adequate images in the
seven reports(1-3, 5-8) is 68% and this is lower than that of
94% in our present study.
   Since the initial clinical application of transesophageal
echocardiography by Frazin et al.(13) only several studies
(9-12,14,15) using this method have been carried out because

of the uniqueness of the technique and also the difficulty to
manipulate the probe. The incorporation of the echo probe into
the tip of a gastroscope in the present study facilitated the
manipulation of the probe and the usefulness of the transesophageal method in exercise echocardiography in various types of
patietnts was documented in the first part of the study. Although
it was difficult to conclude something definite about the response
of left ventricle to exercise in each patient group, some interesting tendencies which led us to the second part of the study were
observed. In the second part of the study decrease in enddiastolic
diameter was shown at the maximal dynamic exercise in normal
subjects and asymptomatic aortic regurgitation indicating good
reserve of left ventricular pump function. In symptomatic aortic
regurgitation no significant decrease was observed in enddiastolic
diameter at maximal exercise revealing decrease in the reserve of
left ventricular pump function. Exercise fractional shortening in
symptomatic aortic regurgitation took different attitude from
that in normal subjects and asymptomatic aortic regurgitation
disclosing the presence of an intrinsic left ventricular dysfunction. Exercise fractional shortening in symptomatic and
asymptomatic aortic regurgitation in the present study showed
the same tendency as the exercise ejection fraction reported
by Borer and associates(16).

In conclusion transesophageal M-mode echocardiography was
useful in the evaluation of left ventricular performance during
supine bicycle ergometry, especially in aortic regurgitation.
The present method seems to offer a useful guide to the prog-
nosis of cardiac diseases.

REFERENCES
1. Stein RA, Michielli D, Fox EL, Krasnow N: Continuous ventricular dimensions
   in man during supine exercise and recovery. Am J Cardiol 41:655, 1978
2. Mason SJ, Weiss JL, Weisfeld ML, Garrison JB, Fortuin NJ: Exercise
   echocardiography: Detection of wall motion abnormalities during ischemia.
   Circulation 59:50, 1979
3. Goldstein RE, Bennett ED, Leech GL: Effect of glyceryl trinitrate on
   echocardiographic left ventricular dimensions during exercise in the
   upright position. Br Heart J 42:245, 1979

236

4. Weiss JL, Weisfeld ML, Mason SJ, Garrison JB, Livengood SV, Fortuin NJ:
    Evidence of Frank-Starling effect in man during severe semisupine
    exercise. Circulation 59:655, 1979
5. Crawford MH, White DH, Amon KW: Echocardiographic evaluation of left
    ventricular size and performance during handgrip and supine upright
    bicycle exercise. Circulation 59:1188, 1979
6. Sugishita Y, Koseki S: Dynamic exercise echocardiography. Circulation
    60:743, 1979
7. Wann LS, Faris JV, Childress RH, Dillon JC, Weyman AE, Feigenbaum H:
    Exercise cross-sectional echocardiography in ischemic heart disease.
    Circulation 60:1300, 1979
8. Morganroth J, Chen CC, David DD, Sawin HS, Naito M, Parrotto C, Meixell L:
    Exercise cross-sectional echocardiographic diagnosis of coronary artery
    disease. Am J Cardiol 47:20, 1981
9. Matsumoto M, Oka Y, Lin YT, Strom J, Sonnenblick EH, Frater RWM: Trans-
    esophageal echocardiography for assessing ventricular performance.
    New York State J Med 79:19, 1979
10. Matsumoto M, Oka Y, Strom J, Frishman W, Kadish A, Becker R, Frater RWM,
    Sonnenblick EH: Application of transesophageal echocardiography for
    continuous intraoperative monitoring of left ventricular performance.
    Am J Cardiol 46:95, 1980
11. Hanrath P, Kremer P, Langenstein BA, Matsumoto M, Bleifeld W:Transöso-
    phageale Echokardiographie. Ein neues Verfahren zur dynamischen Ven-
    trikelfunktionsanalyse. Deutsche Medizinische Wochenschrift 106:523,
    1981
12. Matsuzaki M, Matsuda Y, Takahashi Y, Sasaki T, Toma Y, Ishida K, Yorozu T,
    Kumada T, Kusukawa R: Esophageal echocardiographic left ventricular
    antero-lateral wall motion in normal subjects and patients with coronary
    artery disease. Circulation 63:1085, 1981
13. Frazin L, Talano JV, Stephanides L, Loeb HS, Kopel L, Gunnar RM:
    Esophageal echocardiography. Circulation 54:102, 1976
14. Hisanaga K, Hisanaga A: A new real-time sector scanning system with
    ultrawide angle and real-time recording of entire adult cardiac images.Trans-
    esophageal and transthoracic wall methods. In:White DN, ed. Ultrasound
    in Medicine Vol. 4. New York: Plenum Press, 1978:391
15. Hisanaga K, Hisanaga A, Nagata K, Ichie Y: Transesophageal cross-sectional
    echocardiography. Am Heart J 100:605, 1980
16. Borer JS, Bacharach SL, Green MV, Kent KM, Henry WL, Rosing DR, Seides SF,
    Johnston GS, Epstein SE: Exercise-induced left ventricular dysfunction in
    symptomatic and asymptomatic patients with aortic regurgitation: Assessment
    with radionuclide cineangiography. Am J Cardiol 42:351, 1978

EFFECTS OF ANESTHESIA ON LEFT VENTRICULAR PERFORMANCE
ASSESSED BY TRANSESOPHAGEAL M-MODE ECHOCARDIOGRAPHY

P. Kremer, M.D.
M.K. Cahalan, M.D.

INTRODUCTION. Complex and invasive forms of monitoring play an increasing role in the care of patients with serious cardiac disease. Significant morbidity and (rarely) mortality can result from the monitoring itself. We would welcome equally informative monitoring devices that were non-invasive and hence without risk.

Precordial echocardiography now is a commonplace noninvasive aid to the preoperative assessment of patients with a variety of cardiac disorders. Precordial inaccessability and instability of the position of the echo probe are two inherent problems that prevent the intraoperative application of this technique. We now report that continuous, high quality M-mode and two dimensional (2-D) echocardiograms can be simply and safely obtained from a transesophageal approach.

METHODS. With the approval of our committee on human experimentation and informed consent, we studied 23 ASA I or II adult patients (ages 19 to 63 years) undergoing abdominal or perineal surgery. All patients received identical rapid intravenous induction sequences. Immediately after endotracheal intubation, a gastroscope tipped with a special 3.5 MHz transducer (either M-mode or 2-D) was introduced into the esophagus. The positional controls of the gastroscope allowed the transducer to show multiple and reproducible views of the heart. We selected and maintained a cross sectional view of the left ventrical (LV) through the base of the papillary muscles. Within five minutes after intubation, we established constant end tidal concentrations of 60 per cent nitrous oxide and one of three randomly selected vapors: 0.7 per cent halothane, 1.0 per cent isoflurane, or 1.5 per cent enflurane. Ventilation was controlled to yield an end tidal CO_2 of 30 to 35 torr.

Fifteen minutes following endotracheal intubation (PSIND), immediately before incision (PREINC), and 5 minutes after incision (PSINC) we measured mean arterial pressure (MAP), heart rate (HR), LV end diastolic dimension (EDD), LV fractional shorting (FS), and LV peak circumferential fiber shorting velocity (VCF). MAP and HR were measured by an automated blood pressure cuff (Dinamap model 845).

RESULTS. For the PSIND period our results ($\pm$ 1 SE) are displayed in the following table:

	N	MAP (torr)	HR (bpm)	EDD (mm)	FS (%)	VCF (circ/s)
Hal	6	66.0(3.0)	61.2(3.9)	46.8(1.7)	32.6(1.5)	1.95(.22)
Enf	8	61.5(7.2)	67.8(5.6)	47.3(2.2)	32.7(0.9)	1.73(.09)
Iso	9	72.2(5.7)	76.5(5.1)	48.3(2.3)	33.3(2.0)	2.15(.11)

Similar results were found in the other two periods. Patient ages, weights, fluid infusions, and temperatures were not significantly different for the three groups. Only VCF results showed a significant difference (P=0.045 by analysis of variance).

DISCUSSION. In individuals without myocardial dysfunction, angiographic studies have demonstrated that EDD and FS are reasonable estimators of LV end diastolic volume and ejection fraction respectively.(1) VCF is a derived variable which characterizes LV performance and is strongly dependent on contractility and afterload and to a lesser degree on preload.(2) Our finding that isoflurane has the highest average VCF and enflurane the lowest is consistent with previous studies indicating the least in vivo depression of myocardial function from isoflurane.(3) Since our measures of afterload and preload, MAP and EDD, show no significant differences, we believe that the likely cause for the difference in VCF is greater contractility in the isoflurane group. However, despite this apparently greater contractility no difference is seen in the FS. One possible explanation for this finding is that the velocity of LV contraction might slow without decreasing the extent of contraction and therefore VCF may be a more sensitive marker of global LV function.

In conclusion, we believe that transesophageal echocardiography has great promise as a safe and highly informative intraoperative monitor.

REFERENCES. 1. Teichholz LE et al. Problems in echocardiographic volume determinations. Am J Cardiol 37:7, 1976.
2. Quinones MA et al. Echocardiographic determination of left ventricular stress--velocity relations in man: with reference to the effects of loading and contractility. Circ 51:689, 1975.
3. Stevens WC et al. The cardiovascular effects of a new inhalational anesthetic, Forane, in human volunteers at constant arterial carbon dioxide tension. Anesthesiology 35:8, 1971.

TRANSESOPHAGEAL CROSS-SECTIONAL ECHOCARDIOGRAPHY WITH A MECHANICAL
SCANNING SYSTEM

K. HISANAGA and A. HISANAGA
Department of Internal Medicine, Mitsubishi Nagoya Hospital
Nagoya, Japan

INTRODUCTION

Since B-mode echocardiography has been applied to diagnosis of cardiac
disease, it has proven useful in anatomical and functional assessment of the
heart, and several real-time imaging systems have been developed. However,
thoracic configuration, excessive chest wall tissue, or air containing lung may
often limit the fields of view and resolution. In order to minimize these
limitations. Hisanaga and associates have developed a transesophageal pulsed
Doppler echocardiographic system.[7,8] Although this method is useful, it does
not provide two-dimensional cardiac images.

We have developed many kinds of transesophageal (transgastric) ultrasonic
imaging systems (linear scanner,[6,16] sector scanner,[1,2,16] rotating scanner[9,17]) which
can obtain heart images without hindrance from ribs, sternum, and lung.
Transesophageal echocardiography provides a wider area for study of the heart
than that available using a conventional external system. Heart images are
observed through esophageal tissue in which ultrasound absorption is very
low. Therefore there is little difference in the image quality among various
subjects.

TECHNIQUE

Transesophageal (Transgastric) Rotating Scanner[1,9,14,17]

The scanner consists of a pulse motor, a flexible metal tube containing
a flexible rotating shaft, a small transducer, a small slip ring commutator,
and an oil bag (Figure 1, Figure 2). The specifications of the transducer
are 2.25 MHz or 3.5 MHz, 10 mm diameter, and 7.5 cm focus. The transducer
is mounted in a 12 mm by 20 mm by 6 mm casing with rounded edges for easy
esophageal passage. The transducer and commutator are positioned at the tip
of the flexible rotating shaft and are enclosed in the oil bag (maximum 20 mm
diameter). In order to obtain horizontal or oblique two-dimensional images

240

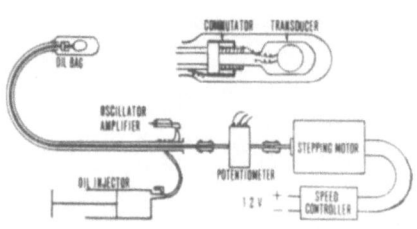

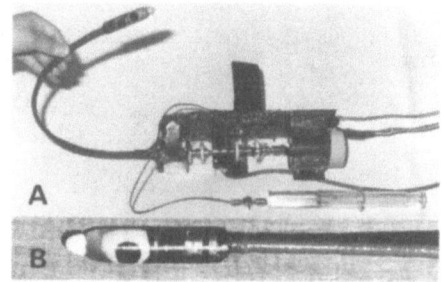

FIGURE 1. Diagrammatic illustration of the transesophageal
(or transgastric) high speed
rotating scanner.[7]

FIGURE 2. Transesophageal high speed
rotating scanner (A). Transducer
and commutator (B).

of the heart, the transducer can be bent at a fixed angle between 5 degrees
and 45 degrees (Figure 4). The flexible rotating shaft is enclosed in the
flexible metal tube (diameter about 7 mm) and the tube is then wrapped with
vinyl chloride tape. Total length of shaft and tube is 40 cm or 70 cm
(The long shaft is used for transgastric examination). The oil bag covering
the transducer can be filled by an injector.

The small transducer in the esophagus is rotated for a full 360 degrees
by the rotating shaft and the motor at a rate of 20 - 50 cycles/sec. The
direction of the transducer in the esophagus is detected continuously by a
potentiometer connected directly to the rotating shaft. The reflected echoces
are transmitted through the commutator and the tube containing the rotating
shaft and displayed on a cathode ray tube as B-mode. Thus the angle of an
individual scanning line is equal
to the angle of the transducer
at the same instant.

In this way, horizontal or
oblique two-dimensional images
of the heart through the
esophageal wall are displayed
on the cathode ray tube at
a rate of 20 - 50 cycles/sec.
Maximum selective pulse repetition frequency is 6.0 KHz.

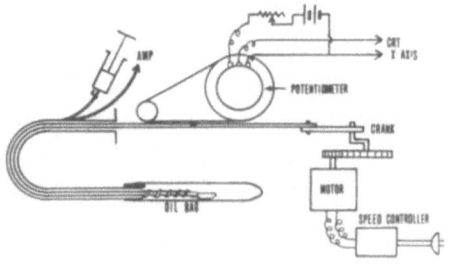

FIGURE 3. Diagrammatic illustration
of the transesophageal high speed
linear scanner.[6,16]

The field of view is 10 - 17 cm deep depending on the pulse repetition frequency. Although the sonographic beam is swept radially, the display angle is fixed at 270 degrees or 180 degrees. In this system, only one commutator is used because the flexible rotating shaft in the flexible tube acts as another commutator. Although the transducer is rotated for a full 360 degrees at a high frequency, the external tube does not itself move but is stable within the stomach. Moreover, the enveloping oil bag minimizes trauma to the esophagus.

Transesophageal Linear Scanner[6,16]

In the linear scanner, a small transducer is moved up and down in the esophagus through a flexible shaft by a motor at a rate of 4 to 10 Hz and vertical two-dimensional heart images are displayed in rectangular format on a cathode ray tube at a rate of 8 - 20 fields/sec (Figure 3). Other specifications are as in the transesophageal rotating scanner.

Insertion of Transducer[14,17]

Prior to examination, the patients' throats were sprayed with 4 % lidocaine liquid. Lidocaine jelly was applied to the oil bag and flexible tube in

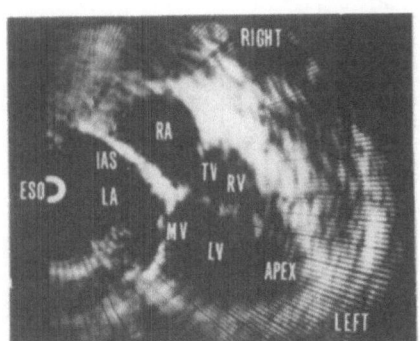

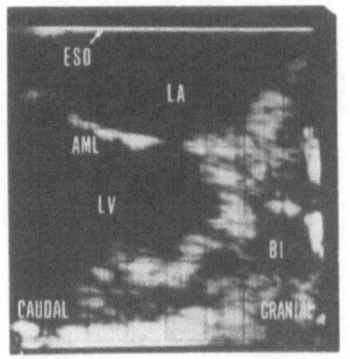

FIGURE 4. Inferior oblique scan through the apex in a normal adult by using the transesophageal high speed rotating scanner. The entire heart including the apex is seen.[11]

FIGURE 5. Vertical scan through the mitral valve in another normal adult by using the transesophageal high speed linear scanner.[6,16]

ESO = esophagus; LA = left atrium; LV = left ventricle; IAS = interatrial septum; MV = mitral valve; TV = tricuspid valve; RV = right ventricle; RA = right atrium; IVS = interventricular septum; BI = bifurcation of pulmonary artery.

242

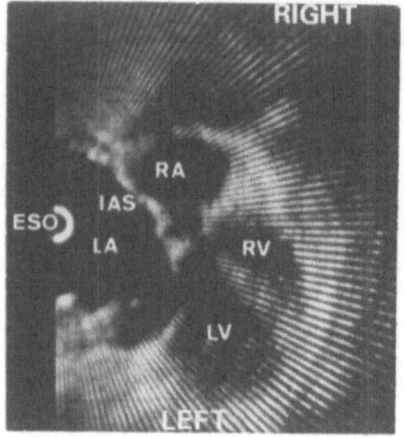

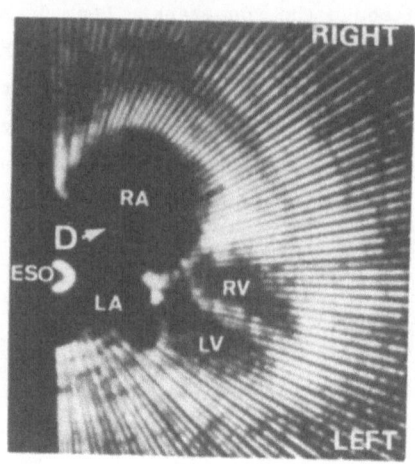

FIGURE 6. Horizontal scan in
a normal adult. A part of aorta
(A) is seen.

FIGURE 7. Horizontal scan at the
level of the mitral valve in a patient
with an secundum atrial septal defect.[17,18]
The large defect (D) is seen.

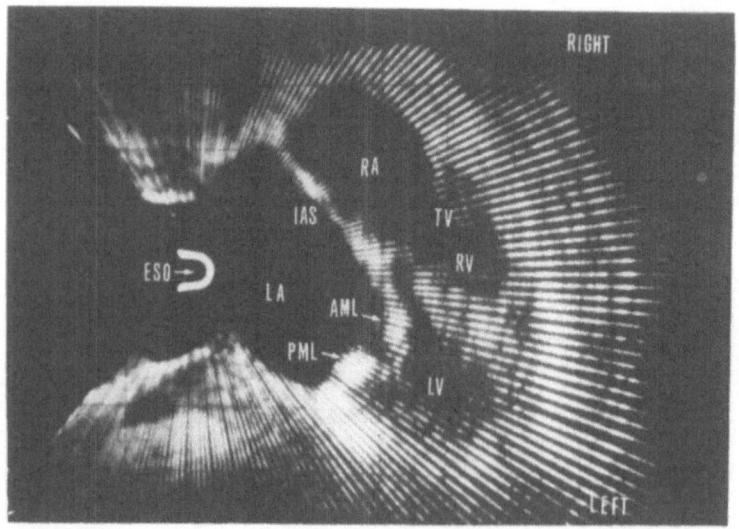

FIGURE 8. Horizontal scan at the level of the mitral valve in a patient with
mitral stenosis.[17] The thickened mitral leaflets and the large left atrium are
seen. AML = anterior mitral leaflet; PML = posterior mitral leaflet.

order to minimize discomfort and the loss of contact with the esophageal wall.

Subjects usually swallowed the oil bag voluntarily and as easily as a commercially available esophageal fiberscope. Oil was then injected into the bag through an external catheter in order to obtain good contact with the esophageal wall.

RESULTS

Transesophageal two-dimensional echocardiographic examinations were performed in more than 200 adult patients. Exampled of transesophageal two-dimensional echocardiograms are shown in Figure 4 to Figure 10.

Normal Adult

Figure 4 shows an inferior oblique scan through the apex in a normal adult. The cross-section is angled downward 35 degrees from the horizontal plane.[11] The entire heart including the apex is observed. The atrial septal echo is much stronger than other echoes, since the atrial septum is almost perpendicular to the sound beam.

Figure 5 shows a vertical scan through the mitral valve in another normal adult.[6,16] Mitral valve and bifurcation of pulmonary artery are seen clearly.

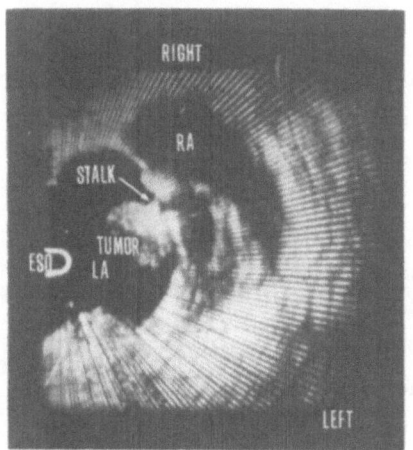

FIGURE 9. Horizontal scan at the level of aorta in a patient with left atrial myxoma. The stalk is seen clearly.

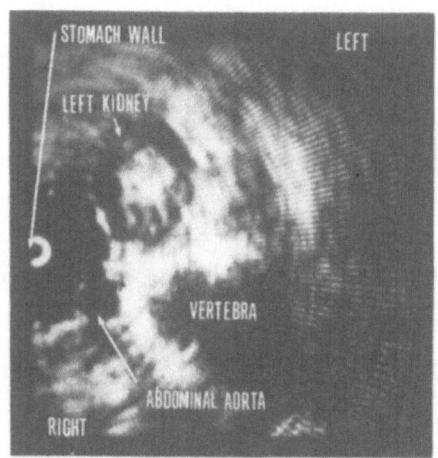

FIGURE 10. Abdominal horizontal scan through the stomach wall at the level of the kidney in a normal adult by using the transgastric high speed rotating scanner.[9,10,12,14]

Figure 6 shows a horizontal scan in a normal adult. A part of the aorta is seen.

Atrial Septal Defect[17, 18]

Figure 7 shows a horizontal scan at the level of the mitral valve in a patient with an secundum atrial septal defect. The large defect is seen. The right atrium is extremely enlarged.

Mitral Stenosis[16, 17]

Figure 8 shows a horizontal scan at the level of the mitral valve in a patient with mitral stenosis. The chambers are side by side and both atria and ventricles are separated the septa and atrioventricular valves. The large left atrium and the thickened mitral leaflets are seen.

Left Atrial Myxoma

Figure 9 shows a horizontal scan in a patient with left atrial myxoma. A large tumor including a short stalk is seen clearly.

Transgastric Sonography[3, 4, 9, 10, 14]

Figure 10 shows a horizontal scan through stomach wall at the level of the kidney in a normal adult. Left kidney and abdominal aorta are seen clearly.

DISCUSSION

We found that insertion of the transducer for recording heart images through the esophageal wall is no more difficult than inserting a commercially available gastrofiberscope. The small flexible tube and transducer are easily swallowed, and the occasional gagging is usually so mild that the examination is hardly interrupted. Although the transducer is moved rapidly, there is no loss of esophageal wall contact or any esophageal trauma, since the oil bag covers the transducer.

In clinical examinations, the amount of oil in the oil bag was slightly decreased before insertion in order to facilitate insertion of the transducer into the esophagus. After insertion, oil was injected into the bag to obtain good contact between the esophageal wall and oil bag. After insertion to the 30 to 40 cm level, cardiac images of high quality were easily obtained. Apart from gagging, no serious complications were encountered. The vibration felt by the patient during the examination decreased so remarkably that the rotation of the transducer was hardly perceived.

Unlike conventional external echocardiography, our system can record cardiac images continuously from base to apex as the transducer is being withdrawn or advanced in the esophagus. In this study the transducer position was usually identified by the mitral or tricuspid valve echo because these echoes were most easily observed in the examination. In this position, so-called four chamber views were obtained, and in all patients both the mitral and tricuspid valves were observed. By withdrawing the transducer from this position, we could observe the aorta, aortic valve and right ventricular outflow tract. In obese or elderly patients, the subcostal and parasternal apical approaches using a conventional scanner have been used, but the quality of results was inferior to that obtained with the esophageal method.

REFERENCES

1. Hisanaga K, Hisanaga A, Nagata K, Yoshida S. A new transesophageal real-time two-dimensional echocardiographic system using a flexible tube and its clinical application. Proceedings of the Japan Society of Ultrasonics in Medicine 32:43-44, 1977.
2. Hisanaga K, Hisanaga A. A new real-time sector scanning system of ultra-wide angle and real-time recording of entire adult cardiac images— Transesophagus and trans-chest-wall methods—. In:White D, Lyons AE, eds. Ultrasound in Medicine. Vol. 4. New York; Plenum Press, 1978:391-402.
3. Hisanaga K, Hisanaga A. A new trans-digestive-tract scanner with a gastro-fiberscope. Proceedings of the 23rd Annual Meeting of American Institute of Ultrasound in Medicine. p.108, November, 1978, San Diego.
4. Hisanaga K, Hisanaga A. A new trans-digestive-tract scanner with a gastrofiberscope. Reflections 4:221, 1978.
5. Hisanaga K, Hisanaga A. A transesophageal real-time sector scanner with an oil filled cell. Proceedings of the 23rd Annual Meeting of American Institute of Ultrasound in Medicine. p.47, 1978, San Diego.
6. Hisanaga K, Hisanaga A, Ichie Y. A new transesophageal real-time linear scanner and initial clinical results. Reflections 4:203, 1978.
7. Hisanaga K, Hisanaga A. A transesophageal pulsed Doppler echocardiographic system and initial clinical results. Proceedings of the Japan Society of Ultrasonics in Medicine 34:9-10, 1978.
8. Hisanaga K, Hisanaga A, Ichie Y, Nishimura K, Hibi N, Fukui Y, Kambe T. Transesophageal pulsed Doppler echocardiography. Lancet 1:53-54, 1979.
9. Hisanaga K, Hisanaga A, Nagata K, Ichie Y. A trans-stomach-wall ultrasonic high speed rotating scanner and initial clinical results. Proceedings cf the Japan Society of Ultrasonics in Medicine 35:115-116, 1979.
10. Hisanaga K, Hisanaga A, Nagata K, Ichie Y. A trans-stomach-wall sector scanner with a gastrofiberscope. Abstract of 2nd WFUMB. p.383, July, 1979, Miyazaki.
11. Hisanaga K, Hisanaga A, Ichie Y. A transesophageal ultrasound sector scanner for oblique scans (abstr). Circulation 60 (suppl II):II-245, 1979.
12. Hisanaga K, Hisanaga A. Pancreatic echography using a trans-stomach wall ultrasound rotating scanner (abstr). Gastroenterology 78:1183, 1980.
13. Hisanaga K, Hisanaga A, Kambe T. An endoscopic ultrasound scanner for abdominal echography (abstr). Gastrointestinal Endoscopy 26:68, 1980.

246

14. Hisanaga K, Hisanaga A, Nagata K, Ichie Y. High speed rotating scanner for transgastric sonography. Am. J. Roentgenol. 135:627-629, 1980.
15. Hisanaga K, Hisanaga A, Kambe T. Detection of atrial septal defect by transesophageal two-dimensional echocardiography (abstr). Circulation 62 (suppl III):III-34, 1980.
16. Hisanaga K, Hisanaga A, Nagata K, Ichie Y. Transesophageal cross-sectional echocardiography. Am. Heart J. 100:605-609, 1980.
17 Hisanaga K, Hisanaga A, Hibi N, Nishimura K, Kambe T. High speed rotating scanner for transesophageal cross-sectional echocardiography. Am. J. Cardiol. 46:837-842, 1980.
18. Hisanaga K, Hisanaga A. Measurement of defect size of atrial septal defect by transesophageal two-dimensional echocardiography. Proceedings of the Japan Society of Ultrasonics in Medicine 38:5-6, 1981.

DETECTION OF ATRIAL SEPTUM DEFECTS BY TRANSOESOPHAGEAL TWODIMENSIONAL ECHOCARDIOGRAPHY WITH A MECHANICAL SECTORSCANNER

N. REIFART, W.D. STROHM

Since 1980 we have had the opportunity to use a transoesophageal mechanical sectorscanner for cardiac imaging. We have now available the third prototype, a conventional flexible gastroscope (Olympus) with a mechanical rotating transducer at its end. Its 10 MHZ probe visualizes a sector of 180 degrees with a depth of 10 cm.

We examined 88 patients with various deseases. The twodimensional endoscopic echocardiography (2DEE) was performed with the patient in supine left lateral position after an i.v. injection of 5-10 mg Diazepam and local anaesthesia of the pharynx with Lidocaine.
There were no problems with insertion of the endoscope. A bidimensional echocardiographic image of the heart could be obtained in all cases. There were no complications due to the procedure. Patients did not complain of the endoscopic manoeuvres and the rotating of the scanner.

Cardiac structures are imaged after 35-40 cm of insertion. After detection of the ascending aorta at the base of the heart a " four chamber view " can be obtained by axial displacement and slight rotation to the right. In this view the left atrium is close to the transducer and all four cavities of the heart with the atrioventricular valves are visualized (Fig.1).
Since the ultrasonic beam is almost perpendicular to the atrial septum it can be seen very clearly.

248

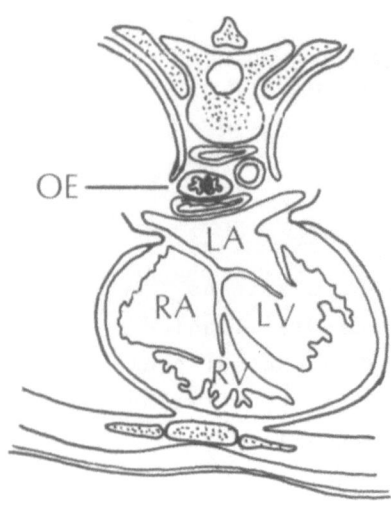

FIGURE 1

Twodimensional transoesophageal (endoscopic) echocardiography revealing a four chamber view. The left
atrium (LA) is close to the oesophageus (OE). Right
atrium (RA), left and right ventricle (LV,RV) and the
atrioventricular valves are visualized.

We performed conventional twodimensional echocardiography (2DE) and transoesophageal (endoscopic) two-
dimensional echocardiography (2DEE) in 18 consecutive
patients with atrial septum defect and a right to left
shunt between 33% and 78%. Three of them had a bidirectional shunt. All were injected with 10 cc of cold
saline in a cubital vein in order to obtain a contrast-
echo of the right heart. Serving as our control-group
were 17 patients without atrial septum defects:
3 ventricular septum defect, 6 mitral stenosis, 2 anomalous pulmonary vein, 2 primary cardiomyopathy and
4 normals. None of the angiographic diagnosis were
known by the investigator.

2DE verified an atrial septum defect in 11/18 patients.
After an i.v. injection of cold saline a right to left
shunt could be detected in 3/3 cases.

A false positive diagnosis was made in 2 out of 17.
In all 18 patients with atrial septum defect 2DEE was
correct (Fig.2). In 6 patients bubbles could be detected
in the left atrium and left ventricle following injection
of cold saline into the cubital vein. Only three out
of this group had an evidence of right to left shunt by
angiograhy and indicator dilution. In none of the control
group (0/17) was a false positive diagnosis made by 2DEE.

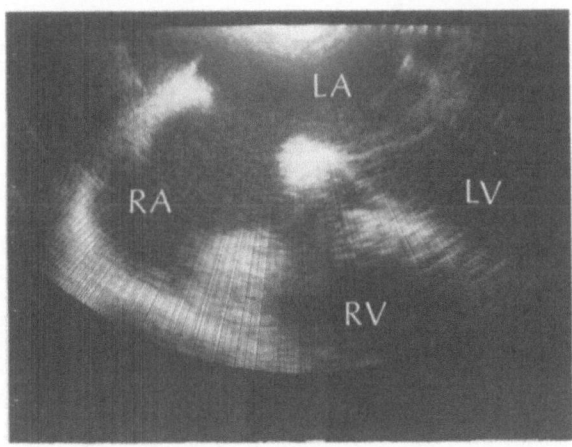

FIGURE 2

Transoesophageal twodimensional echocardiographic four
chamber view. A large septum defect is shown between
left and right atrium (LA,RA). Left and right ventricle
(LV,RV) are visualized below.

   Allthough our experience is still limited, we anti-
cipate 2DEE is a reliable method to detect atrial septum
defects. Its sensitivity and specificity is 100%.
Conventional echocardiography (2DE) is less sensitive
(61%) and specific (88%). Bidirectional shunts can be
visualized after injection of cold saline into a cubital
vein. The findings however are not specific.

References

King D.L.: Cardiac ultrasonography: cross-sectional
ultrasonic imaging of the heart. Circulation, 47:843,1973

Frazin L, Talano J.V., Stephanides L., Loeb H.S., Kopel L.
Gunnar R.M.: Esophageal echocardiography. Circulation
1976; 54:102-8

Hisanaga K., Hisanaga A., Hibi N., Nishimura K., Kambe T.
High speed rotating scanner for transesophageal cross-
sectional echocardiography. Am.J.Cardiol. 46: 837-842
1980.

Strohm W.D., K.Jessen, J. Phillip und M. Classen:
Endoskopische Ultraschalltomographie des oberen Ver-
dauungstraktes. Dtsch. Med. Wschr. 106, 714-717, 1981

PHASED ARRAY TRANSDUCER TECHNOLOGY FOR TRANSESOPHAGEAL IMAGING OF THE HEART: CURRENT STATUS AND FUTURE ASPECTS

JACQUES SOUQUET, Ph.D
ADVANCED TECHNOLOGY LABORATORIES, INC.
DIVISION OF CARDIOLOGY
13208 NORTHUP WAY
BELLEVUE, WA 98008-0639   U.S.A.

1. INTRODUCTION

The field of ultrasound imaging has entered a phase of product development and clinical investigation in which ultrasound devices are used to image areas of the body through surfaces other than the skin. The various projects involved in internal applications as seen through the publications include mechanical sector scanners, linear arrays and phased arrays. Any of these devices may be used for several applications including: upper gastrointestinal (endoscopic or non-endoscopic); lower gastrointestinal (transrectal or colonoscopic); and direct application (intraoperative or endoscopic, for example laparoscopy).

In the case of two dimensional echocardiography compromised image quality is due to abnormal chest wall configuration, small intercostal space, obesity, emphysema, chronic obstructive pulmonary disease. Since 1972 some attempts have been made to record important parameters of the heart through the esophagus using an endoscope, the main advantage being lungs and ribs do not intervene resulting in clean and stable recordings.

More recently, the advent of real time ultrasound imaging has led to esophageal ultrasonic imaging units, some using a mechanically scanned transducer[1,2] and another a high resolution linear array system[3]. A mechanically scanned system requires an oil pouch surrounding the transducer and thus leads to some discomfort to the patients. The linear array system has a rigid tip 80 mm long which makes it difficult to swallow and to obtain good contact with the esophagus without the use of a waterbag.

We wanted to build a transducer array as small as possible in order to minimize discomfort to the patient. This led us to

type of 2D cross section obtained. In the following sections we
will describe in more detail the design of the transducer array,
various endoscopic phased array already built and some potential
future design and present some clinical results.

2. TRANSDUCER ARRAY

   The transducer is a 32-element linear array of PZT-5A material with a center frequency of operation of 3.5MHz (wavelength =
0.43 mm). The spacing between adjacent elements is 0.28 mm, resulting in a total aperture of approximately 9 mm. The elevation
dimension was also chosen equal to 9 mm. Thirty-two flexible
phono wires (AWG 30) were soldered on each individual element of
the transducer array, a bigger wire was used for the returning
ground. The bundle of 33 wires had an outer diameter of 0.3 mm
and was connected to a printed circuit board located in the control unit of the gastroscope. Another cable connects then the
gastroscope to the phased array electronic system. While the
main emphasis in the design of the esophageal array was to reduce
its size for comfortable insertion, it remained necessary to provide high efficiency along with good bandwidth in order to achieve
good signal-to-noise ratios as well as adequate depth resolution.
   Detailed consideration of the above factors, along with the
desire for low spurious response, led us to design employing a
front matching layer and a mismatched backing.[4] The matching
layer used is a composite material with an acoustical impedance of
about 4×10^6 kg/m^2 sec, and the backing is a very lossy "home-
made" material with an acoustical impedance of approximately
1×10^6 kg/m sec. Figure 2 shows the theoretical and experimental
results for the electrical impedance for such an array. The
measurement has been performed with all the 32 elements connected
together and the simulation has assumed the same configuration.
In the theoretical simulation, the Mason model is used for the
transducer with the load considered as a complex impedance due to
the small element width. Agreement between theory and experiment
can be seen from these curves. The impulse response for an element of this array is shown on Figure 3, demonstrating only a
small amount of ringing. This impulse response has been obtained

choose a phased array system where, by appropriately phasing the individual elements of the transducer array, one can obtain real time images over a 90° sector whose apex is located at the transducer.

Among various applications of transesophageal ultrasonic imaging systems are:

- Left ventricular performance during exercise: the stability of this new technique might replace radionucleid techniques in clinical cardiology.
- Intraoperative monitoring of the left ventricule with the hope of being able to quantify cardiac output.
- Postoperative observation of the heart.

For the realization of the transesophageal scanhead a multi-element phased array transducer was incorporated into the distal end of a commercially available gastroscope in order to facilitate the introduction of the transducer and allow for the transducer position and orientation via external control. Figure 1 shows a typical array gastroscope position in the esophagus as well as the

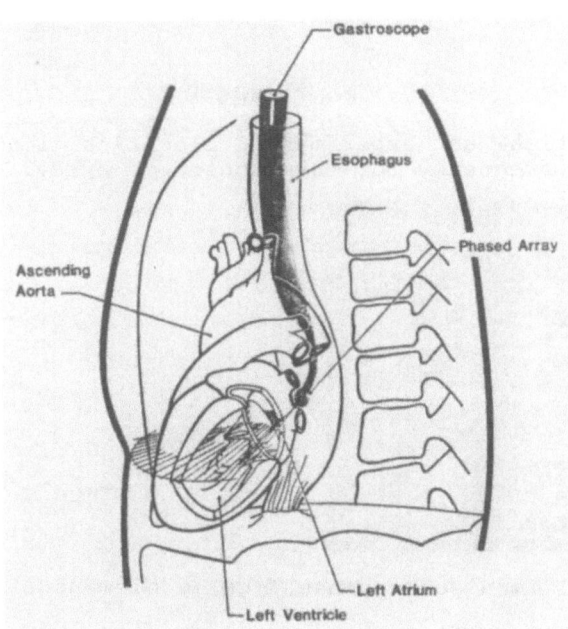

FIGURE 1. Orientation of array and gastroscope with respect to the heart.

by reflecting from a flat target in a lossy medium.

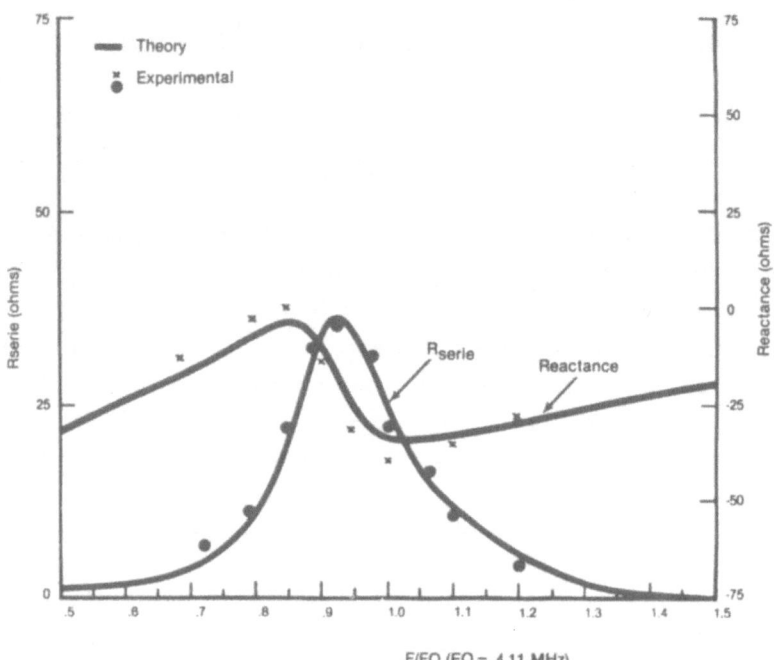

FIGURE 2. Theoretical and experimental electrical impedance
versus frequency for the endoscopic array.

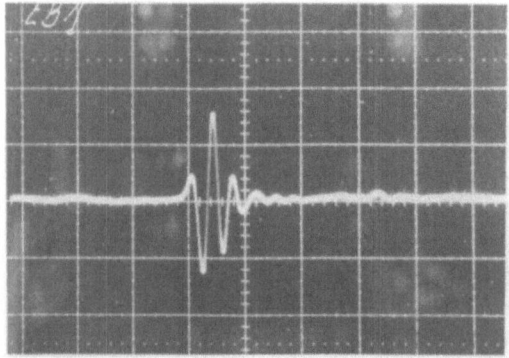

FIGURE 3. Typical impulse response from an element of the
array.

In a phased array system, a wide acceptance angle of the transducer elements is important. As can be seen from Figure 4, we achieved a ±45° acceptance angle at -5 dB, which agrees quite well with the theoretical radiation pattern of a single element.[5] The acceptance angle measurement was performed with the array slotted and its protective lens on place by isolating one element and leaving the adjacent elements of the array open. The agreement between theory and experiment shows the low level of acoustical cross-coupling through the protective lens.

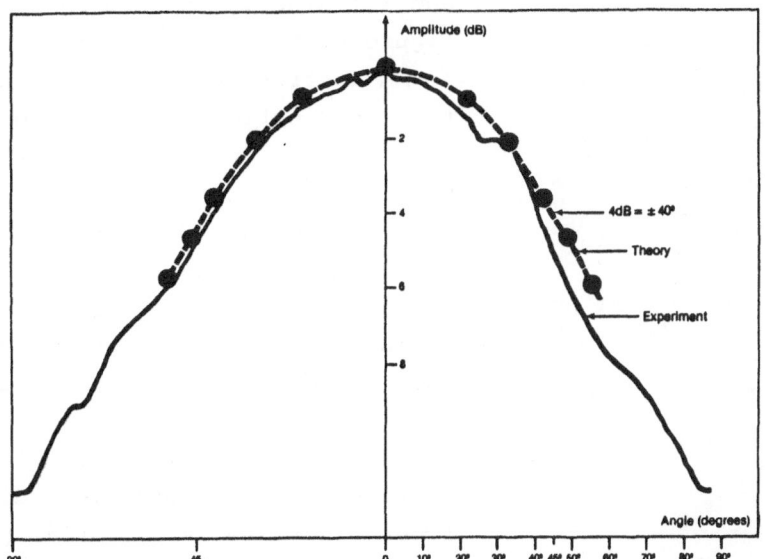

FIGURE 4. Acceptance angle of simple element of the array.

Finally, for the contacting surface of the transducer we choose a spherical lens made of a low velocity material. The optics were designed to give a depth of field from 2 to 10 cm in front of the array. With such a lens the -6dB beamwidth measured at 50 mm in front of the array was equal to 3 mm in azimuth and elevation. The -6dB pulse width indicates an axial resolution of about 1 mm.

3. CURRENT STATUS AND FUTURE ASPECTS

Three different types of esophageal probes have already been built and tested in clinical settings.

Figure 5 shows the first of the three kinds. The completed array is fitted on the distal end of an Olympus gastroscope. The

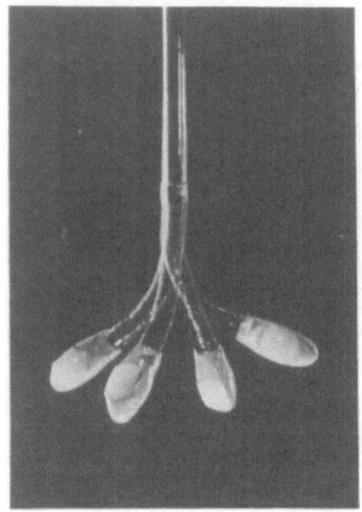

FIGURE 5. Esophageal phased array fitted on the Olympus gastroscope.

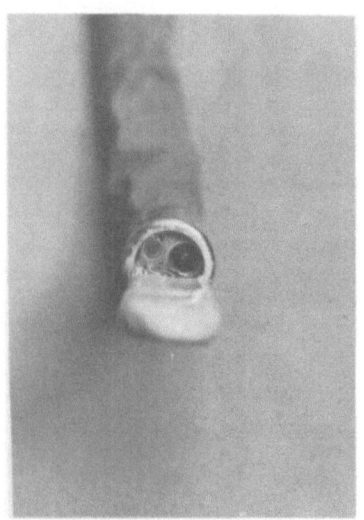

FIGURE 6. "Thin" phased array on ACMI gastroscope with optic channels on plate.

outside diameter of the gastroscope is 9 mm and the outer dimensions of the array are the following: 35 mm long, 15 mm wide and 16 mm thick. For this first prototype model the fiber optics components for viewing and illumination have been removed. Figure 6 shows a new design with a 13 mm gastroscope from ACMI where the fiber optic channels have been kept. The biopsy channel has been used for passing the cables through the endoscope to the control unit. In this design the transducer backing has been reduced to 5 mm. From an initial investigation it appears that the optical fibers do not seem to be essential for the application mentioned previously in the introduction. Furthermore, including the fibers increases substantially the cost of the instrument.

Being able to image different cross sections of the heart without moving the gastroscope is of great interest, essentially, if one wants to evaluate cardiac output. Figure 7 shows our first attempt to solve this problem. Two phased array at right angle are mounted on the distal end of the gastroscope. Thus, if on the electronic one, implements a commutation to switch from one array to the other, the doctor is able to visualize two scan plane at right angle (i.e., short axis and long axis) without moving the gastroscope. This has been tested clinically and gave very good results.

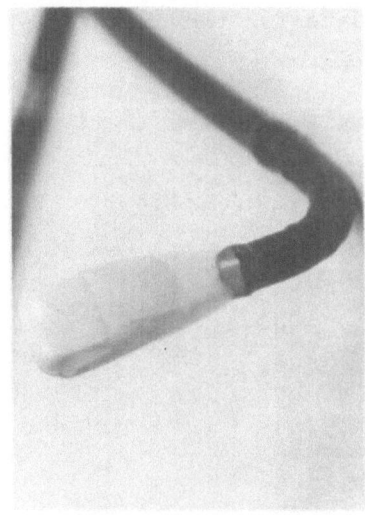

In the system previously described, only 2 right angle scan plane can be obtained, and by switching between the two, we go through a "dead" zone which can not be imaged. Future work will compensate for this drawback and a new probe will provide continuous manual rotation over 90° with a single phased array. Future probes might also include a microphone for phonocardiogram recording as well as pressure sensors.

FIGURE 7. Olympus gastroscope fitted with 2 phased array transducers at right angle.

4. CLINICAL RESULTS

The main clinical results have been reported in this book already. One Hundred patients have been scanned in surgery using this technique and close to 200 conscious patients underwent a transesophageal echocardiography (TEEC) examination.[6] Some of the most spectacular results have been obtained for the following cases:
- Mitral valve prolapse (Figure 8).
- Atrial septal defects.
- Excellent cross sectional view of the apex of the heart.
- Observation of air trapping following open heart surgery.
- Excellent recording of RV with tricuspid valve.
- Good cross section of aortic valve.

5. CONCLUSION

Although the transesophageal technique implies some discomfort to the patient and some skill is required to introduce the gastro-

258

scope into the esophagus, the high imaging quality due to the close anatomical relationship between the esophagus and the heart, and the visualization of the heart in planes which cannot be obtained from the external approach compensate for the disadvantages.

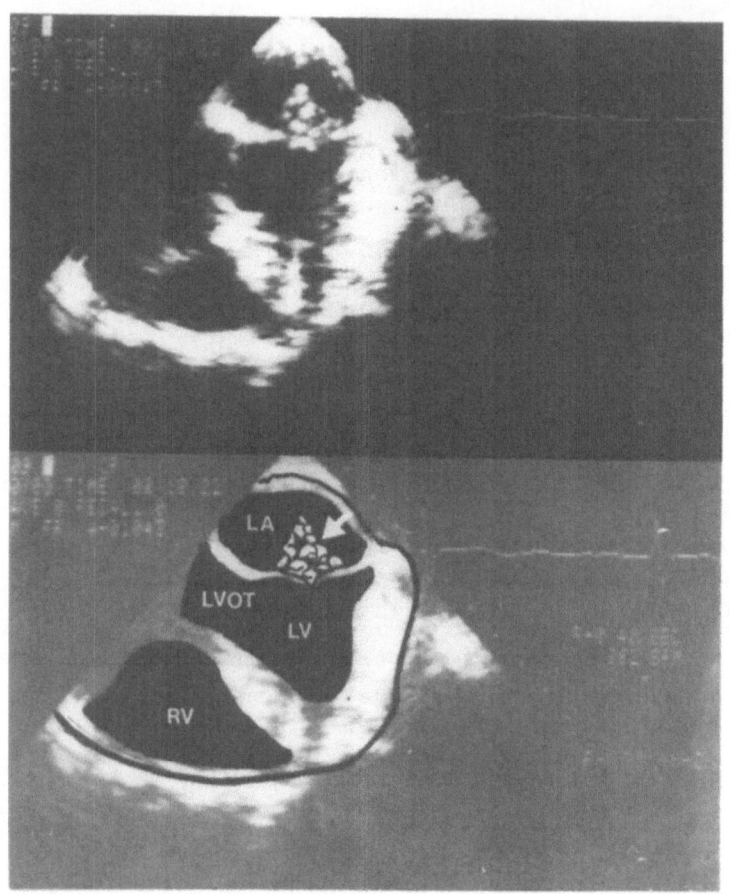

FIGURE 8.   Mitral valve prolapse.

REFERENCES

1. W.D. Strohm, J. Phillip, F. Hagenmuller, M. Classen:
   Ultrasonic Tomography by means of an Ultrasonic
   Fiberendoscope.
   Endoscopy, vol. 12, No. 5, Sept., 1980.
2. K. Hisanaga, A. Hisanaga, N. Hibi, K. Nishimura, T. Kambe:
   High Speed Rotating Scanner for Transesophageal Cross-
   Sectional Echocardiography.
   The American Journal of Cardiology, vol. 46, 837-842,
   Nov., 1980.
3. B. Rajogopolan, E. P. DiMagno, J. F. Greenleaf, P. T. Regan,
   J. Buxton, P. S. Green, J. W. Whitaker:
   Transesophageal ultrasonic imaging of the heart.
   Proceedings of the 9th International on Acoustical Imaging,
   1979.
4. J. Souquet, P. DeFranould, J. Desbois:
   Design of low-loss wide-band ultrasonic transducers
   for noninvasive medical application.
   IEEE SU, vol. SU-26, No. 2, 75-81, March 1.
5. A. R. Selfridge, G. S. Kino, B. T. Khuri-Yakub:
   A theory for the radiation pattern of a narrow-strip
   acoustic transducer.
   Appl. Phys. Lett., vol. 37, No. 1, July 1, 1980.
6. Kremer, P., P. Hanrath, B. A. Langenstein, M. Matsumoto,
   C. Tams, W. Bleifeld:
   The evaluation of left ventricular function at rest and
   during exercise by transesophageal echocardiography in
   Amer. J. Cardiol. 47: 412, 1981 (Abstract).

ON THE DESIGN AND CONSTRUCTION OF A TRANSESOPHAGEAL
SCANNER

C.T. LANCEE, C.M. LIGTVOET and N. DE JONG

1. INTRODUCTION

The interest in ultrasound scanning from positions
located inside the human body has remained after the first
proposals some 10 years ago (1, 2). The number of workers
in this particular field has been, however, rather low.
This may be explained by the high success rate of ultrasound in standard non-invasive applications. Still there
exists a clinical demand for alternative scanning
procedures for some specific applications. The prostate,
for instance, is hard to scan successfully from locations
outside the patient and therefore intra-rectal scanning
has become an accepted procedure.

The heart is another organ which sometimes ($\pm$ 20 %
of all patients) presents difficulties when scanned per-
cutaneously, whether it be scanned from a parasternal,
suprasternal, subcostal or apical position. Transesophageal scanning could then be a useful alternative.
This alternative, however, is certainly not fully
compatible with the totally atraumatic standard procedure. One should always balance the induced strain of
a gastroscopic examination (in relation to the patient's
condition) against the potential yield of additional
clinical information. In the case of open chested cardiac
surgery transesophageal scanning is almost the only
practical way of obtaining anatomic and functional
information with ultrasound, while at the same time the
gastroscopic procedure is performed without inconvenience
for the patient. Another promising field is the scanning
of the pancreas from the duodenum.

As a result of the above mentioned considerations we decided to develop an electronic sector scan probe mounted at the tip of a standard gastroscope (Olympus GIF P3). The feasibility of such a project has already been proven by Jacques Souquet and Peter Hanrath (3). Other trans-esophageal scanners have been reported over the last years based on a mechanically rotated transducer assembly with the paramount disadvantage of relatively large overall scanhead dimensions (4, 5, 6).

2. ACOUSTICAL DESIGN

The most critical design parameter of a phased array sector scanner is the center to center distance of the individual elements. In order to reduce unwanted grating lobe effects this distance should be less than the wave-length of the ultrasonic center frequency in the medium of observation. For a phased array with a working frequency of 3.1 MHz the associated wavelength in soft tissue is 0.5 mm and an interelement spacing of 0.4 mm was selected.

Previous work (7,8) has shown that an optimal resonant behaviour of each element will occur when there is a specific relation between the width w and the thickness T of an element. The ratio $\frac{w}{T}$ should be in the order of 0.8 or less. At 3.1 MHz the thickness of the material used (PZT 5H) is .48 mm. Optimal performance may be expected at a maximum width of $\simeq$ .38 mm. Since the cutting procedure allows for a sawing cut of no less than 0.1 mm, as will be explained elsewhere, the actual element width obtained is .3 mm.

3. BACKING AND MATCHING

In order to obtain maximum sensitivity a combination has been chosen of a quarter-wavelength front layer and a backing material with a very low acoustic impedance. The backing material consists of a two-component foam. This material exhibits three distinct advantages:

a) because of its low impedance it acts as an almost
perfect reflector yielding a high acoustic output;
b) because of the large content of air the absorption
is extremely high, therefeore backing echoes are virtually
non-existent; c) due to its mechanical stiffness it acts
as a mechnical support for the array.

The matching layer consists of a mixture of araldite
and fine carborundum powder. Its density ρ and com-
pressibility K are chosen such that the acoustical
impedance $\sqrt{K.\rho}$ is close to $\sqrt[3]{2.z_1^2 z_2}$, where z_1 is the
acoustical impedance of soft tissue and z_2 that of the
ceramic material in its final form after cutting (7, 8).

Since the longitudinal propagation velocity in the
quarter wavelength layer after the cutting process is
hard to predict, the thickness of this layer is determined
by measuring the complex electrical impedance. The
matching layer is ground down to its optimal thickness,
while the modulus and the argument of the element
impedance is continuously being monitored. Following this
procedure optimal impulse response is ensured, independent
of small variations in the composition of the matching
layer mixture.

Finally, control of the thickness of the scanning plane
is obtained by using a thin spherical silicone lens. The
focal distance F of this lens is set to meet the following
equation: $F = 0.34 \frac{H^2}{\lambda}$ (9). H is the height of the array
(and of the individual elements) and λ is the wavelength
associated with the center frequency f_c. For H = 10 mm
and λ = 0.5 mm (f_c = 3.1 MHz) this results in F =
68 mm.

4. ANATOMIC DESIGN

The esophagus makes a small angle with the long axis
of the left ventricle. In order to obtain as much clinical
information as possible from the transesophageal scanner
we decided to mount the scanner in such a way that the

scanning plane is perpendicular to the axis of the
gastroscope. In principle short axis views of the heart
will be obtained. Because of the extreme mobility of the
tip of the Olympus GIF P3 other cross-sections such as
the four chamber view are possible (3).

Another advantage of the flexible tip is that it is
no longer necessary to use a fluid filled balloon to
ensure acoustic contact with the anterior esophageal wall.
The probe can be pressed gently against it using the
posterior wall for balancing the gastroscope. This led
us to mount the array at an angle of 15° relative to the
long axis of the gastroscope.

In order to make the use of the scanner as atraumatic
as possible we decided that the physical dimensions of the
array should not differ too much from the diameter of the
gastroscope tip, i.e. 8 mm. This means that the length L
of the array should be of the same order of magnitude. The
resolution to be obtained is a direct function of L. At
the focal point F (the array is supposed to focus
electronically both in the transmit and the receive mode)
the total width of the main lobe is given by the equation:
$\delta = 2 \cdot \lambda \cdot \frac{F}{L}$. Putting F = 60 mm; λ = 0.5 mm and L = 8 mm
yields δ = 7,5 mm. Increasing L to 10 mm yields δ = 6 mm,
which value has been chosen as a compromise.

The height H of the array is less critical since this
dimension is orientated along the long axis of the
gastroscope. However, H defines the length of the
unflexible tip and should therefore not be too long. A
physical restriction acting upon both H and L is the depth
of the near-field area. If unambiguous echoes from the
left ventricular posterior wall are required, then the
value for both H and L of 10 mm is maximal.

The thickness of the complete array assembly i.e. lens,
matching layer, ceramic and backing material has also to
be kept in the order of 8 mm. Because of the acoustic
characteristics of the previously described backing

material this requirement is easily met. A backing thickness of only 2 mm is sufficient to eliminate spurious
backing echoes.

5. THE ACTUAL DESIGN

The final parameters of the array are:
- 24 elements
- 300 μm element width
- 100 μm element spacing
- 9.5 mm length of the array
- 10 mm height of the elements
- 15° inclination relative to gastroscope long axis
- 3.1 MHz center frequency
- 2 MHz bandwidth
- 60 mm fixed focus in the tangential plane by means of
  a silicone lens
- 90° maximum sector angle.

6. THE MANUFACTURING PROCEDURE

Step 1 - The ceramic material is being cut from a plate
with electrodes on both sides.

Step 2 - A small strip is soldered on one electrode
using low melting-point solder. This strip will be the
common earth connection for the array.

Step 3 - The ceramic is placed in the bottom part of
a mold. The upper part of the mold has a space in the
form of the eventual transducer assembly.

Step 4 - After the mold is assembled, the two-component
foam is mixed and poured into the mold.

Step 5 - After the foam has stabilized the mold is
turned upside down and the top is removed. The mold now
functions as a mechanical support in the next steps.

Step 6 - A flexible printed circuit is bonded on the
backing material against one side of the ceramic. The
copper pattern on the print has the same pitch (.4 mm) as
the specified array.

Step 7 - The top electrode of the ceramic is soldered to all copper strips with low melting-point solder.

Step 8 - The matching layer compound is applied over the top electrode and is allowed to harden.

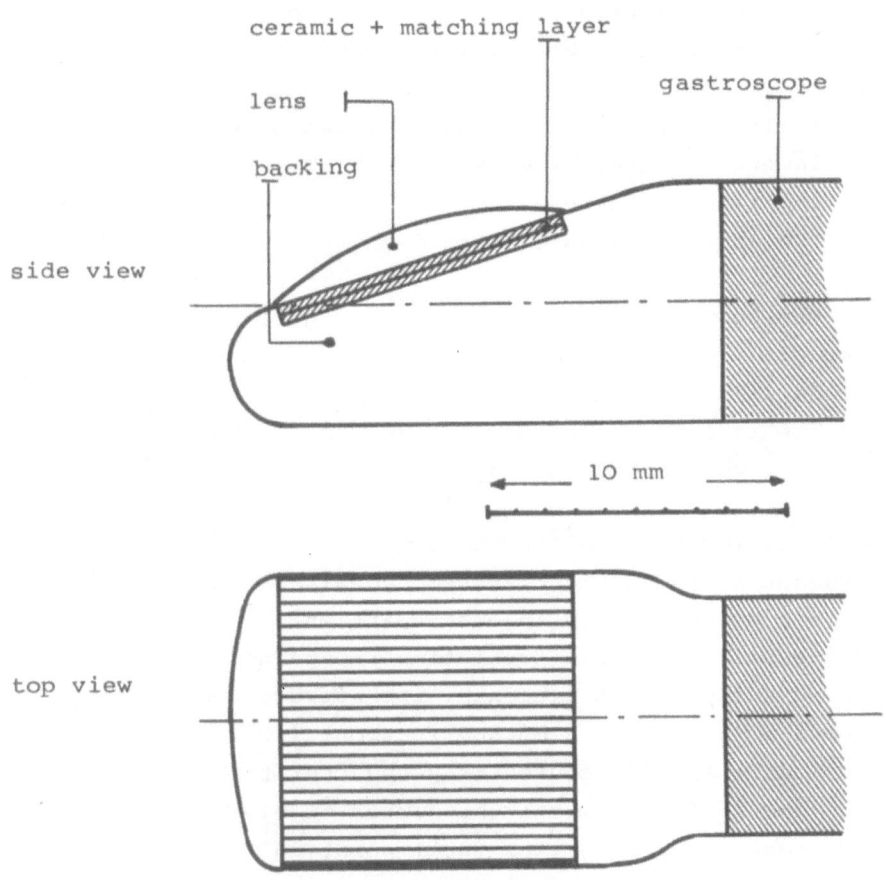

Fig. 1. Schematic drawing of the transesophageal transducer assembly

Step 9 - The matching layer material is ground down to slightly oversize.

Step 10 - The assembly is placed under a multiple wire-saw. The wires run parallel .4 mm spaced apart. Precise positioning is obtained by using the copper pattern on the printed circuit as a reference.

Step 11 - The wires will cut through the matching layer and the ceramic until the common earth strip is reached. At the same time the soldered connections between the top electrode and the copper pattern will be separated from their neighbours.

Step 12 - While monitoring the frequency response of a reference element the quarter wave matching layer is now tuned to its final thickness.

Step 13 - The acoustic lens is bonded on top of the array.

Step 14 - The 24 wires are fed through the gastroscopic tube together with a common ground wire and are connected to the flexible print.

Step 15 - The assembly is bonded to the tip of the gastroscope and a thin epoxy coating is applied.

7. DESCRIPTION OF THE DRIVING ELECTRONICS

The instrument to which the transesophageal scanner is connected has been designed in our department. Although originally intended for use as "real-time" compound scanner with an array of 256 elements, its micro-processor control enables a wide variety of applications (10). In order to accomodate the miniature array the operator introduces by means of a terminal the number of elements, the center to center distance, the focal point in transmission, the focus in reception and the number of scan angles. After an initialization time of only 15 seconds the machine has set up all the required control sequences for the time delay section and the digital scanconvertor.

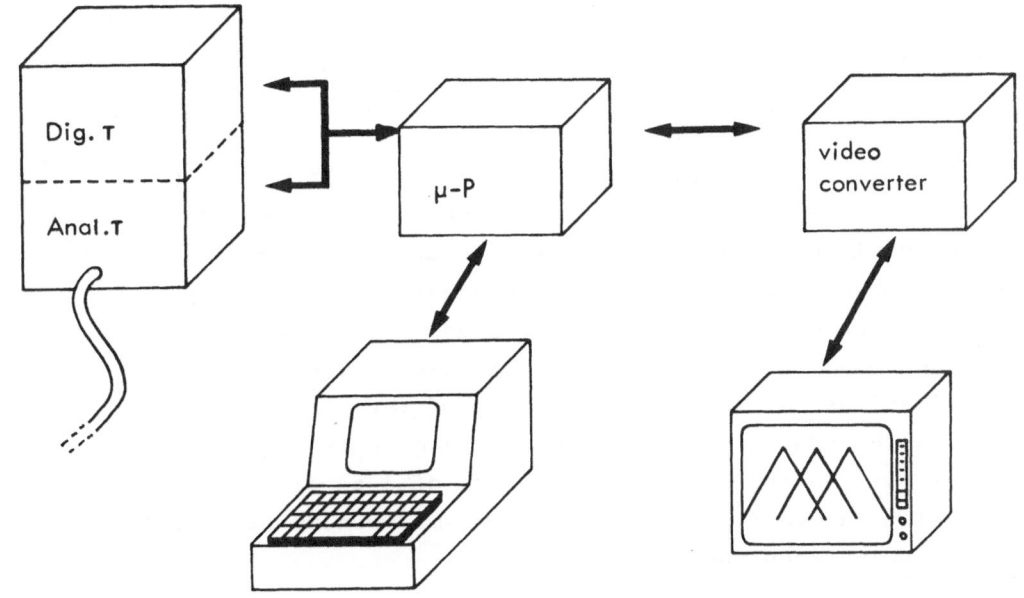

Fig. 2. Schematic representation of the electronic system

As indicated in figure 2 the time delay section
consists of two different parts. In the analogue part
small time delays of multiples of 40 μsec are preselected, then 4 channels are combined and fed through a
TGC amplifier into a 6 bit A to D convertor. The digitized
signals are further delayed in steps of 80 μsec and then
combined into one 8 bit digital signal which is rectified
and read into a video scanned digital memory.

The flexible (software) control of the array not only
allows for optimal setting of the beamsteering electronics
but also provides the operator with several scanning

modes. Apart from the normal sector scan mode the operator may select one or more M-mode lines everywhere in the 90° sector with adjustable repetition frequencies.

Even with an array this small, a compound image may be selected, for instance two overlapping sectors from two subarrays of 16 elements each, 8 elements spaced apart (i.e. 3,2 mm).

8. POTENTIAL APPLICATIONS

In this stage of development in vivo results are yet to be obtained. If in vivo experiments prove to be successful we are inclined to expect at least two different applications. Transesophageal echocardiology will be one of them, while upper abdominal scanning from the duodenum is within the possibilities. Other applications may arise from the use of the miniature array alone. The transducer assembly can be made as small as to fit within the finger compartment of a surgical glove. Manually guided transrectal scanning may become feasible using this technique.

ACKNOWLEDGEMENT

The authors are obliged to give full credit to A. den Ouden for his valuable contributions to the design of the manufacturing procedure and to L. Bekkering for his continuous efforts to make and improve our transducers. They are both from the Research Workshop of the Medical Faculty. Furthermore we wish to thank our secretary Corrie de Bruijn for the careful preparation of the manuscript.

REFERENCES

Other transesophageal transducers:
1. Ebina T et al. 1967. Japanese Heart Journal Vol. 8 No. 4: 331-353.
2. Eggleton RC and Weidner AW. 1973. US patent 3,779,234.
3. Hanrath P and Souquet J. 1981.Presentation at the 4th Symposium on Echocardiology, Rotterdam.
4. Frazin LI. 1978. Journal of Applied Radiology Vol. 7: 108-113.

5. Misanaga K and Misanaga A. 1978. Ultrasound in Medicin
    Vol. 4: 391-402 (Eds White D and Lyons EA), Plenum
    Press, New York.
6. Fearnot NE, Babbs CF, Bourland JD and Geddes LA. 1980.
    Ultrasonic Imaging Vol.2: 78-83.

Transducers:
7. Souquet J, Defranould P and Desbois J. 1979. IEEE
    Trans. on Sonics and Ultrasonics Vol. SU-26 No.2: 77-
    81.
8. Defranould P and Souquet J. 1979. Echocardiology (Ed.
    Lancée CT): 395-412. Martinus Nijhoff Publishers, The
    Hague/Boston/London.
9. Marini J and Rivizez J. 1974. Ultrasonics: 251-256.

Driving electronics:
10. Ligtvoet C and Eversdijk CH. 1981. Recent Advances
    in Ultrasound Diagnosis (Eds Kurjak A and
    Kratochwil A): 51-55. Excerpta Medica, Amsterdam/
    Oxford/Princeton.

ESOPHAGEAL PHASED-ARRAY SECTOR ECHOCARDIOGRAPHY: AN ANATOMIC
STUDY

James B. Seward, M.D., Abdul J. Tajik, M.D.,
and Eugene P. DiMagno, M.D.

1. INTRODUCTION

Esophageal echocardiography has received limited attention
over the past few years. M-mode esophageal echocardiography,
although promising as a means of monitoring myocardial function,
has been limited in its usefulness for assessment of cardiac
anatomy.[1-6] More recently, mechanical sector scanners have been
developed which permit two-dimensional esophageal imaging.[7-9]
These instruments are characteristically encumbered by a
mechanical linkage to a rotating crystal. Other potential
endoscopic functions, such as fiberoptics, suction, and universal
control of crystal angulation, are made difficult and require
an inordinate increase in the size of the endoscope.

This report describes the use of a phased-array wide-angle
two-dimensional echocardiographic esophageal system. Because
there are no moving parts and no obligatory electro-mechanical
coupling, the endoscope and the crystal elements can be placed
in a much smaller housing. The objective of this technology
is to develop small, versatile imaging devices that will permit
relatively nontraumatic transesophageal imaging. Such instrumentation is most promising for the diagnosis of cardiac and
mediastinal pathology and for intraoperative or critical-care
monitoring of myocardial anatomy and function.

The particular purpose of this communication is to describe
our initial experience in the animal model with the use of an
84-degree wide-angle phased-array esophageal sector scanner.
This prototype instrument was utilized to show the versatility
of such technology in demonstrating detailed intracardiac and
mediastinal anatomy in the animal model.

2. METHODS

Adult mongrel dogs, all weighing in excess of 20 kg, were utilized. General anesthesia was achieved with 0.5 ml/kg of intravenous 6% pentobarbital. No respiratory assist or other support was utilized during the endoscopic procedure.

Two endoscopic instruments were utilized (Fig. 1). One was a 100-cm, 8.5-mm-diameter conduit with a phased-array element. No suction, tip flexibility, or fiberoptics were available in this particular device. A second instrument, with identical phased-array electronics, was a 100-cm, 12.5-mm-diameter American Cystoscopic Makers, Inc. (ECMI) endoscope with flexible tip, fiberoptics, and suction. One biopsy port served as a passageway for the electronics, which was a 32-element, 3.5-MHz phased-array epoxy-imbedded crystal at the tip of the endoscope. An 84-degree sector field with 7 cm of depth was utilized. On the endoscope, the active element extended approximately 2 cm from the end of the instrument. The crystal was designed so that it would lie flat against the esophageal wall, its active

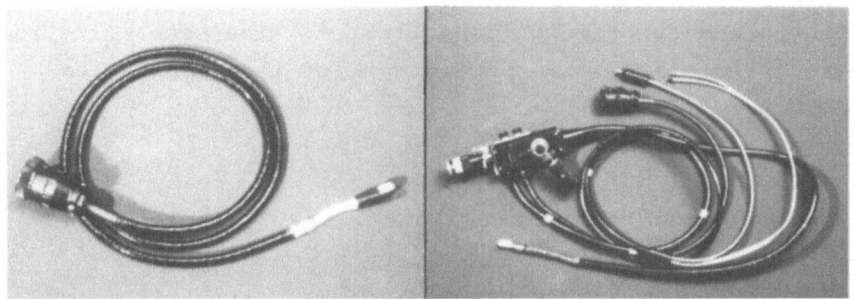

FIGURE 1. a) Two-dimensional echocardiographic phased-array endoscope, 8.5 mm in diameter and 100 cm in length. The rigid tip is approximately 3 cm long, and the diameter of the active element is 12 mm. A 32-element phased-array crystal is embedded in epoxy cement at the tip of the instrument. The resulting plane of section is horizontal to the long axis of the body. b) Same electronics are incorporated into a 12.5-mm-diameter, 100-cm-long American Cystoscopic Makers, Inc. endoscope. Fiber-optics, flexible tip, and suction capabilities are available in this instrument.

elements needing no liquid interface. The resultant plane of
section was horizontal to the long axis of the body, with the
image oriented so that it displayed the cardiac structures in
an anatomic format (as though looking down on a frontal projec-
tion--i.e., option 1 of the American Society of Echocardiography[10]).
The endoscope had a hand-controlled, flexible tip, which permitted an approximately 30-degree superior and inferior tilt
from the neutral position. Multiple oblique horizontal planes
of section were thus feasible. For views lateral to the neutral
position, the endoscope was rotated. The phased-array endoscopic
unit was interfaced with a Varian (Diasonics) 3400 phased-array
sector echocardiography instrument.

   The endoscope was advanced into the esophagus with the use of
a jelly lubricant. Although fiberoptics were available, they
were usually not necessary, and the endoscope was advanced under
echo visualization. With utilization of cardiac pulsations as
a means of localizing the heart, the cardiac chambers and
mediastinal great arteries could be visualized in each animal.
Occasionally, contact with the esophagus was hampered by gas
distal to the endoscope; this was eliminated by simple suction
through an existing port.

   Images were recorded onto a 3/4-inch video cassette system
with slow-motion and stop-action capabilities. The echo illustra-
tions in this article are 35-mm photographs of the stop-action
video images.

3. RESULTS

   In each animal, major cardiac structures were consistently
imaged. Left and right atrium, atrial septum, and left ventricle were imaged in each instance, and these serve as landmark
structures (Fig. 2 and 3). More detailed inferior and superior
scanning usually permitted short-axis and oblique four-chamber
views of the cardiac chambers from the midventricle to the base
(Fig. 3). At the base of the heart, short-axis views of the
aortic valve, right ventricular outflow tract, pulmonary valve,
and proximal pulmonary arteries could be obtained (Fig. 2 and 4b).
Other mediastinal structures imaged included the ascending aorta

(Fig. 4a), aortic arch, and descending thoracic aorta (Fig. 4c).
At the esophageal junction, portions of the liver, hepatic veins,
and inferior vena cava were imaged (Fig. 5).

The resulting images permitted comparison of cardiac chambers,
study of valve motion, and visual assessment of cardiac function.
Simultaneous M-mode capabilities were also available. This

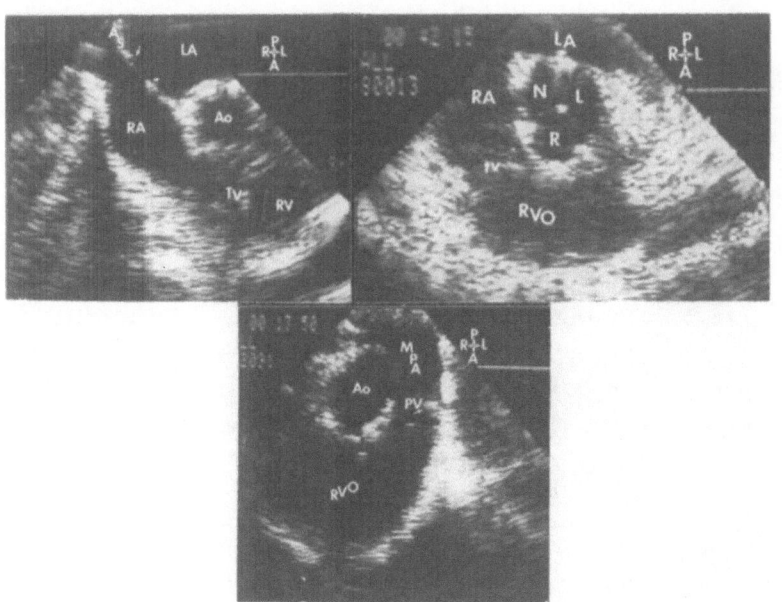

FIGURE 2. Short-axis scans at the base of the heart. a) The
transducer lies closest to the left atrium (*LA*); the atrial
septum (*AS*) separates the right atrium (*RA*) from the left atrium.
The valve of the fossa ovalis (*small arrows*) appears as a
thinned segment in the atrial septum. The aorta (*Ao*) is a
central structure and serves as a landmark. The tricuspid
valve (*TV*) is anterior and leftward on the image. b) The three
aortic cusps--i.e., left (*L*), right (*R*), and noncoronary
(*N*)--are visualized. The right ventricular outflow tract (*RVO*)
is anterior to the aorta and encircles from left to right.
Other abbreviations as above. c) The pulmonary valve (*PV*) is
to the viewer's right and lies next to the aorta (*Ao*), separating
the right ventricular outflow tract (*RVO*) anteriorly from the
posteriorly located main pulmonary artery (*MPA*). P = posterior;
R = right; L = left; A = anterior. *RV* = right ventricle.

report concentrates on anatomic detail and our ability to visualize particular cardiac structures from the retrocardiac transducer position. Described below are the major observations of this series of examinations.

3.1. Left ventricle

From the esophagus, an oblique horizontal (i.e., four-chamber) plane of the left atrium, mitral valve, and left ventricle was consistently obtained (Fig. 3a). The septal and lateral portions

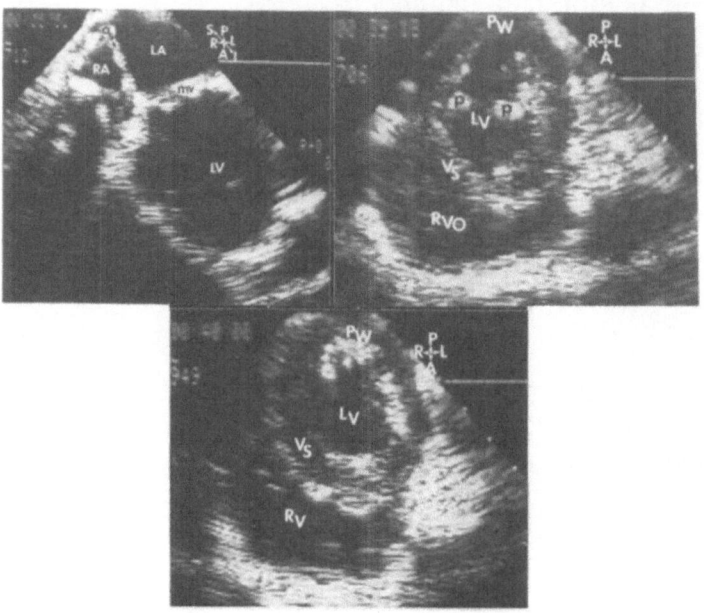

FIGURE 3. Oblique and short-axis tomographic views of the left ventricle. a) Oblique four-chamber view of the left atrium (LA), right atrium (RA), and left ventricle (LV). The atrial septum (as) separates the left and right atria. Portions of the anterior leaflet of the mitral valve (mv) separate the left atrium from the left ventricle. b and c) Tilt of the transducer beneath the cardiac structure permits short-axis views of the left ventricle. The posterior wall (PW) is closest to the transducer, whereas the right ventricle (RV) and right ventricular outflow tract (RVO) lie anterior to the left ventricle (inferior on the image). Papillary muscles (p) can be visualized within the ventricle cavity. The ventricular septum (VS) separates the left (LV) and right ventricles. P = posterior; L = left; A = anterior; R = right; S = superior; I = inferior.

of the anterior mitral leaflet separated the left atrium and the left ventricle. Superior and inferior tilt of the transducer best assessed leaflet coaptation and the valve support apparatus. Superior and inferior translation and tilt of the transducer produced short-axis and oblique views of the left ventricle. Positions of the papillary muscles, myocardial thickness, and overall global function could be assessed visually or scanned by simultaneous M-mode echocardiography.

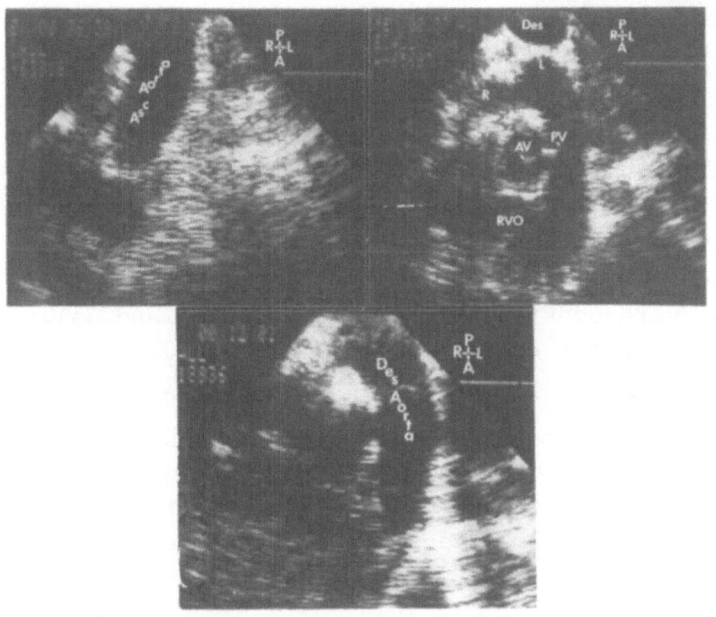

FIGURE 4. Sequential views at the base of the heart, illustrating visualization of the ascending and descending thoracic aorta and its anatomic relationships. a) An oblique scan in the frontal projection at the base of the heart permits visualization of the ascending (Asc) aorta. b) With slightly posterior tilt, the ascending aorta anteriorly joins the aortic root at the level of the aortic valve (AV) and pulmonary valve (PV). The proximal bifurcation of the left and right pulmonary arteries is also visualized. The proximal right (R) and left (L) pulmonary arteries lie between the aortic root from the upper descending thoracic aorta (Des). RVO = right ventricular outflow tract. c) With posterior tilt of the transducer, an oblique tomographic section of the descending (Des) thoracic aorta is visualized. P = posterior; L = left; A = anterior; R = right.

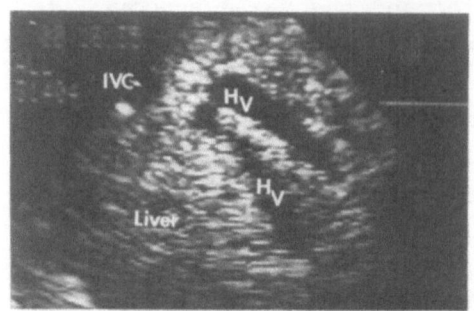

FIGURE 5. With the transducer at the gastroesophageal junction and tipped toward the liver, portions of the liver, hepatic veins (*HV*), and inferior vena cava (*IVC*) are visualized.

The right ventricle was less consistently imaged; it appeared to be out of the plane in many of the dog models. However, the right and left atria were consistently imaged (Fig. 2a and 3a). Anatomic detail of the atrial septum could be viewed by superior and inferior scanning, which allowed recognition of the valve with the fossa ovalis (Fig. 2a).

3.2. Left atrium

The most consistently imaged chamber was the left atrial cavity. The structure was found directly against the esophagus and was the cavity easiest to image (Fig. 2a and b and 3a).

3.3. Right atrium

The right atrial cavity was consistently visualized although not as completely as the left atrium (Fig. 2a and b and 3a). The atrial septum separating these two chambers was always visualized, and details of the intra-atrial anatomy were consistently imaged.

3.4. Semilunar valves

Aortic and pulmonary valves were imaged in the horizontal plane with superior scanning from the body of the left ventricle (Fig. 2 and 4). The horizontal sections were viewed as though in looking down on the tomographic horizontal plane. This placed the aorta as the central structure, the tricuspid valve to the

viewer's left, and the pulmonary valve anterior and slightly to
the right, with the main pulmonary artery to the viewer's right
and the right pulmonary artery encircling the aorta posteriorly.
The descending thoracic aorta was visible posterior to the
right pulmonary artery, passing between the bifurcation of the
right and left pulmonary arteries (Fig. 4b).

3.5. Aorta

The aorta could be imaged from multiple transducer positions,
starting from the aortic valve to the ascending aorta, aortic
arch, and descending thoracic aorta and into the abdomen past
the gastroesophageal junction (Fig. 4). The dimension of the
aorta and its anatomic relationships were easily appreciated.
Unique views of the posterior mediastinal vascular anatomy could
be obtained.

3.6. Pulmonary veins

Assessment of pulmonary venous drainage was not consistently
obtained; however, with high-resolution instruments, this particular observation seemed to be more feasible.

4. DISCUSSION

Increasing numbers of reports on the use of esophageal
echocardiography are appearing in the literature. M-mode echocardiography is confined to left ventricular function.[1-6] As with
its external application, esophageal M-mode echocardiography has
limited usefulness in the assessment of cardiac anatomy.
Mechanical esophageal two-dimensional echocardiography is also
encumbered by the necessity of having a movable coaxial linkage
to the crystal elements, which requires a larger, less versatile
endoscope. Electronic scanners that utilize crystal elements
connected via wire bundles without a mechanical interface introduced the possibility of a small wide-angle two-dimensional
echocardiographic esophageal imaging device. In addition,
other modalities that are commonly used in endoscopy, including
flexible tip, suction, and fiberoptics, are more easily incorporated with the phased-array technology.

A prototype phased-array esophageal instrument was used in
this study to illustrate its application in the visualization

of detailed cardiac anatomy. Additional modalities inherent to the endoscope which were helpful for more complete examination included a flexible tip and suction. Fiberoptic direction of the endoscope was found not to be necessary; instead, ultrasonic direction was used. We foresee the development of endoscopes of pediatric size in the very near future. This type of adaptable instrumentation would markedly broaden the feasibility and increase the cardiologic application of esophageal imaging.

The utility of this technique appears to be varied. Precordial two-dimensional echocardiography is a very adaptable examination, which results in few incomplete studies.[11] However, there are unique applications of the esophageal echocardiography which cannot be achieved from the precordial position, in particular mediastinal and retrocardiac anatomy. Visualization of posterior heart structures, including pulmonary vein, left and right atria, and great arteries, is feasible. Obtaining detailed ultrasonic assessment of the thoracic aorta is far more feasible by means of the transesophageal approach. This may add some advantage over the present contrast and computed radiography techniques for the differentiation of aortic aneurysm and aortic dissection.

A role for esophageal echocardiography would appear to be in the determination of cardiac anatomy and function during operative procedures or in the intensive critical-care facility. In these circumstances, the heart is difficult or impossible to image by conventional means. Esophageal echocardiography would be ideal not only for monitoring ventricular function and dimension but also for assessing pertinent cardiac anatomy. During surgery, the recognition of residual defects or complications of operative repair would be facilitated by esophageal imaging.

This experience in a dog model illustrates the utility of the transesophageal approach to cardiac imaging. Potential small size, absence of the need for mechanical linkage, and versatility of the phased-array instrumentation make it superior to existing esophageal echocardiographic instruments. The detailed assessment of mediastinal and also cardiac and retrocardiac structures will make this technique clinically applicable. Further

development of instrumentation and rational applications of the
technique are to be developed.

REFERENCES

1. Frazin L, Talano JV, Stephanides L, et al.   1976.   Esophageal
   echocardiography.   Circulation   54:102-108.
2. Matsumoto M, Oka Y, Lin YT, et al.   1979.   Transesophageal
   echocardiography: for assessing ventricular performance.
   NY State J Med   79:19-21.
3. Matsuzaki M, Yorozu T, Fukagawa K, et al.   1978.   Assessment
   of left ventricular anterior wall motion: a new application
   of esophageal echocardiography.   J Cardiography   8:113-124.
4. Matsumoto M, Oka Y, Strom J, et al.   1980.   Application of
   transesophageal echocardiography to continuous intraoperative
   monitoring of left ventricular performance.   Am J Cardiol
   46:95-105.
5. Fukagawa K.   1981.   Prediction of left anterior descending
   coronary artery disease by esophageal echocardiography.
   Jpn Heart J   22:173-183.
6. Matsuzaki M, Matsuda Y, Ikee Y, et al.   1981.   Esophageal
   echocardiographic left ventricular anterolateral wall motion
   in normal subjects and patients with coronary artery disease.
   Circulation   63:1085-1092.
7. Hisanaga K, Hisanaga A.   1978.   A new real-time sector
   scanning system of ultra-wide angle and real-time recording
   of entire adult cardiac images: transesophagus and trans-
   chest-wall methods.   In Ultrasound in medicine.   Vol 4.
   Edited by D White, EA Lyons.   New York, Plenum Press,
   pp 391-402.
8. Hisanaga K, Hisanaga A, Hibi N, et al.   1980.   High speed
   rotating scanner for transesophageal cross-sectional echocardiography.   Am J Cardiol   46:837-842.
9. Hisanaga K, Hisanaga A, Nagata K, et al.   1980.   Transesophageal cross-sectional echocardiography.   Am Heart J   100:
   605-609.
10. Henry WL, DeMaria A, Gramiak R, et al.   1980.   Report of the
    American Society of Echocardiography Committee on Nomenclature
    and Standards in Two-Dimensional Echocardiography.   Circula-
    tion   62:212-217.
11. Bansal RC, Tajik AJ, Seward JB, et al.   1980.   Feasibility of
    detailed two-dimensional echocardiographic examination in
    adults: prospective study of 200 patients.   Mayo Clin Proc
    55:291-308.

TRANSESOPHAGEAL HORIZONTAL AND SAGITTAL IMAGING OF THE
HEART WITH A PHASED ARRAY SYSTEM. INITIAL CLINICAL RESULTS.

P. HANRATH, M. SCHLÜTER, B.A. LANGENSTEIN, J. POLSTER,
S. ENGEL

INTRODUCTION

Ultrasonic imaging of the heart and its motion can
provide valuable diagnostic information. However, cardiac
imaging from the standard transducer locations on the
thorax is frequently compromised, mainly by the interposition
of ribs and air-containing lung tissue into the ultrasound
beam. Two-dimensional sector scanning of the heart is therefore
generally restricted to certain planes which may not allow
to identify all cardiac structures and regions of interest.
In order to overcome these limitations, Frazin et al. (1)
introduced cardiac imaging from the esophagus in 1976. They
and others (2-6) have demonstrated the value of transesophageal
M-mode echocardiography. The feasibility of transesophageal
cross-sectional imaging of the heart with a mechanical sector
scanner was first reported on in 1978 (7). In this paper we
describe transesophageal cardiac imaging in humans with a
specially designed miniature phased array transducer system
incorporated into the tip of a commercially available gastroscope (8).

TRANSDUCER DESIGN AND TRANSESOPHAGEAL IMAGING TECHNIQUE

Two prototypes of endoscopic ultrasound systems were
used in our laboratories (Fig. 1). One consists of a 3.5 MHz
transducer array of 32 elements attached to the flexible tip
of a standard gastroscope (Fig. 1, right hand side) which
obtains cardiac cross-sections in a horizontal plane, while
the 3.5 MHz transducer head of the second system holds two adjacent 32-element arrays mounted at right angles to each other

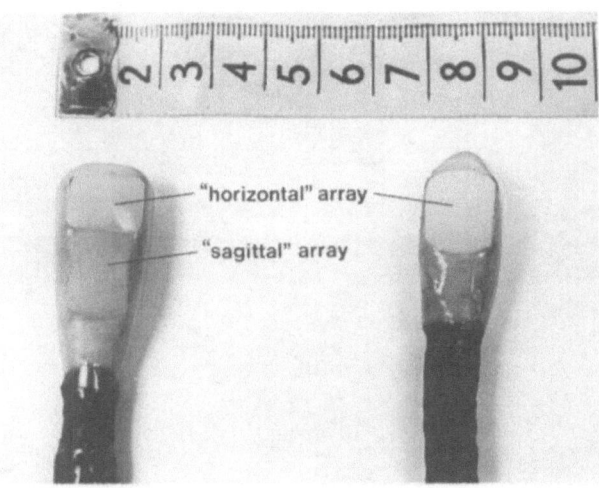

FIGURE 1. Transducer heads of two prototype ultrasonic
gastroscope systems. Head on the right contains single
array of 32 elements for horizontal cross-sectional
imaging. Head on the left holds two adjacent arrays,
one for horizontal and one for sagittal imaging.

for horizontal as well as sagittal cross-sectional imaging
of the heart (Fig. 1, left hand side). The only rigid parts
of both systems are represented by the outer dimensions of
the transducer heads which are (length x width x thickness)
35 mm x 15 mm x 16 mm and 40 mm x 17 mm x 15 mm, respectively.
Gastroscope diameter is 9 mm in both instruments. Further
technical information concerning transducer technology was
described in detail elsewhere (9).

Investigations with the ultrasonic gastroscopes are
similar to routine endoscopic examinations. The patient is
lying in a supine position, he was fasted for about 8 hours
and received 10 mg diazepam i.v. for sedation and .5 mg
atropine sulfate subcutaneously to avoid hypersalivation
and bradycardia. Since the fiber optics system was replaced
by the electrical connections for the transducer arrays, the
gastroscope is introduced blindly. Thus, an x-ray examination
must be performed prior to the ultrasound investigation in
order to rule out a diverticulum of the esophagus.

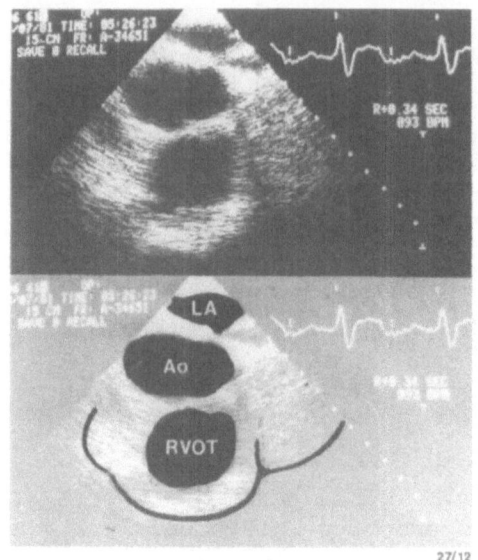

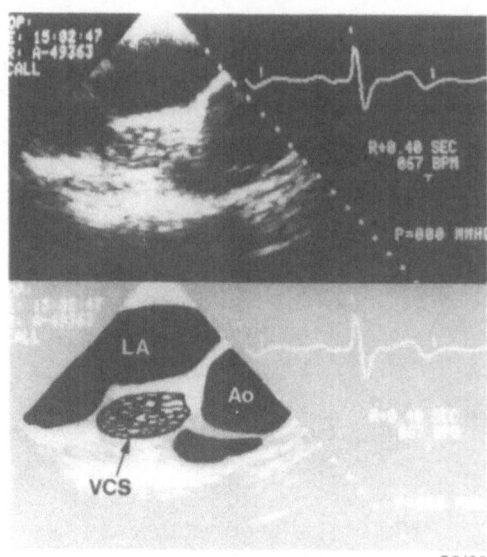

FIGURE 2. Transesophageal horizontal view of aorta ascendens
(Ao), left atrium (LA), and
right ventricular outflow tract
(LVOT).

FIGURE 3. Transesophageal horizontal view with left atrium
(LA), vena cava superior (VCS)
and aorta (Ao). VCS is filled
with echo contrast due to peripheral venous injection of
saline.

IDENTIFICATION OF ANATOMICAL STRUCTURES

The gastroscope is inserted with the transducer array
facing anteriorly. At a depth of about 40 cm from the patient's
teeth the aorta ascendens at a level above the leaflets can
usually be seen (Fig. 2). Clockwise rotation of the endoscope
will image the vena cava superior (Fig. 3) which can easily
be identified by peripheral venous injections of echogenic
agents such as agitated saline. Further insertion of about
1 cm enables the identification of the ostia of the right
coronary artery (Fig. 4) and, by counter-clockwise rotation
of the gastroscope at roughly the same level, of the left coronary
artery (Fig. 5). A short-axis view of the aortic root with
the three cusps of the aortic valve in diastole is shown on
Fig. 6. The right ventricular outflow tract is outlined
anteriorly to the aorta.

283

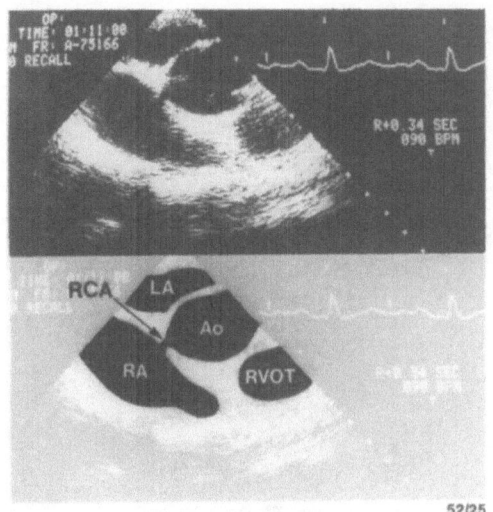 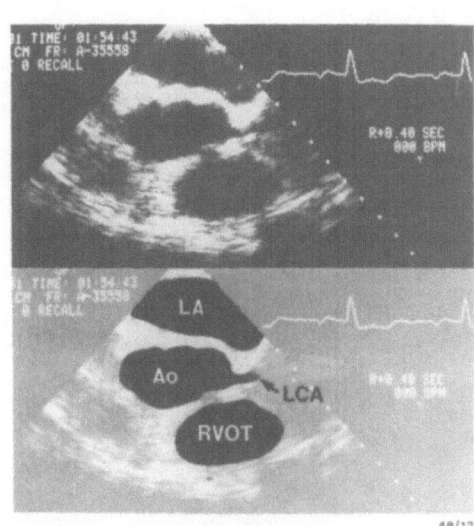

FIGURE 4. Transesophageal horizontal view showing ostium of
right coronary artery (RCA). Ao:
aorta. LA: left atrium. RA: right
atrium. RVOT: right ventricular
outflow tract.

FIGURE 5. Ostium of left coronary artery (LCA) in transesophageal horizontal view. Left
atrium (LA), aorta (Ao), and
right ventricular outflow tract
(RVOT) are also shown.

The left ventricular outflow and inflow tracts can be
visualized (Fig. 7) by slightly pushing the gastroscope down
the esophagus from the aortic root level and rotating
counter-clockwise. At various lower esophageal levels of the
transducer short-axis views of the left ventricle can be
obtained, e.g. at the papillary muscles (Fig. 8) or at the
cardiac apex. Turning the endoscope to the right heart will
image both ventricles in a horizontal plane (Fig. 9).

If the double-array system is used for the investigation,
horizontal and sagittal cross-sections of the heart can be
obtained from the same esophageal transducer position by
activating the respective transducer array. A sagittal image
of the left ventricle corresponding to the horizontal view
of Fig. 8 is shown on Fig. 10. The apical region is to the
left and the mitral valve area to the right of the sector
image.

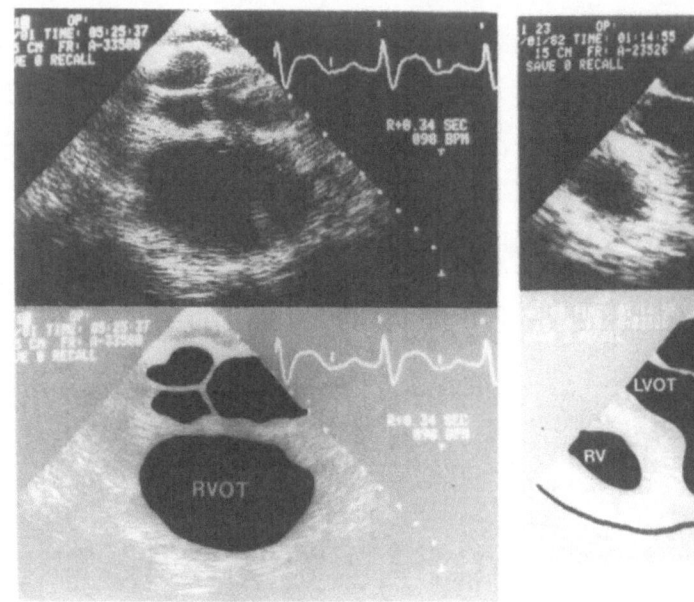

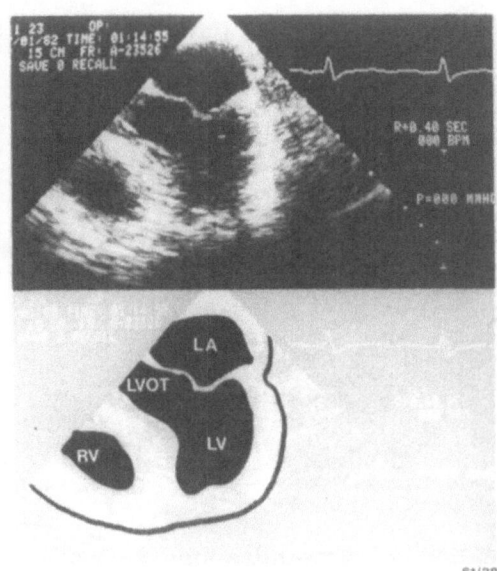

FIGURE 6. Aortic root with all three cusps in transesophageal short-axis view. Abbreviations as before.

FIGURE 7. Transesophageal horizontal view at the level of the atrioventricular junction with left atrium (LA), mitral leaflets, left ventricle (LV) and left ventricular outflow tract (LVOT), interventricular septum, and right ventricle (RV).

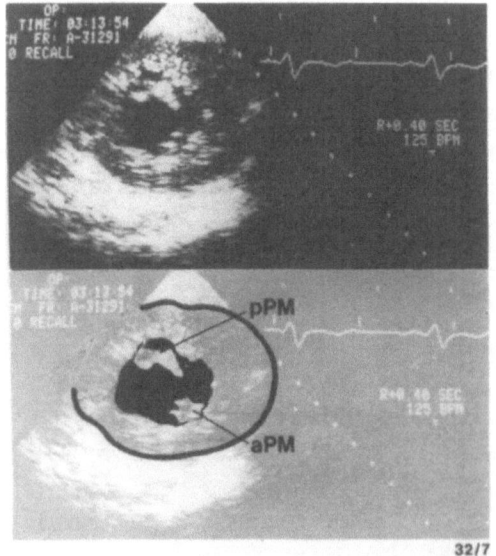

FIGURE 8. Transesophageal short-axis view of left ventricle at the level of the papillary muscles. aPM: anterior papillary muscle. pPM: posterior papillary muscle.

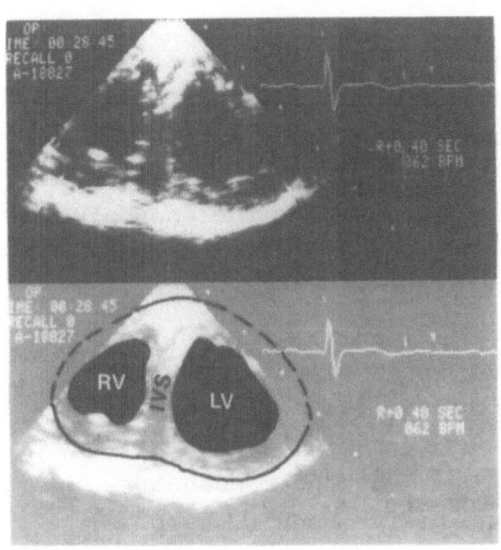

FIGURE 9. Transesophageal horizontal view of left (LV) and right ventricle (RV) with interventricular septum (IVS).

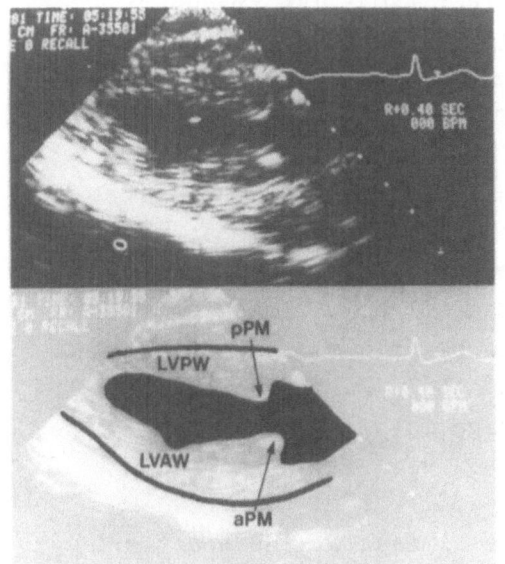

FIGURE 10. Transesophageal sagittal view of left ventricle at the level of the papillary muscles. Apical region to the left, mitral region to the right of figure. LVAW: left ventricular anterior wall. LVPW: left ventricular posterior wall. aPM: anterior papillary muscle. pPM: posterior papillary muscle.

DISCUSSION

Transesophageal two-dimensional imaging of the heart adds a new dimension to the diagnostic application of cardiac ultrasonography. Outlines and motion of valves, cavities, and great vessels can be clearly identified by choosing the correct depth and transducer orientation within the esophagus. The proximity of the heart to the esophagus permits the use of high-frequency transducers resulting in cardiac cross-sections of high spatial resolution.

Interest in transesophageal cardiac imaging is presently increasing and various types of ultrasonic imaging devices for esophageal use have already been presented. Hisanaga and coworkers (10) used single-element rotatable scanners to obtain horizontal cross-sections of the heart, while Eggleton et al. (11) and Fearnot et al. (12) developed multi-element rotatable scanning systems for the same purpose. Sagittal cross-sections in animals obtained with a linear array system were reported by DiMagno et al. (13). All these devices suffered either from a rigid tip too large to allow use in man (12, 13) or from mechanical vibrations which might cause discomfort to the patient (10). The frequent incorporation of an inflatable oil bag surrounding the transducer to secure esophageal wall contact is also liable to cause mechanical irritation of the esophagus or adjacent cardiac regions such as the left atrium.

A miniature phased array transducer fixed to the distal end of a flexible gastroscope, on the other hand, has the advantages of being small in size and eliminating the need for mechanically moving parts or an oil bag. Close contact between transducer surface and esophageal wall is established in this system by transducer angulation. Furthermore, the line density within the sector image is higher than in mechanical scanners and the field of view is considerably larger than in the linear array system.

Transesophageal two-dimensional images of the heart are generally less familiar than those obtained from transthoracic transducer locations. Since the long axis of the heart is

oblique to the axis of the esophagus in the frontal as well
as in the lateral plane and since the ultrasonic plane is
either perpendicular or parallel to the esophageal axis,
true long-axis views of the heart cannot be obtained with
present esophageal imaging systems, while short-axis views
at various left ventricular levels are possible with the
horizontal phased array by transducer angulation. It is
desirable to examine the heart at angles oblique to the
esophagus, i.e. parallel to the cardiac long axis, and we
believe that this can be achieved with an esophageal phased
array system which can be rotated about its normal axis.

Cardiac imaging from the esophagus is particularly indicated
in patients with obesity, emphysema, or barrel chests, and
it is generally advantageous in investigations of cardiac
anatomy which is hard or not at all accessible from the
precordium, such as the interatrial septum, the vena cava
superior, the pulmonary artery, or apical regions. With the
availability of a rotatable phased array transducer able
to collect true short-axis and long-axis scans the functional
and morphological assessment of the left ventricle from an
esophageal transducer position should be greatly enhanced.

REFERENCES

1. Frazin L., Talano J.V., Stephanides L., Loeb H.S., Kopel L.,
   Gunnar R.M.: Esophageal echocardiography.
   Circulation 54: 102, 1976
2. Matsumoto M., Oka Y., Lin Y.T., Strom J., Sonnenblick E.H.,
   Frater R.W.M.: Transesophageal echocardiography for
   assessing ventricular performance.
   N.Y. State J. Med. 79: 19,1979
3. Matsumoto M., Oka Y., Strom J., Frishman W., Kadish A.,
   Becher R., Frater W.M., Sonnenblick E.H.: Application of
   transesophageal echocardiography for continuous intra-
   operative monitoring of left ventricular performance.
   Am. J. Cardiol. 46: 95, 1980
4. Hanrath P., Kremer P., Langenstein B.A., Matsumoto M.,
   Bleifeld W.: Transösophageale Echokardiographie.
   Dtsch. med. Wschr. 106: 523, 1981
5. Kremer P., Hanrath P., Langenstein B.A., Matsumoto M.,
   Tams C., Bleifeld W.: The evaluation of left ventricular
   function at rest and during exercise by transesophageal
   echocardiography in aortic insufficiency (abstr.).
   Am. J. Cardiol. 47: 412, 1981

6. Matsuzaki M., Matsuda Y., Yoshinobu I., Takahashi Y., Sasaki T., Toma Y., Ishida K., Yorozu T., Kumada T., Kusukawa R.: Esophageal echocardiographic left ventricular anterolateral wall motion in normal subjects and patients with coronary artery disease.
Circulation 63: 1085,1981
7. Hisanaga K., Hisanaga A.: A new real-time sector scanning system of ultra-wide angle and real-time recording of entire adult cardiac images: Transesophagus and trans-chest-wall methods.
In: White D., Lyons E.A., eds.: Ultrasound in Medicine, Vol. 4. New York: Plenum Press, 1978: 391
8. Schlüter M., Langenstein B.A., Polster J., Kremer P., Souquet J., Engel S., Hanrath P.: Transesophageal cross-sectional echocardiography with a phased array transducer system - technique and initial clinical results.
Br. Heart J.: in press
9. Souquet J., Hanrath P., Zitelli L., Kremer P., Langen-stein B.A., Schlüter M.: Transesophageal phased array for imaging of the heart.
IEEE Trans. Biomed. Eng.: in press
10. Hisanaga K., Hisanaga A., Hibi N., Nishimura K., Kambe T.: High speed rotating scanner for transesophageal cross-sectional echocardiography.
Am. J. Cardiol. 46: 837, 1980
11. Eggleton R.C.: Ultrasonic visualization of the dynamic geometry of the heart.
Proc. 2nd World Congr. on Ultrasonics in Medicine, Excerpta Medica, Intl. Congr. Series 277: 10, 1973
12. Fearnot N.E., Babbs C.F., Bourland J.D., Geddes L.A.: Dynamic intraesophageal imaging of the heart with ultrasound.
Ultrasonic Imaging 2: 78, 1980
13. DiMagno E.P., Buxton J.L., Regan P.T., Hattery R.R., Wilson D.A., Suarez J.R., Green P.S.: Ultrasonic endoscope.
Lancet 1980: I, 629

Evaluation of Cardiac Function during Surgery by Transesophageal
2-Dimensional Echocardiography

Nelson B. Schiller

The surgical patient with advanced or unstable cardiac disease is at
increased risk for developing complications in the intraoperative and
postoperative periods. Traditional monitoring methods such as heart rate
or blood pressure by sphygmomanometer provide incomplete information
about cardiovascular status during surgery. In the last decade flow
directed pulmonary artery catheters have been shown to provide a highly
effective albeit invasive form of intraoperative monitoring. By sampling
intracardiac pressures and by measuring flow by thermodilution the
anesthesiologist can quickly detect common complications such as hypo-
volemia or depressed left ventricular performance. Unfortunately the
use of these expensive "disposable" catheters carries the risk of morbidity or even mortality.
Transthoracic 2-dimensional echocardiography is an effective totally
noninvasive method which can preoperatively evaluate the presence and
severity of a variety of cardiac disorders. Its safety and reliability
would make it an ideal method for intraoperative monitoring. However,
during surgery the precordium is usually inaccessible to transducer
placement and it is impossible to maintain stable transducer positions
for long periods of time. In this communication we describe a new
method of obtaining 2-dimensional and M-mode echocardiograms which is
suitable for intraoperative monitoring. This new method is called
transesophageal echocardiography (TEE) and is accomplished by intro-
ducing a gastroscope mounted with an echocardiographic transducer into
the esophagus and using the resultant high resolution images to monitor
left ventricular function and size continuously during surgical pro-
cedures(figure 1).
Method: 60 patients undergoing elective abdominal, perineal or cardiac
surgery were selected after gaining informed consent. After induction
of anesthesia and endotracheal intubation a special 3.5 MHz phased

array transducer afixed to the end of a commercially available gastroscope is inserted into the esophagus. The external dimensions of the
transducer are 35 mm length, 15 mm wide and 16 mm thick. The positional
controls of the gastroscope allow an easy atraumatic introduction and
manipulability. By rotation, advancement, withdrawal and slight tip
angulation high quality recordings of the left ventricle can be obtained.
Once this position is achieved the control end of the gastroscope is
-ocked and clamped to a rigid pole. Heart rate and arterial pressure
were simultaneously obtained and recorded.

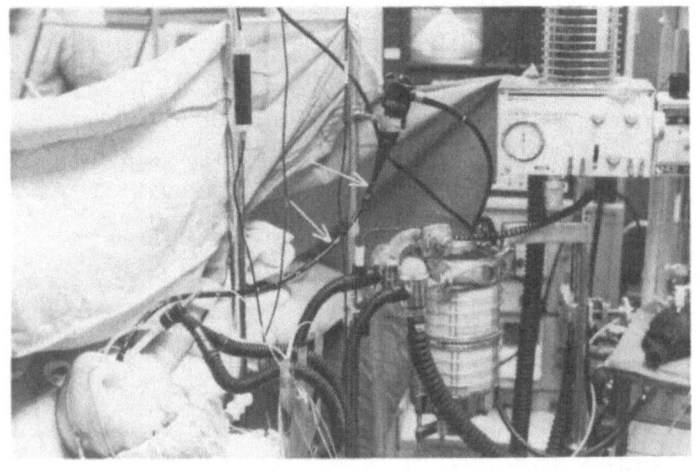

Results: In all 60 patients high quality images of the left ventricle
were obtained in the short axis view (figure 2). It was possible to
monitor these patients continuously for up to 12 hours while maintaining a stable transducer position. Comparison between the echocardiographic images and simultaneous clinical or hemodynamic data
revealed that accurate assumptions about contractility was always
possible from the qualitative information provided by the real-time
echocardiographic image. In most cases it was possible to estimate
shifts in central blood volume from the echocardiographic image.However,
such estimations were frustrated by the inability to easily compare a
given image with earlier recorded images.For this purpose simultaneously
generated M-mode data was extrmely useful. In general, subtle or early

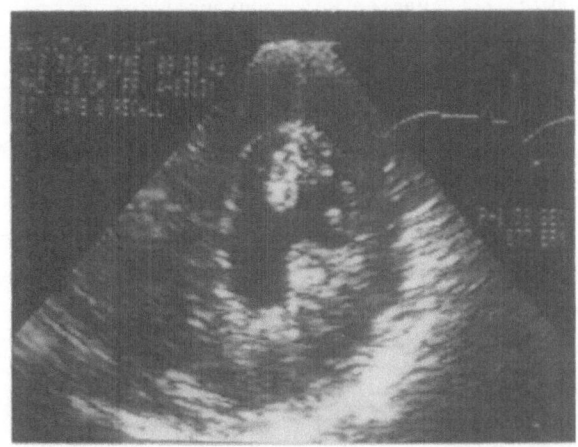

changes in circulating volume are difficult to detect by the qualitative
method employed in this study. No complications have occured in asso-
ciation with intraoperative TEE in our patient series.

Illustrative cases: A 42 year old female with endstage renal failure
and symptomatic coronary artery disease undergoing renal transplantation
had frequent episodes of severe hypotension during surgery. It was
unclear to the attending anesthesiologist as to the cause of hypotension.
Evaluation of global LV performance by intraoperative TEE revealed
an adequate ejection fraction of 60% without segmental wall motion
abnormalities.Based directly on this information the anesthesiologist
chose to administer additional parenteral fluid which resulted in
immediate restoration of normal arterial pressure. Concomitant with
the rise in blood pressure there was a visible increase in the size
of the LV and a further increase in ejection fraction.

A 55 year old female underwent mitral valve replacement because of
mitral valve stenosis. Attempts to discontinue cardiopulmonary bypass
were frustrated by low cardiac output and hypotension. Comparison of the
intraoperative TEE taken in period immediately preceding cardiopulmonary
bypass with the one at the end of surgery demonstrated major new wall
motion abnormalities involving the entire free wall and most of the

interventricular septum (figure 3-6). In contrast the inferior and posterior LV walls were hyperdynamic. ECG changes were nonspecific and consisted of T wave inversions. Based on the TEE a diagnosis of intraoperative myocardial infarction was made and led to aggressive use of positive inotropic agents. These agents partially restored blood pressure and enabled the termination of cardiopulmonary bypass.

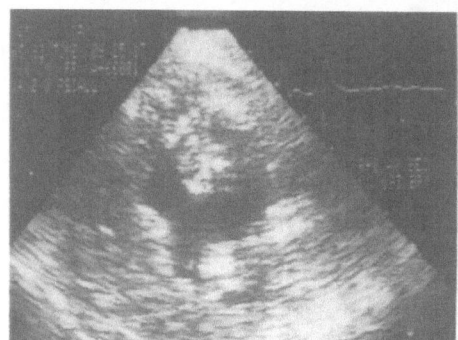 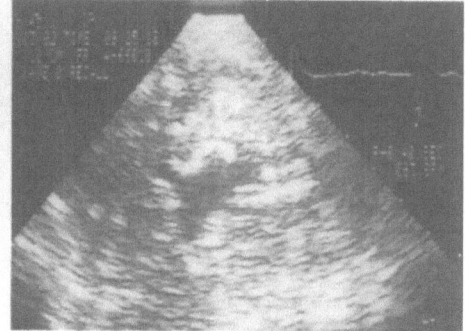

Enddiastolic (left) and endsystolic (right) LV short axis before cardiopulmonary bypass

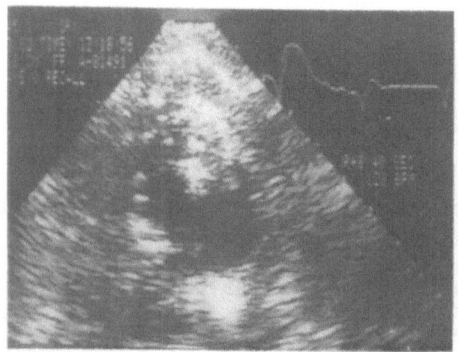 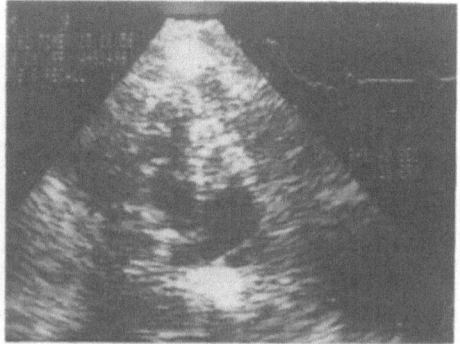

Enddiastolic (left) and endsystolic (right) LV short axis after cardiopulmonary bypass

Mitral and aortic valve replacement requires entrance into the cardiac
chambers. This implies the introduction of relative large quantities
of air into the LV chamber. There are many maneuvers which are aimed at
removing this air from the ventricle at the termination of the procedure.
In spite of these maneuvers, TEE has demonstrated that all patients
undergoing valve replacement have numerous large contrast targets
at the time of defibrillation. The clinical significance of these
targets is currently under study but they imply that "air maneuvers"
may be inadequate(figure 7).

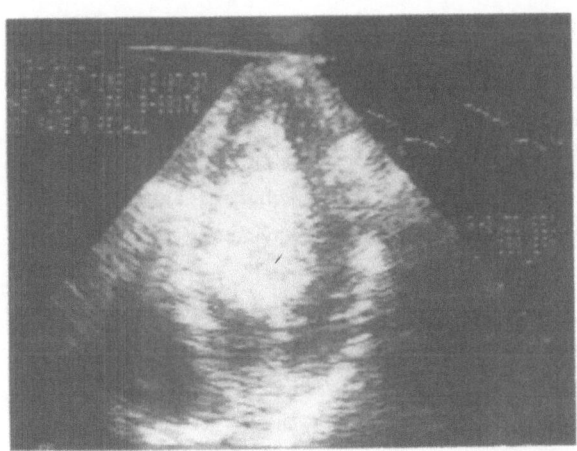

Conclusions: TEE is an exciting new method of intraoperative cardiac
monitoring. Our initial experience with 60 cases suggests that it is
simple, safe and effective. Although the initial cost of the instrumentation is high, this equipment can be used indefinately. The acceptance
of this technique by our surgical and anesthesia colleages suggest
that they prefer it to hemodynamic monitoring and that TEE may well
become a standard technique in the "high risk" surgical patient.

APPLICATIONS OF TWO-DIMENSIONAL ECHOCARDIOGRAPHY DURING OPEN HEART SURGERY IN HUMANS FOR EVALUATION OF ACQUIRED AND CORONARY HEART DISEASE

D.J. SAHN

Echocardiography, both M-mode and two-dimensional, has seen recent application in the operating room for evaluation of valvular and ischemic heart diseases [1-4]. Our own recent efforts and those of others have been directed toward using intraoperative echocardiography as a method to assess coronary artery disease and its physiologic implications [4-8]. The safety and efficacy of this recent work using ultrasound for scanning of open chest humans has suggested that ultrasound scanning will have a real and meaningful place during heart surgery. The purpose of this paper is to review our own experience in open chest imaging performed for valvular, congenital and coronary artery disease. Our techniques were initially explored in conjunction with Sir Brian Barratt-Boyes, Mr. Alan Kerr, Mr. Ken Graham, Mr. David Hill, and Drs. Peter W.T. Brandt and Antony Roche, all of the CardioThoracic Unit at Green Lane Hospital, Auckland, New Zealand and our studies have been continued in conjunction with Dr. Jack Copeland at the University of Arizona.

While at Green Lane Hospital, we performed over 150 open chest human imaging studies without electrical or infectious complication. These studies generated data to support the clinical utility of ultrasound during surgery for valvular disease, as well as its potential importance in research applications for coronary disease.

TECHNIQUES FOR STUDY OF VALVULAR AND CONGENITAL DISEASE

The studies we performed in New Zealand for valvular and congenital disease were performed with a 2.4 MHz electronically focused phased array with a specially damped transducer configuration and with a 3.5 MHz mechanical wide angle sector scanner. The rotary mechanical sector scanner was difficult to gas sterilize without bubble formation; bubbles could be removed by adding sterile oil, but this required a significant amount of time and effort. All our probes underwent cold gas sterilization with ethylene oxide and 24 hours de-gassing at a negative evacuation pressure of 1 atmosphere. With similar gas sterilization, the phased array transducers, when compared with control transducers, underwent no detectable deterioration. One transducer was damaged by mechanical abrasion against a surgical instrument during scanning. All our instruments were separately and specially grounded for use in open chest humans. Transducers were periodically tested for electrical leakage and integrity of the scan face.

Quantitative Doppler interrogation was not available to us in New Zealand; nonetheless, we believe (based on our recent experience) that Doppler will be of significant importance for intraoperative evaluation of residual valvular disease after reconstructive valve procedures. As an alternative to Doppler for detection of residual shunts and for valve studies, we used intraoperative contrast echocardiography, usually direct injection of saline bubbles or indocyanine green dye by needle into the aorta, left atrium, right or left ventricle. The following utilities were evaluated and proved quite promising in this experience.

VALVULAR DISEASE

In our 20 New Zealand mitral stenosis cases, intraoperative echocardiography showed close correlation to direct operative observations for mitral valve orifice measurement ($r = +0.96$). In addition, intraoperative echocardiography provided excellent detail for subchordal thickening and fusion, a significant degree of which makes the patient a poor candidate for valvotomy. In studies performed after cardiopulmonary bypass but with the chest still open after mitral valvotomy, contrast echo provided excellent information regarding the integrity of the valve, the size of the wash-in, and the presence or absence of significant mitral insufficiency (Figure 1). Pre- and postoperative ultrasound scanning and aortic contrast injections were extremely useful in defining the extent of residual aortic insufficiency postoperatively and degree of aortic valve opening after commissurotomy (Figure 1). The effect and results of mitral Carpentier ring annuplasty and chordal shortening for dominant mitral insufficiency or mitral valve prolapse and residual mitral insufficiency could be quite accurately assessed using contrast two-dimensional echocardiography. In our patients with mitral or aortic valve disease, intraoperative ultrasound scanning, as well as

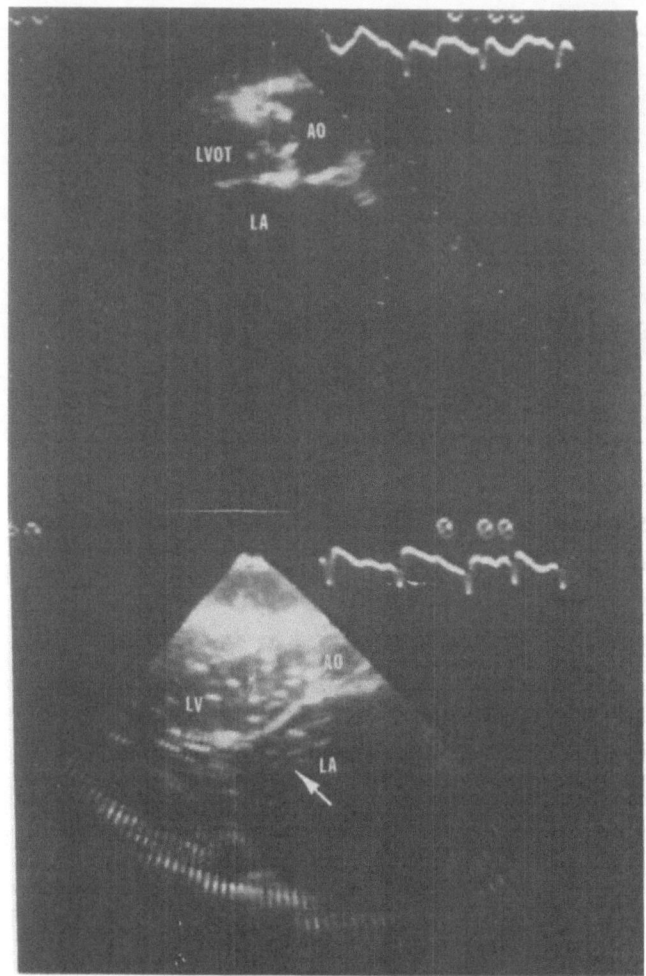

Figure 1:   In the upper panel, a domed stenotic aortic valve is shown.
In the lower panel, the patient, after having undergone aortic valvulo-
tomy and mitral reconstruction, is still found to have gross aortic regurgitation, as shown by the reflux of bubbles (arrow) into the left
ventricle after injection into the aorta. Mitral regurgitation is also
present with reflux of bubbles into the left atrium as well. The amount
of aortic regurgitation in conjunction with hemodynamic data suggested
the need for replacement of the aortic valve.

hemodynamic measurements, led to a suggestion of the need for at least

two valves to be replaced after plastic repair did not seem to produce

adequate results as judged by hemodynamic measurements as well as ultra-

sound imaging information.   Unsuspected tricuspid valve disease in

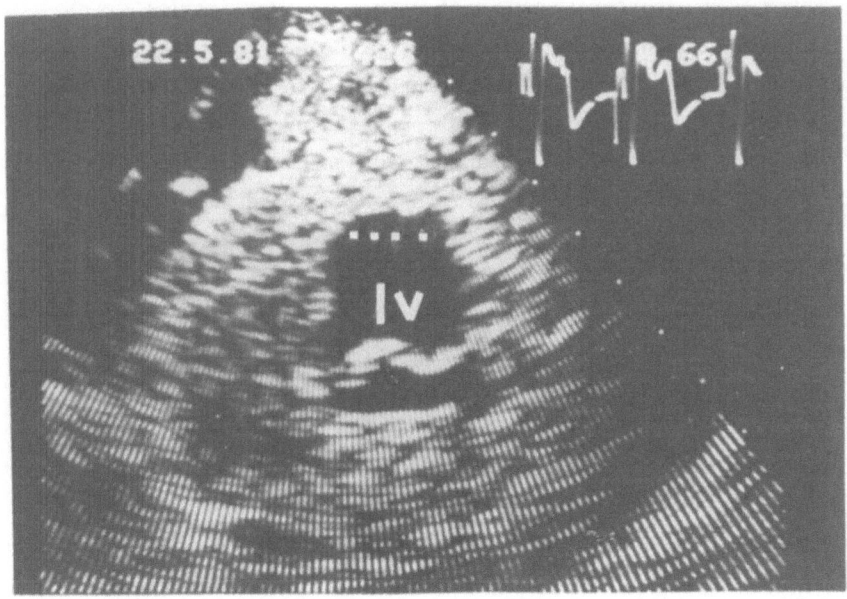

Figure 2: Short axis view shows the area resected during a myotomy-my-ectomy for IHSS. Systolic anterior motion is no longer seen. The tunnel of muscle resection within the septum is easily visualized.

patients whose tricuspid valves were poorly imaged on external echo was detected in at least two patients. Intraoperative scanning through the right atrioventricular junction or through the right atrium provided a unique view of the right ventricular inflow tract and tricuspid valve morphology, and was quite helpful in assessing unsuspected and silent tricuspid stenosis, and for assessing the effects of the tricuspid an-nuloplasty for tricuspid insufficiency.

IDIOPATHIC HYPERTROPHIC SUBAORTIC STENOSIS (IHSS)

Our experience in IHSS likewise supports the importance of intraop-erative echocardiography. The technique appeared useful for defining the tunnel of muscle resected during myotomy-myectomy, for defining the absence of residual systolic anterior motion in conjunction with hemody-namic measurements, and for assessing immediate intraoperative adequacy of the resection (Figure 2).

CONGENITAL HEART DISEASE

The standard phased array instrumentation which we employed did not have the resolution capable of providing detailed information about very small pediatric hearts. It was also of interest, in view of the deep hypothermia (below 23° C.) employed for complex heart repairs in infants in New Zealand, that a radical change in myocardial appearance took place which produced poor image quality in general on echocardiograms. This precluded efforts which we entertained at the time of our sabbatical leave for evaluating Mustard repairs and right ventricular outflow after tetralogy repairs. The small parts high frequency scanning transducer (which will be described in the coronary section of this paper) was unwieldy for adequate imaging of small pediatric patients; the probe was just too large to fit adequately in the chest cavity. Nonetheless, we were quite successful at imaging ventricular septal defects and feel that external localization by scanning with the transducer placed immediately over a ventricular septal defect, such as the muscular one shown in Figure 3, was quite helpful in reducing the size of the ventriculotomy. The adequacy of valve repair for atrioventricular valve defects and overriding and straddling valves likewise appeared to be a promising area for evaluation in the operating room for assessing the integrity of repair of such complicated malformations. Beyond this, our pediatric scanning experience was quite limited.

It was obvious to us that the instrumentation to be used for valvular and congenital intraoperative scanning required significant portability, large screen displays, and pedal operation for most functions so that a surgeon alone could operate the instrumentation and be able to see the display from across the table. This requires scan conversion capability, small sophisticated video tape decks which can be played back at variable speeds so that review of ultrasound images can be obtained on line. Multiplexing for digital recording on the same image of intraoperative hemodynamic data is likewise of importance. Probe arrays will have to be small and flat, capable of fitting on the surgeon's fingers. Such second generation dedicated surgical instruments are now being designed by our group in collaboration with several manufacturers.

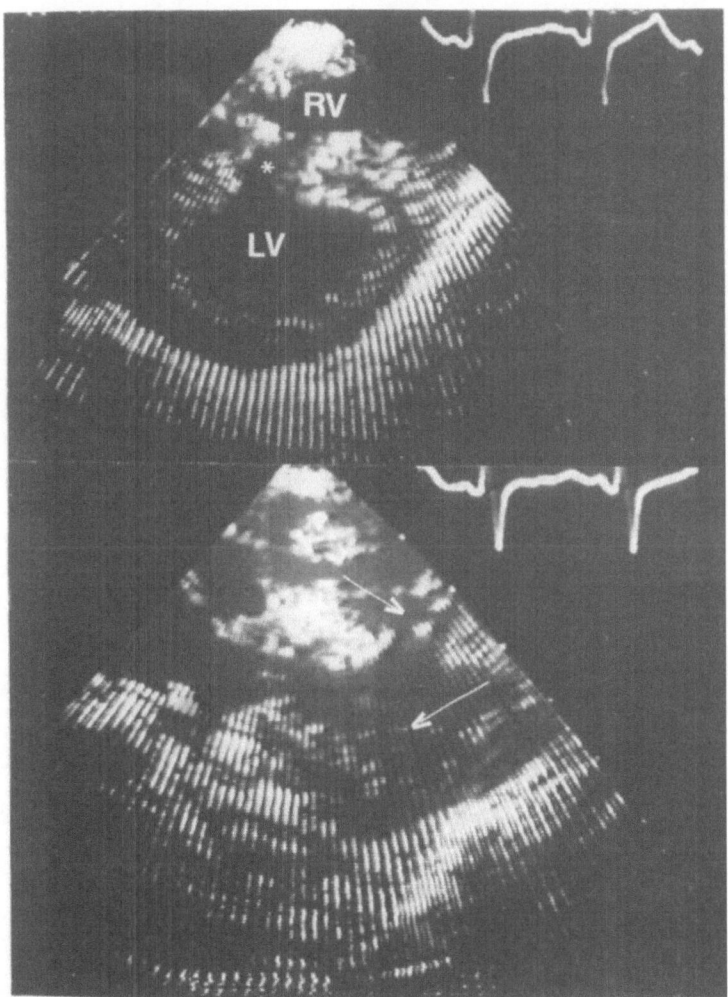

Figure 3: An oblique short axis, almost four chamber view shows the position of a mid-muscular ventricular septal defect (VSD) beneath the moderator band. In the lower panel, a contrast injection has been performed and bubbles are shown within the VSD.

CONTRAST ECHO OBSERVATIONS

A sidelight observation resulting from our scanning efforts was that gross amounts of contrast echo targets, probably small bubbles, appeared within the left heart cavities after cardiopulmonary bypass.

Even with meticulous bypass technique and no obvious air in the pump lines, our immediate post-pump scanning showed gross evidence of contrast echo targets, so dense, in fact, that we often had to wait 5-10 minutes for the "spontaneous" contrast to clear before we were able to perform a contrast injection. In reviewing the surgical literature, it appears that such bubbles probably hide within the pulmonary venous radicals, or the interstitium and trabeculations of the left ventricles, and are liberated into the left-sided circulation once intracardiac flow is re-established. They do not appear to be associated with clinical sequalae, and, as such, probably do not represent gross air embolization [9].

CORONARY SCANNING

Intraoperative coronary artery imaging had never been performed prior to our experience in New Zealand. The availability to us of vascular scanning ultrasound scanning technology at 9 MHz with excellent lateral resolution (the BioDynamics BioSound [R] system) suggested such capabilities. We worked closely in collaboration not only with the BioDynamics Company, but with William Glenn, Ph.D., New York Institute of Technology Research and Development Center, Dania, Florida, who had developed the water path scanner. The BioDynamics system is a 9 MHz electronically focused water path system. The scan head configuration of this device is now widely known. Ultrasound energy is electronically focused from an array and is then further focused and steered by an oscillating mirror within the water path. The sound travel time occurring within the 4 cm. water path is subtracted from the electronic imaging, therefore, the imaging begins immediately at the contact surface without any electronic switching noise, allowing scanning of the area directly under the transducer with very high resolution. Three open chest sheep were studied and gave a graphic impression of the potential capability of the technique for imaging coronary arteries. Nonetheless, the probe, which is 5 x 6 cm in volume, proved quite unwieldy for scanning small vessels and for achieving access to the diaphragmatic and posterior surface of the heart.

We found scanning of the coronary arteries most dramatic during normal cardiac contraction and relaxation. Nonetheless, the gross motion of the coronary arteries across the scan plane (which is quite narrow in the BioDynamics system) required slow motion and stop frame play

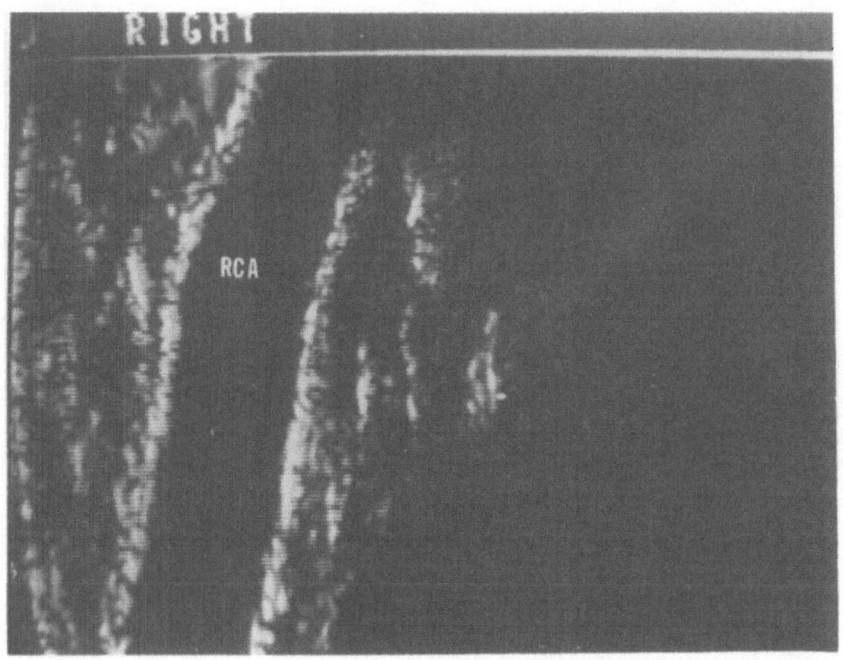

Figure 4: A normal right coronary artery is shown. The proximal portion is at the bottom of the image, the distal portion at the top of the image. The image is inverted because of the unwieldy configuration of the probe requiring its inversion, being placed over the atrioventricular sulcus. There is, however, good endothelial resolution.

back for achieving adequate understanding of the coronary artery images and the lesions imaged. After cardiopulmonary bypass and cardioplegia, the lack of physiologic distension of the coronary arteries made lesions, while imageable, difficult to assess in terms of severity.

A normal right coronary artery is imaged by our system as shown in Figure 4. The excellent endothelial resolution and the large display and imaged vessel size were quite reassuring. The variety of angiographic/ultrasonic correlates which we have obtained for over 150 imaged lesions provides a spectrum of ultrasonic appearances for imaged atherosclerotic lesions. The lesions shown in Figure 5 can be seen to cast an ultrasonic shadow, while that shown in Figure 6 appears to represent an organized thrombus within a coronary lesion. Both lesion appearances have been documented pathologically. The ultrasonic appear-

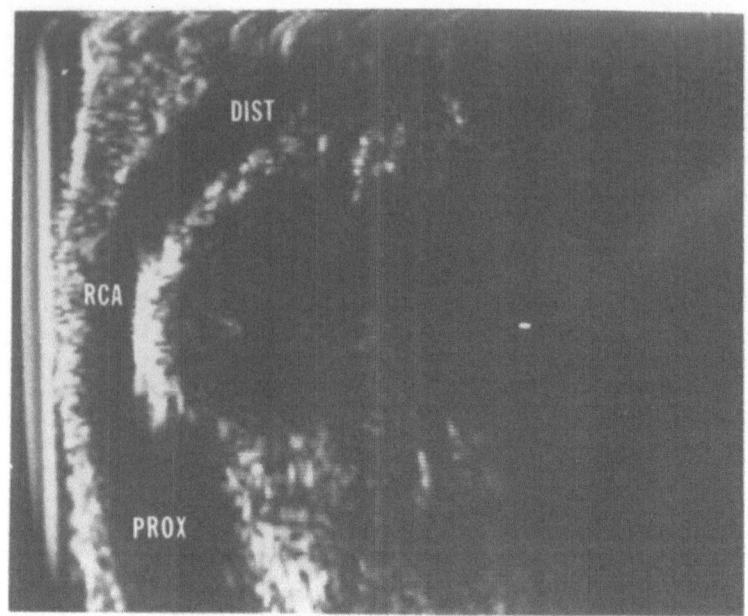

Figure 5: A right coronary artery lesion in the proximal portion of the vessel indents the vessel from what appears to be posteriorly and casts an ultrasonic shadow. The image corresponds to an 80-85% angiographic obstruction. The faint lines of the image (a 2 mm graticule) give an idea of the small size of all these vessels.

ance of what correlates to minimal angiographic change or endothelial irregularity usually appears much more dramatic than the angiogram. It is our impression, based on pathologic examination of specimens obtained from patients who did not survive bypass surgery, and others in Arizona whose hearts were harvested for pathological examination because they received cardiac transplants after scanning, that the ultrasonic detail of coronary artery lesions exceeds the detail provided by current day standard coronary angiographic techniques and bears a close relationship to the anatomy. We believe, as do others, that angiography may not be the appropriate "gold standard" for coronary artery disease (10). Our experience in this regard is ongoing in Arizona.

Most of the difficulty we encountered was with probe configuration. Therefore, in conjunction with Dr. Glenn, a dedicated surgical imaging probe was designed to function at 13 MHz with an examination depth of 2 cm, and a configurational change was made so that the water path is con-

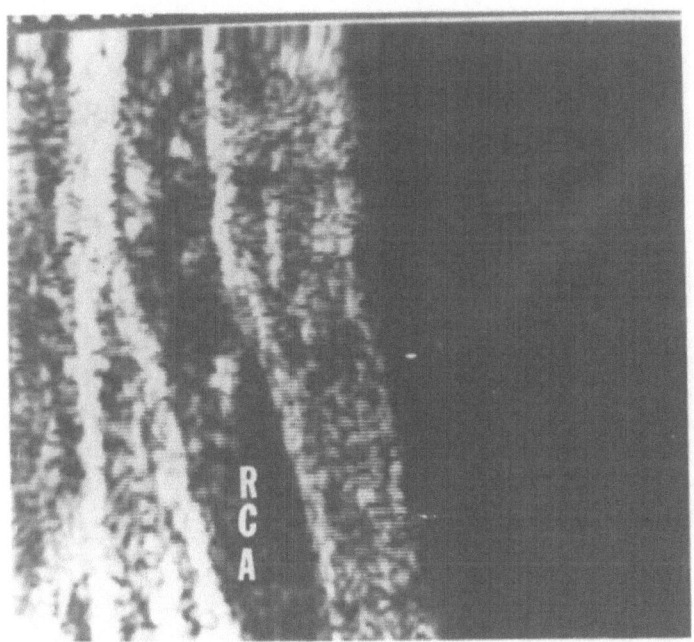

Figure 6: Organized thrombus within an obstructed coronary vessel is imaged within the right coronary circulation. The appearance corresponds with complete obstruction on the coronary angiogram.

tained within a long cylinder about the size of a large crayon, a probe achieving the overall size and configuration of an electric toothbrush. This new probe is significantly easier to manipulate on the surface of the heart. It allows us to obtain biplane ultrasound images for most lesions. It also allows access to small diagonal septal perforating vessels, as well as detailed imaging of the arteries to the sinus node and the atrioventricular node, and has allowed access to vessels on the acute marginal surface of the heart and along the course of the posterior descending circulation. Figure 7 gives an idea of the resolution capabilities of the new probe for imaging a diseased diagonal coronary artery which was subjected to intraoperative balloon dilation under ultrasound guidance. The BioDynamics system and the new surgical probe contain Doppler interrogation capabilities; these are, however, difficult to exercise with the heart moving the vessels across the scan plane. The Doppler interrogation capabilities of the system are most

304

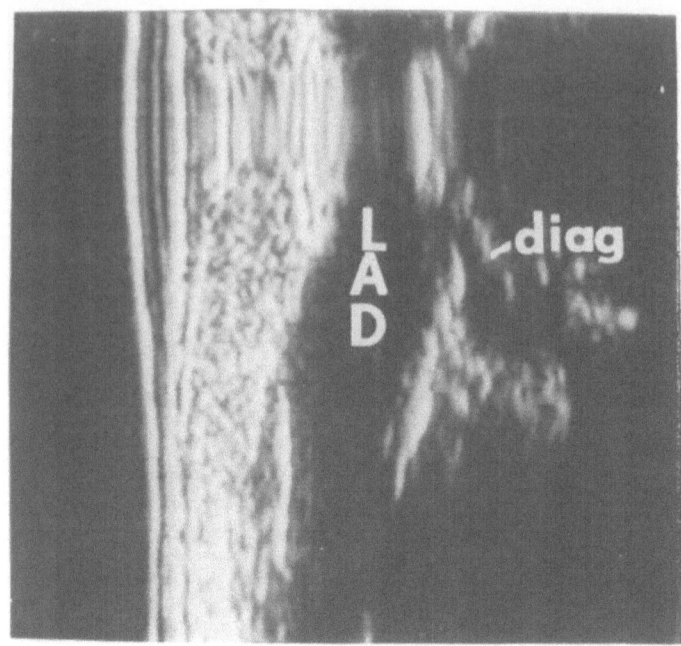

Figure 7: The new 13 MHz probe can be utilized to image very small diagonal and septal perforating vessels. Here, an image of a diseased diagonal with a somewhat bright, atherosclerotic lesion at its orifice gives an idea of the resolution capabilities of the system.

useful for assessing flow in grafts. The ultrasonic imaging system has likewise been used for assessing proximal and distal anastomotic insertions of coronary vein bypass grafts. Coronary artery imaging techniques appear to provide information in addition to that provided angiographically in patients whose proximal coronary circulations are occluded by severe disease, and in whom distal circulations may not be well visualized. We have imaged lesions which have progressed since angiography and provided a way for the surgeon to localize lesions which had been demonstrated adequately by prior coronary angiograms. We have imaged lesions missed or poorly visualized angiographically, including left main orifice lesions sometimes not well visualized on angiography. Our surgeons tell us that we provide a method for them to judge the appropriate site, especially for the distal site of insertion, of distal

coronary vein grafts, and to assess the adequacy of graft insertion and
graft flow.

Based on this feedback from surgeons that we have worked with both
in New Zealand and Arizona, we believe that coronary artery imaging with
Doppler interrogation will find an ongoing place in coronary bypass surgery and that the ultrasound imaging that it provides will allow the
surgeon to feel more at ease about intraoperative dilation of lesions
which are not accessible to catheter dilation in the cardiac catheterization suite because they are too distal. The opportunity of intraoperative dilation of such lesions may avoid the need to provide these additional bypass grafts, especially if our method proves acceptable for
allowing the surgeon to judge whether the dilation is adequate. This
represents an acute need for the surgeon, since angiography performed
in the operating room is unwieldy and difficult to arrange. At present,
we are collaborating with Dr. Glenn and with commercial enterprises in-
terested in development of dedicated coronary vascular imaging devices.

SUGGESTIONS TO ENGINEERS

We would like to say a final word about transducer configurations
which we believe would be most useful for intraoperative use. We do
not see the feasibility for providing detailed coronary imaging without
at least some sort of water path standoff which would therefore have
some bulk to the transducer scan head configuration. We believe such
scanners should function at 9 to 15 MHz and have Doppler capability.
In valvular and congenital heart disease, we believe that the surgeon
should be given not a full phased array transducer but just the front
end of the array itself to wear as a ring or mounted on a handle like a
dental mirror. Many of these small arrays being built for esophagoscop-
ic use, if mounted for a surgeon to be worn in a condom or on a ring,
will allow him to run his finger over the heart to achieve the plane of
scanning which he desires. We believe that in patients with valvular
and congenital heart disease whose chests are open, direct application
of a gas sterilized ultrasound scanning transducer to the heart by the
surgeon is an easy, safe and fast way of achieving the necessary imaging, and in fact can be achieved more rapidly than trying to do the same
from an esophagoscope. The surgeons find it easy to learn to do ultrasound scanning, and of course easy to orient the transducer with reference to the heart, since they are looking at it.

306

We have found that esophageal imaging in patients whose chests are open takes a longer time and provides less adequate information about anatomical detail than direct scanning by the surgeon. We do suggest, however, that for monitoring patients at times that the surgeon is not scanning, and especially for providing information about cardiac function, cardiac filling, pressure/volume loops and other indices of pump function, esophageal echocardiography will find its place in patients whose chests are not opened, but who may be undergoing prolonged neurologic, reconstructive, and microvascular surgery, or surgery for neoplastic lesions requiring prolonged dissection. Such a monitoring technique would also be highly applicable in sedated patients in a chronic coronary or intensive care unit setting.

We expect, as a result of our work and the work of others in intraoperative and esophageal echocardiography, that a new generation of ultrasound scanners will be developed in the next several years which will make all of these types of images easier to obtain, and that the ease of obtaining such images by the surgeon will be the impetus for further widespread application of ultrasonic techniques for intraoperative imaging during cardiac surgery.

REFERENCES

1. Spotnitz HM, Young CYH, Spotnitz AJ, et al: Intraoperative left ventricular performance evaluated by two-dimensional ultrasound. Circulation 62:329, 1980
2. Wong CYH, Spotnitz HM: Effect of nitroprusside on end diastolic pressure-diameter relations of the human left ventricle after periocardiotomy. Am J Cardiol 45:393, 1980
3. Spotnitz HM: Two-dimensional ultrasound and cardiac operations. J Thoracic Cardiovasc Surg 83:43, 1982
4. Sahn DJ: Intraoperative applications of two-dimensional and contrast two-dimensional echocardiography for evaluation of congenital, acquired and coronary heart disease in open-chested humans during cardiac surgery. In Echocardiology, edited by Rijsterborgh H, The Hague, Martinus Nihjoff Publishers, 1981
5. Wright C, Doty D, Eastham C, et al: A method for assessing the physiologic significance of coronary obstructions in man at cardiac surgery. Circulation 62(I):111, 1980
6. Sahn DJ, Brandt PWT, Barratt-Boyes B, et al: Ultrasonic/angiographic correlations for imaging of coronary atherosclerotic lesions in open chested humans during surgery. Circulation 64:205, 1981

7. Sahn DJ, Barratt-Boyes B, Graham K, et al: Cross-sectional ultrasonic imaging of the coronary arteries in open chested humans: The evaluation of coronary atherosclerotic lesions at surgery. Am J Cardiol 47:403, 1981

8. Likoff M, Reichek N, Macoviak J, et al: High frequency epicardial echo mapping of segmental myocardial performance at multiple sites of right and left ventricles. Am J Cardiol 47:403, 1981

9. Padula RT, Eisenstat E, Bronstein MH, et al: Intracardiac air following cardiotomy-location, causative factors, and a method for removal. 62:73, 1971

10. Isner JM, Kishel J, Kent KM, et al: Accuracy of angiographic determination of left main coronary arterial narrowing. Angiographic-histologic correlative analysis in 28 patients. Circulation 63:1056, 1981

ENDOSCOPIC ULTRASONOGRAPHY, A NEW HORIZON?

Eugene P. DiMagno, M.D.

INTRODUCTION

Conventional abdominal ultrasound examinations may be compromised by inadequate image resolution and gas within the gastrointestinal tract. As examples, pancreatic cancer (1) or metastatic neoplasms to the liver (2), which are smaller than 2 cm in diameter, are infrequently visualized with routine ultrasonography and gas within the gastrointestinal tract prevents ultrasonic visualization of the pancreas in approximately 13% of examinations (3). In transcutaneous cardiac ultrasonography, it is difficult to obtain cardiac images of diagnostic quality in patients with chronic obstructive pulmonary disease or obesity and even under ideal circumstances it is impossible to image all parts of the heart because the ribs introduce artifacts. Unfortunately, it is unlikely that resolution can be enhanced significantly with transcutaneous abdominal ultrasonography, since ultrasound frequencies greater than 5 MHz cannot be used because they do not penetrate deeply enough to image intra-abdominal organs in most adult patients.

To alleviate these problems, a new ultrasonic imaging system consisting of a high-frequency transducer mounted on the tip of a gastroduodenal scope was developed (4). With this instrumentation, the transducer can be placed within the esophagus, stomach or duodenum in close proximity to thoracic and intra-abdominal organs. Because this positioning creates short acoustic paths, high frequency ultrasound (10

MHz) can be used, which in conjunction with electronic focusing, provides provides high-resolution images. Another extremely valuable feature of endoscopic ultrasonography is that gas within the upper gastrointestinal tract can be readily aspirated through the endoscope. Thus, interference with imaging by ultrasonic shadowing secondary to bowel gas is not a problem.

Description of the Instruments

Thus far, two instruments have been developed by the Bioengineering Research Center of SRI International, Menlo Park, California. In both, endoscopic components from American Cystoscope Manufacturers, Inc. were used. We have previously reported our work in animals (4,5) in which we used a prototype instrument which had an 80-mm long, rigid tip. It is these studies I will discuss in detail. However, we have used a second prototype ultrasonic endoscope, which has a 35 mm rigid tip as an integral part of an endviewing ACMI model FX-8 endoscope, in preliminary pre-clinical human studies (6-8). The long-tipped animal endoscope (Fig. 1) is based on the ACMI FX-5 model which has a side-viewing capability. Modifications of this endoscope were made to house the transducer and its electrical cabling so that the cabling was routed through the FX-5's suction channel and the air/water channel was modified so that it could also be used for suction.

The ultrasonic probe of both instruments is a 10 MHz, 64-element linear array which is integrated into the end of the endoscopes. The resulting length of the ACMI FX-5 ultrasonic endoscope was 80 mm (which in our opinion precluded human studies) and was 13 mm in diameter. The ultrasound system generates a real-time field of view which is 3 cm wide and 4 cm deep, at a rate of 35 frames/second. Dynamic focusing is used on both transmission and reception to provide resolution of less than

1 mm in both dimensions over the entire image. A fixed acoustic lens provides focusing in a direction orthogonal to the point of the image. A digital-scan converter is used to provide a NTSC standard television format so that the gray scale of the image can be operator adjusted and videotaped.

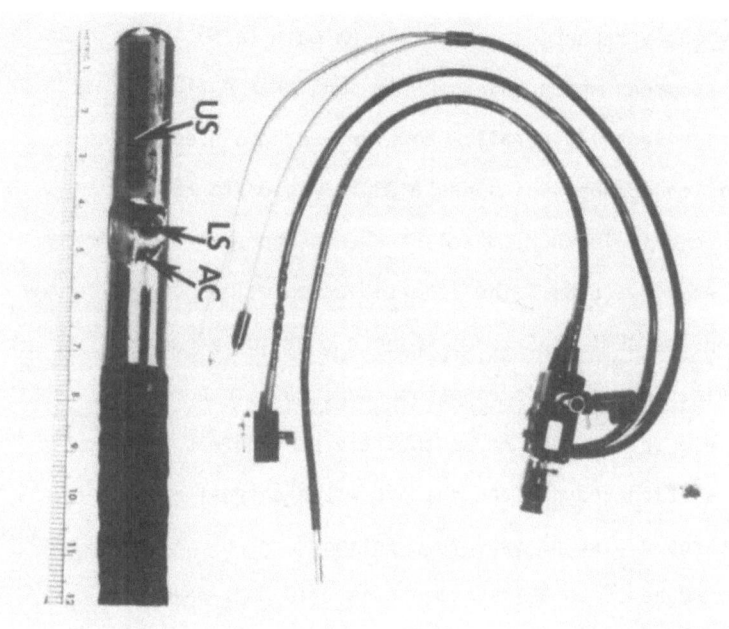

FIGURE 1. The ultrasonic endoscope used in canine experiments. A modified ACMI FX-5 side viewing endoscope and (below) 80-mm rigid tip with ultrasonic probe (US), light source (LS) and aspiration channel (AC) (scale in cm). (Reprinted with permission from DiMagno, E.P., Buxton, J.L., Regan, P.T., Hattery, R.R., Wilson, D.A., Suarez, J.R., and Green, P.S.: The ultrasonic endoscope. Lancet 1:629-631, 1980).

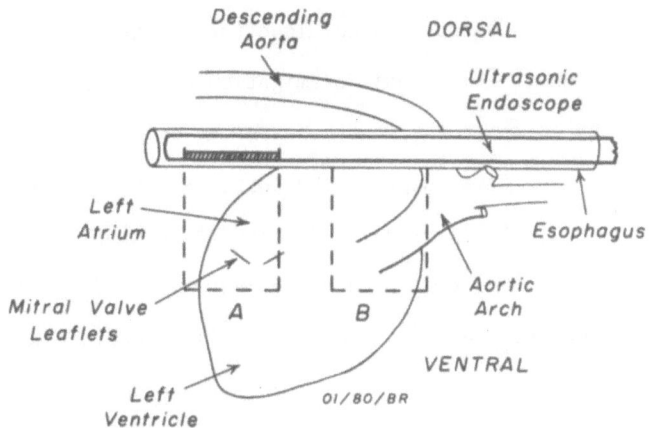

FIGURE 2. Schematic diagram of a longitudinal view from the esophagus of the canine heart using the ultrasonic endoscope. Frames A and B correspond to scans from two different regions of the esophagus. (Reprinted with permission from Rajagopalan, B., DiMagno, E.P., Greenleaf, J.F., Regan, P.T., Buxton, J., Green, P.S., and Whitaker, J.W. Transesophageal ultrasonic imaging of the heart. Acoustical Imaging 9:555-567, 1980).

Animal Studies

In our original animal experiments, 30 endoscopic examinations were performed in dogs anesthetized with sodium pentobarbital. After the endoscope was inserted into the esophagus and stomach and endoscopic visualization of the mucosa of the upper gastrointestinal tract was performed, acoustic images were obtained by aspirating air from the esophagus or stomach. Thus, in a single examination, we could visually examine the esophagus, stomach and duodenum and ultrasonically examine organs and vasculature adjacent to the upper gastrointestinal tract. For example, when the mid esophagus was entered the pulsatile descending aorta was immediately recognizable (Fig. 2 diagrammatically represents the anatomical relationship among the canine esophagus, aorta and heart). The aorta (Fig. 3) was then traced proximally and the cardiac valves identified (Fig. 4,5). Next, the aorta was traced distally, the diaphragm identified and the endoscope passed along the greater curvature of the stomach for the ultrasonic examination of the spleen and left kidney. Then, by rotating the endoscope posteriorly, the abdominal aorta, inferior vena cava, hepatic and portal veins, and liver substance (Fig. 6) were sequentially visualized. The porta hepatitis and gallbladder (Fig. 7) were seen as the endoscope was advanced along the lesser curvature of the stomach. Gastric mucosal folds could also be seen ultrasonically.

To further validate the ultrasonic images of the cardiovascular, renal and gastrointestinal structures, we performed several other canine experiments in which indocyanine green was injected into the cardiac chambers to identify the right (Fig. 4) and left chambers of the heart, mitral valve, aortic bulb (Fig. 5) and pulmonary artery (5). In five dogs, the ultrasonic contrast medium was introduced into the aorta or left ventricle by means of a catheter placed in the femoral artery or into the right ventricle by means of a catheter introduced through the femoral vein. In these studies, we ultrasonically defined the cardiac anatomy (left and right chambers of the heart, mitral value, aorta, aortic bulb, and pulmonary artery) and enhanced myocardial, splenic and renocortical imaging. Similarly, ultrasonic images detected from within the gastrointestinal tract could be enhanced by increased backscattering produced by the contrast agents.

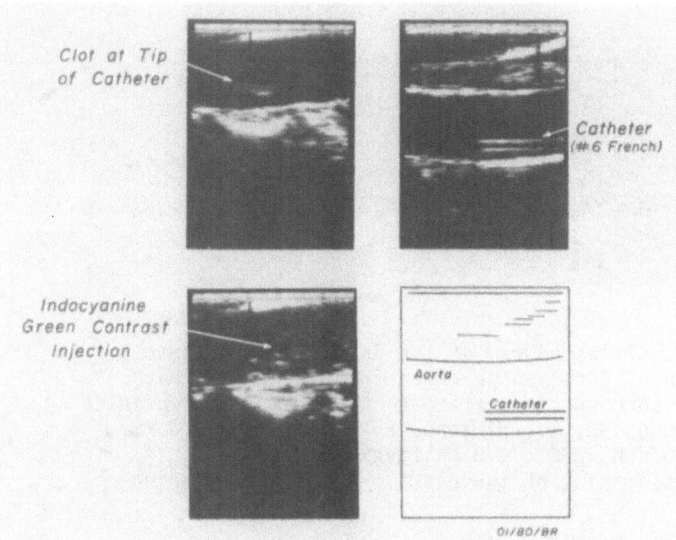

FIGURE 3. Transesophageal ultrasonograms of the in vivo canine aorta. The top right frame shows the catheter in the aorta. The image on the top left shows a clot which formed on the end of the catheter. The bottom left panel shows the intense backscattering from contrast injected into the aorta. (Reprinted with permission from Rajagopalan, B., DiMagno, E.P., Greenleaf, J.F., Regan, P.T., Buxton, J., Green, P.S., and Whitaker, J.W. Transesophageal ultrasonic imaging of the heart. Acoustical Imaging 9:555-567, 1980).

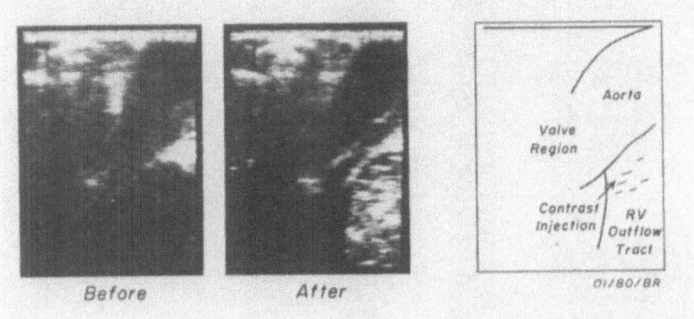

FIGURE 4. Transesophageal ultrasonograms of the canine heart in vivo before and after injection of indocyanine green into the right ventricle. The views correspond to frame B in Figure 2. (Reprinted with permission from Rajagopalan, B., DiMagno, E.P., Greenleaf, J.F., Regan, P.T., Buxton, J., Green, P.S., and Whitaker, J.W. Transesophageal ultrasonic imaging of the heart. Acoustical Imaging 9:555-567, 1980).

314

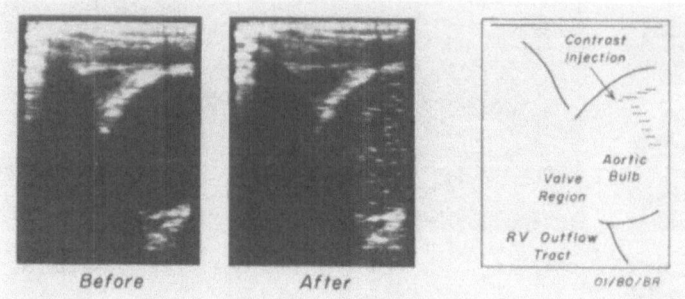

Before   After   01/80/BR

FIGURE 5. Transesophageal ultrasonogram of the in vivo canine heart
before and after injection of indocyanine green into the aortic bulb.
These views approximately correspond to frame B in Figure 2. (Reprinted
with permission from Rajagopalan, B., DiMagno, E.P., Greenleaf, J.F.,
Regan, P.T., Buxton, J., Green, P.S., and Whitaker, J.W.
Transesophageal ultrasonic imaging of the heart. Acoustical Imaging
9:555-567, 1980).

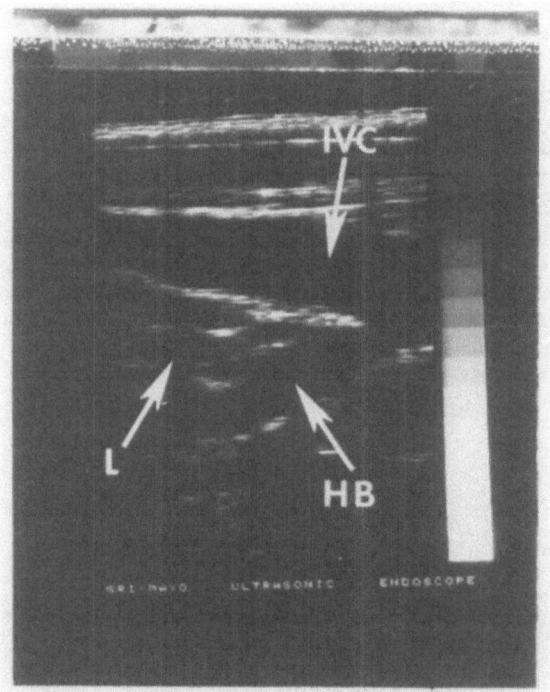

FIGURE 6. Transgastric coronal section of canine liver parenchyma (L)
surrounding the inferior vena cava (IVC) and branch of hepatic vein
(HB). (Reprinted with permission from DiMagno, E.P., Buxton, J.L.,
Regan, P.T., Hattery, R.R., Wilson, D.A., Suarez, J.R., and Green, P.S.:
The ultrasonic endoscope. Lancet 1:629-631, 1980).

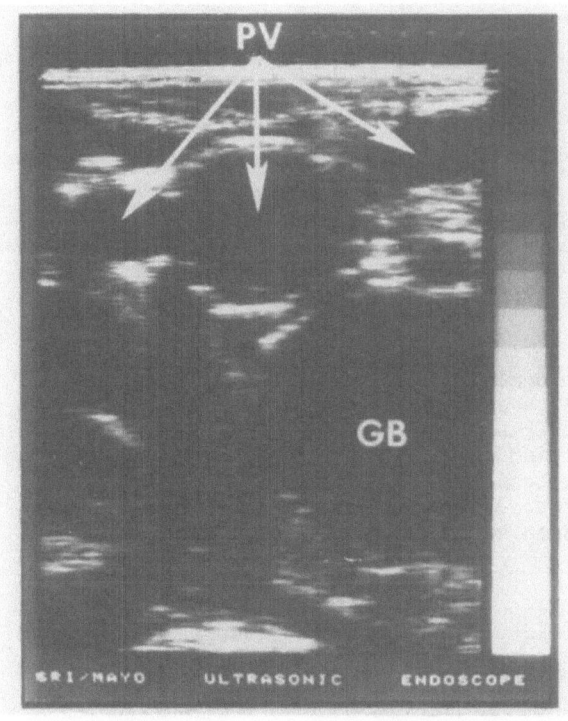

FIGURE 7. Transgastric coronal section through the porta hepatis showing the gallbladder (GB) and branches of portal vein (PV). (Reprinted with permission from DiMagno, E.P., Buxton, J.L., Regan, P.T., Hattery, R.R., Wilson, D.A., Suarez, J.R., and Green, P.S.: The ultrasonic endoscope. Lancet 1:629-631, 1980).

To evaluate contrast ehnancement within the myocardium, green dye was injected into the aortic root. Piror to injection, the endo- and epicardial boundaries of the left atrium were only faintly visible but were clearly distinguishable post-injection (Fig. 8). To image different longitudinal cross sections, the heart was stopped by vagal stimulation and sections were obtained by rotating the endoscope about its axis at the approximate success of 6° turns (Fig. 9). With a more precise orienting mechanism, it should be possible to reconstruct 3-dimensional images.

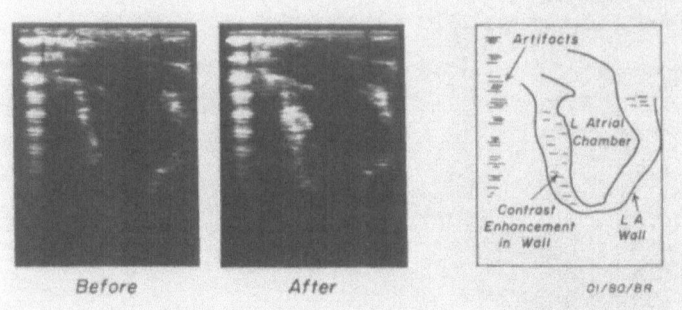

FIGURE 8. Transesophageal ultrasonogram of the in vivo canine left
atrium before and after the injection of indocyanine green at the aortic
root. These pictures correspond to Frame A of Figure 2. Enhancement of
the backscattering from the myocardium is seen in the image on the right
(Reprinted with permission from Rajagopalan, B., DiMagno, E.P.,
Greenleaf, J.F., Regan, P.T., Buxton, J., Green, P.S., and Whitaker,
J.W. Transesophageal ultrasonic imaging of the heart. Acoustical
Imaging 9:555-567, 1980).

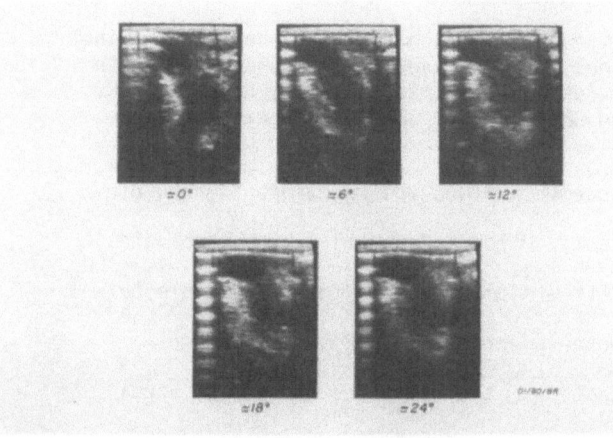

FIGURE 9. Transesophageal ultrasonogram of the vagally blocked in vivo
canine left atrium obtained with incremental rotations about the axis of
the ultrasonic endoscope. The approximate angles of clockwise rotations
are given under each frame. The 0° picture approximately corresponds to
Frame A of Figure 2. (Reprinted with permission from Rajagopalan, B.,
DiMagno, E.P., Greenleaf, J.F., Regan, P.T., Buxton, J., Green, P.S.,
and Whitaker, J.W. Transesophageal ultrasonic imaging of the heart.
Acoustical Imaging 9:555-567, 1980).

In an additional five dogs (9), laparotomies were performed so that the ultrasonic endoscope could be manually manipulated into the duodenum from the stomach. The pancreatic and gallbladder ducts were then cannulated and injected with indocyanine green. This procedure permitted ultrasonic opacification of the bile and pancreatic ducts and enhanced imaging of the contents of the gallbladder.

These canine studies accomplished two goals: first, we demonstrated the feasibility and even the ease of intrathoracic and intragastric imaging. We found no difficulty in maintaining good acoustic contact and little difficulty imaging structure of and near the gastrointestinal tract; second, we demonstrated the safety of the instrumentation.

Recently, a short-tipped endoscope has been constructed and we have performed preliminary studies in humans (6-8). This shorter-tipped instrument does allow positioning of the endoscope within the esophagus, stomach, through the pylorus and into the second and third portions of the duodenum of humans. In preliminary studies, we have been able to visualize the intrathoracic vasculature, spleen, pancreas, kidney, liver and upper gastrointestinal mucosa in both normal humans and in patients with upper gastrointestinal disease.

DISCUSSION

With these instruments, we have developed an imaging system of unprecedented quality which should lead to increased diagnostic capabilities for both intrathoracic and intra-abdominal diseases--a topic we are now actively investigating with the "human", relatively short-tipped ultrasonic endoscope. Already in preliminary studies in patients with diseases, we have been able to visualize pancreatic adenocarcinomas, cystadenocarcinomas islet cell carcinomas pseudocysts, liver metastases less than 1 cm in diameter, and dilated pancreatic ducts secondary to obstruction (7,8). We have also shown in animal experiments that visualization of cardiovascular structures, the myocardium, pancreatic ducts, bile ducts and gallbladder can be enhanced by injection of indocyanine green (5,9). In addition, three-dimensional reconstruction is theoretically possible with this instrumentation (5). Each of these studies demonstrate the potential clinical applicability of intra-cavity endoscopic ultrasonography. That is, ultrasound images can be obtained within the gastrointestinal tract, peritoneum, bile ducts, pancreatic ducts, intravascular spaces or other body cavities. Therefore, it is not surprising that already clinical applications of this technique have been used to detect stones within the biliary tract (10) and to detect prostatic lesions (11).

It should be stressed that an advantage of endoscopic ultrasonography is that endoscopic visualization of the gastrointestinal tract and ultrasound examination of extraluminal organs can be obtained during a single procedure. Thus, in one setting it should be possible to determine whether a disease process is mucosal, intramural, or extraluminal. This advantage alone could potentially decrease time and expense in obtaining a diagnosis. An additional feature of our instrument is that its endoscopic capability eliminates the need for x-ray fluoroscopic positioning of the ultrasonic probe, a requirement for some other instruments (12,13).

There are certain other features of this current instrument that deserve some emphasis. Although even the current "human" endoscope has a relatively long, rigid tip of 35 mm, we have not encountered difficulties in maneuvering the instrument within the esophagus and stomach. But in approximately 25% of studies we were unable to insert the endoscope into the second or third part of the duodenum. In some studies, this has compromised our ability to visualize the pancreas and the biliary system. Currently, we are altering the design of the ultrasonic endoscope to circumvent this minor difficulty.

Poor acoustic contact apparently has been the problem with some ultrasonic endoscopes (14) and as a consequence the ultrasonic probe of these instruments has been immersed within an oil-containing sleeve. We have had no difficulty in maintaining good acoustic coupling from the transducer to the mucosal surface since aspiration of upper gastrointestinal gas through the endoscope collapses the mucosa of the gastrointestinal tract around the transducer and the mucus and fluid naturally present within the esophagus, stomach and duodenum provide an excellent medium for contact.

A potential problem, particularly when one begins to use the ultrasonic endoscope, is the small field of view. In contrast to transcutaneous ultrasonic examinations, our instrument only images to a depth of 4 cm. Thus, a large number of vascular landmarks cannot be identified and aid in positively identifying organs. However, since our 10 MHz ultrasound transducer provides excellent tissue discrimination, the liver, spleen, kidneys, and pancreas are readily identifiable and serve as landmarks for anatomical orientation within the abdomen.

Our initial studies have demonstrated that the intrathoracic, intragastric, and intraduodenal ultrasonic imaging is not only possible but this technique produces images of superior quality which allow differentiation between normal and disease states. Although our results have been very encouraging, it must be recognized that our studies have not proven the medical usefulness of this technique. The diagnostic accuracy of endoscopic ultrasonography for a variety of diseases and the

comparison of this technique with other diagnostic tests needs to be
determined. Lastly, our studies have stimulated widespread interest and
currently other laboratories are investigating this technique.
Undoubtedly, the instrumentation will continue to improve.

REFERENCES

1. Leopold GR. 1979. Ultrasound. In: Alimentary Tract Radiology
    Abdominal Imaging, Alexander R. Margulis and H Joachim Burhenne,
    eds., C.V. Mosby Co., St. Louis, MO, Vol. 3, pp. 275-310, 1979.
2. Taylor KJW, Rosenfield AT. 1979. Ultrasound. In: Alimentary
    Tract Radiology Abdominal Imaging, Alexander R Margulis and
    H Joachim Burhenne, eds., C.V. Mosby Co., St. Louis, MO, Vol. 3,
    pp. 183-247.
3. DiMagno EP, Malagelada J-R, Taylor WP, Go VLW. 1977. A
    prospective comparison of current diagnostic tests in pancreatic
    cancer. New Engl J Med 297:737-42.
4. DiMagno EP, Buxton JL, Regan PT, Hattery RR, Wilson DA, Suarez JR,
    Green PS. 1980. The ultrasonic endoscope. Lancet 1:629-631.
5. Rajagopalan B, DiMagno EP, Greenleaf JF, Regan PT, Buxton J, Green
    PS, Whitaker JW. 1980. Transesophageal ultrasonic imaging of the
    heart. Acoustical Imaging 9:555-567.
6. Buxton JL, DiMagno EP, Regan PT, Wilson DA, James ME. 1980. The
    ultrasonic endoscopic examination of humans: preliminary
    experience. Proceedings of the 25th Annual Meeting of American
    Institute of Ultrasound in Medicine, New Orleans, Louisiana,
    September 15-19.
7. DiMagno EP, Regan PT, James ME. 1980. Visualization of the normal
    and abnormal human pancreas with the ultrasonic endoscope, National
    Pancreatic Project Newletter 5:34.
8. DiMagno EP, Clain JE, James EM. 1981. Human endoscopic examination:
    Preliminary study of diseases of the upper gastrointestinal tract.
    Gastroenterology 80:1136.
9. DiMagno EP, Buxton JL, Regan PT, Hattery RR, Wilson DA, Suarez JR,
    Green PS. 1980. The ultrasonic endoscope: Preliminary human
    studies. Gastroenterology 78:1157.
10. Lane RJ, Glazer G. 1980. Intraoperative B-Mode ultrasound scanning
    of the extrahepatic biliary system and pancreas. Lancet 2:334-337.
11. Harada K, Igari D, Tanahashi Y. 1979. Gray scale transrectal
    ultrasonography of the prostate. J Clin Ultrasound 7:45-49.
12. Lutz H, Rosch W. 1976. Transgastroscopic ultrasonography. Endoscopy
    8:203-205.
13. Strohm WD, Phillip J, Hagenmuller F, Classen M. 1980. Ultrasonic
    tomography by means of an ultrasonic fiberendoscope. Endoscopy
    12:241-244.